ATLAS OF
CANINE
AND FELINE
CYTOLOGY

ATLAS OF CANINE AND FELINE CYTOLOGY

ROSE E. RASKIN, D.V.M., PH.D.

Diplomate, A.C.V.P.
Associate Professor, Clinical Pathology
Service Chief, Clinical Pathology Laboratory
Department of Physiological Sciences
College of Veterinary Medicine
University of Florida
Gainesville, Florida

DENNY J. MEYER, D.V.M.

Diplomate, A.C.V.I.M., Diplomate, A.C.V.P.
Director, Pathology
Life Sciences
Gilead Sciences, Inc.
Boulder, Colorado

W.B. SAUNDERS COMPANY
A Harcourt Health Sciences Company
Philadelphia   London   New York   St. Louis   Sydney   Toronto

W.B. SAUNDERS COMPANY

A Harcourt Health Sciences Company

The Curtis Center
Independence Square West
Philadelphia, Pennsylvania 19106

Library of Congress Cataloging-in-Publication Data

Atlas of canine and feline cytology/[edited by] Rose Raskin, Dennis J. Meyer.—1st ed.

p. cm.

ISBN 0–7216–6335–4

1. Dogs—Diseases—Atlases. 2. Cats—Diseases—Atlases. 3. Veterinary
    cytology—Atlases. I. Raskin, Rose. II. Meyer, Dennis J.

SF991.A85 2001
636.7′089607582—dc21   00-049270

Acquisitions Editor: Raymond R. Kersey
Developmental Editor: Denise LeMelledo

ATLAS OF CANINE AND FELINE CYTOLOGY   ISBN 0–7216–6335–4

Printed in the United States of America.

Last digit is the print number: 9   8   7   6   5   4   3   2   1

"To be and remain true to oneself and others is to possess the noblest attribute of the greatest talents."

Johann Wolfgang von Goethe

Rose thanks her family and friends. I could not have accomplished my life's goals without your continued love and support. I especially wish to dedicate this book to my daughter Hannah, brother Richard, father, and memory of my mother.

Denny dedicates this work to his wife, Jae, who continues to support the solitude on weekends and evenings required for this extracurricular activity—you are special . . . and to Chris and Jen, his favorite son and daughter, for continuing to be an integral component of my life's experiences and, along with Jae, make it all seem worthwhile.

Contributors

CHAP 5 / RESPIRATORY TRACT

**Mary Jo Burkhard, D.V.M., Ph.D.,
Diplomate A.C.V.P.**
Assistant Professor of Clinical Pathology
Microbiology, Pathology, and Parasitology
College of Veterinary Medicine
North Carolina State University
Raleigh, North Carolina

Amy Valenciano, D.V.M., M.S.
Clinical Pathologist
IDEXX Veterinary Services, Inc.
West Sacramento, California

**Anne Barger, M.S., D.V.M.,
Diplomate A.C.V.P.**
Veterinary Clinical Pathologist
Antech Diagnostics
Alsip, Illinois

CHAP 6 / BODY CAVITY FLUIDS

**Sonjia M. Shelly, B.S., D.V.M.,
Diplomate A.C.V.P.**
Head Clinical Pathology, Western Region
IDEXX Veterinary Services, Inc.
West Sacramento, California

CHAP 7 / ORAL CAVITY,
GASTROINTESTINAL TRACT, AND
ASSOCIATED STRUCTURES

**Claire B. Andreasen, D.V.M., Ph.D.,
Diplomate A.C.V.P.**
Associate Professor
Department of Veterinary Pathology
College of Veterinary Medicine
Iowa State University
Ames, Iowa

**Albert E. Jergens, D.V.M., M.S.,
Diplomate A.C.V.I.M.**
Associate Professor
Department of Veterinary Clinical Sciences
College of Veterinary Medicine
Iowa State University
Ames, Iowa

CHAP 9 / CYTOLOGIC EXAMINATION OF
THE URINARY TRACT

**Dori L. Borjesson, D.V.M., M.P.V.M.,
Diplomate A.C.V.P.**
Department of Microbiology and Pathology
School of Veterinary Medicine
University of California–Davis
Davis, California

CHAP 11 / REPRODUCTIVE SYSTEM

**Kristin L. Henson, D.V.M., M.S.,
Diplomate A.C.V.P.**
Graduate Research Assistant
Clinical Pathology Instructor
College of Veterinary Medicine
University of Florida
Gainesville, Florida

CHAP 12 / MUSCULOSKELETAL SYSTEM

**David J. Fisher, D.V.M.,
Diplomate A.C.V.P.**
Veterinary Clinical Pathologist
IDEXX Veterinary Services, Inc.
West Sacramento, California

CHAP 13 / CYTOLOGY OF THE CENTRAL
NERVOUS SYSTEM

Kathleen P. Freeman, D.V.M., M.S., Ph.D.
Pathologist
IDEXX Laboratories
Wetherby, West Yorkshire
United Kingdom

CHAP 15 / ENDOCRINE SYSTEM

A. Rick Alleman, D.V.M., Ph.D.
Assistant Professor of Clinical Pathology
College of Veterinary Medicine
University of Florida
Gainesville, Florida

CHAP 16 / ADVANCED DIAGNOSTIC
TECHNIQUES

*Janice M. Andrews, D.V.M., Ph.D.,
Diplomate A.C.V.P.*
Veterinary Laboratory Director
Veterinary Laboratory Service of Rex
Healthcare
Raleigh, North Carolina

David E. Malarkey, D.V.M., Ph.D.
Assistant Professor of Pathology
College of Veterinary Medicine
North Carolina State University
Raleigh, North Carolina

Preface

The *Atlas of Canine and Feline Cytology* is designed to provide the user easy access to the vast and emerging information related to the diagnostic application and interpretation of cytology and cytopathology in veterinary medicine. It is intended to be a "bench book" to which the reader can turn when confronted with problematic microscopic findings or to affirm an initial diagnostic impression. It covers a wide range of diseases that affect multiple organ systems. The information for each organ system reflects the expertise of an individual well-versed in its diseases and attendant pathology and its evaluation by the microscopic examination of a cytologic specimen. Emphasis is placed on those areas in which the application of cytology has the greatest diagnostic value. In some organ systems, histology is provided to demonstrate the histologic or histopathologic corollary of the cytologic findings. The objective is to emphasize the complementary role of both and, in some cases, the interpretative limitations of relying solely on cytology for assessing the disease process.

The photomicrographs are derived from an enormous collection of cytologic specimens that span many collective decades of clinical experience. Each one has been carefully selected to best represent the normal cytomorphologic features and the notable cytopathologic findings. Nonetheless, the contributors labored with the frustrations of trying to select a single photomicrograph that adequately reflected the impressions gained from scanning multiple slide preparations in arriving at a diagnostic interpretation. We believe the final choices were worth the interrogative deliberation but realize that an atlas cannot address all the visual nuances associated with the use of diagnostic cytology and yet be kept to a manageable size.

Each author has focused on the anticipated needs of the reader in compiling this atlas and sincerely hopes that the final product has achieved that goal. Our only reward is the satisfaction of the reader. It may be the student struggling to sort out the initial myriad visual distractions, the veterinarian who requires a quick confirmation of cytologic findings in the evaluation of a patient, or the academic cytologist who values this atlas as a useful reference and teaching source. We acknowledge that it is incomplete but have striven to support the clinical dictum that "common things occur commonly." To paraphrase the admonition of Sherlock Holmes, we hope that this atlas illustrates most of the important and unimportant microscopic findings that are commonly seen and highlights those that deserve additional interrogative observation in formulating a diagnostic impression.

Denny & Rose

Acknowledgments

"One must attend in medical practice not primarily to plausible theories, but to experience combined with reason."

Hippocrates

We are greatly indebted to the chapter authors who contributed generously of their time and expertise to assist in the timely completion of this Atlas. We also acknowledge the contribution of the many veterinarians in both private and academic practices who provided the cytologic specimens and their clinical relevance.

Denny acknowledges the impact that Dr. Vic Perman, the father of modern veterinary cytology, had on him as a student at the University of Minnesota. That influence resulted in the development of this Atlas more than a quarter of a century later. Admittedly, the content of the Atlas pales in comparison to Vic's knowledge of diagnostic cytology. He also acknowledges the many clinical and anatomical pathologists that contributed to the development of his microscopic ability during his tenures at the University of Florida, Colorado State University, and IDEXX Veterinary Services.

Rose acknowledges the guidance provided by her pathology mentors while as a student and resident. She also acknowledges the powerful influence on veterinary cytology by the American Society for Clinical Pathology, especially through its publication *Veterinary Clinical Pathology* and its annual case review.

Lastly, the Atlas could not have become a reality without the continued support of Mr. Ray Kersey, Executive Editor at W.B. Saunders Company. We are grateful for his guidance and patience.

Contents

CHAPTER 1

The Acquisition and Management of Cytology Specimens

Denny J. Meyer

Sapere vedere—"Learn to see."

Leonardo da Vinci

The classification of events that depend on the accuracy of observation is limited by the ability of the observer to describe and of the interpreter to decipher.

Michael Podell, M.Sc., D.V.M.

For the microscopic examination of tissue, another limiting factor that affects the accuracy of observation is specimen management. The successful use of aspiration cytology depends on several interrelated procedures: acquisition of a representative specimen, proper application to a glass side, adequate staining, and examination with a quality microscope. A deficiency in one or more of these steps will adversely affect the yield of diagnostic information. The objective of this chapter is to provide general recommendations for successful sample management in support of its diagnostic interpretation.

GENERAL SAMPLING GUIDELINES

Prior to executing any sampling procedure, a cytology kit should be prepared and dedicated for that purpose. An inexpensive plastic tool caddie works well. Suggested contents are listed in Table 1–1. Six or more slides are placed on a firm flat surface such as a surgical tray immediately prior to the sampling procedure. The surface of the glass slide should be routinely wiped with a paper towel, or at least on a shirtsleeve, to remove "invisible" glass particles that interfere with the spreading procedure.

TABLE 1–1	Contents of the Cytology Kit

Syringes: 6 to 12 cc

Needles: 1- and 1½-inch—20- to 22-gauge; 2½- or 3½-inch spinal needle with stylet

Scalpel blades: #10 and #11

Box of precleaned glass slides with frosted end

Tubes: EDTA (purple top) and serum (red top without separator)

Rigid, flat surface on which 6 to 10 slides can be spread out

Intravenous extension tubing

Permanent black marker (Sharpie)

4% sterile EDTA

Hair dryer

Table 1–2 lists suggested indications for the application of diagnostic cytology. The collection of specimens for cytologic evaluation from cutaneous and subcutaneous tissues and abdominal organs and masses in smaller animals is generally accomplished with a 20- or 22-gauge, 1- to 1½-inch needle firmly attached to a 6- or 12-cc syringe. For more difficult to reach internal organs, a 2½- to 3½-inch spinal needle is used. The added length amplifies the area for cell collection and enhances the diagnostic yield. Literally, cores of hepatic tissue have been obtained with the use of a longer needle. The stylet can be left in place as the cavity is entered to avoid contamination during the "searching" process of locating the tissue of sampling interest. Coating the needle and syringe hub with sterile 4% disodium EDTA prior to aspiration biopsy sampling of vascular tissues, notably bone marrow, reduces the risk of clot formation that will compromise the quality of the cytologic specimen. For the relatively inexperienced, this may be a practice to consider routinely when sampling any tissue. Clotted speci-

mens are a frequent cause of cytologic preps of poor quality.

The general steps for obtaining a cytologic specimen are illustrated in Figure 1–1. The tip of the needle is inserted into the tissue of interest, the plunger is retracted slightly (½ to 1 cc of vacuum), the needle advanced and retracted in several different directions, the plunger released, the needle withdrawn, and the specimen placed on a glass slide or in an EDTA (purple-topped) tube as appropriate. If fluid is obtained, the site is completely drained, the needle withdrawn, the fluid placed in an EDTA tube, and the procedure repeated with a new needle directed at firm tissue. Both specimens are examined microscopically. To enhance operator flexibility, intravenous extension tubing (Extension Set, Abbott Laboratories) can be used to attach the needle and syringe. Positioning and redirection of the needle is easier and accommodates for patient movement.

Aspiration is not a prerequisite for obtaining a cytologic specimen. A technique that is based on the principle of capillarity,

TABLE 1–2	General Indications for the Use of Diagnostic Cytology

Effusions—thoracic and abdominal

Urine sediments, urinary bladder washing

Prostate—direct aspirate, washing

Lymphadenopathy—focal, generalized

Examination for metastatic disease

Diffuse organomegaly—liver and kidney

Cutaneous/subcutaneous mass, ulcerative lesion

Conjunctival/vitreous/aqueous cytology

Pulmonary/nasal aspirates/brushings, bronchoalveolar/nasal washing/lavage

Unidentified abdominal mass

Evaluation of a mass or lesion discovered intraoperatively

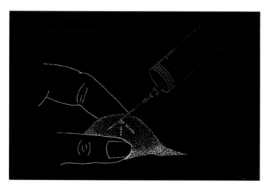

FIGURE 1-1. General concept of the fine-needle aspiration biopsy technique. The needle is inserted into the tissue and redirected three or four times using either an aspiration or a nonaspiration technique. The same concept generally applies to the use of the technique for sampling sites within the thorax or abdomen. (Reprinted with permission from Meyer DJ: The management of cytology specimens. Compend Contin Educ Pract Vet 1987; 9:10–17.)

referred to as "fine-needle capillary sampling," is performed by placement of a needle into the lesion with or without a syringe attached (Mair et al., 1989; Yue and Zheng, 1989). The technique has been shown to have diagnostic sensitivity similar to that of aspiration biopsy when used to sample a variety of tissues. The major advantage of the technique is a reduction of blood contamination from vascular tissues such as liver, spleen, kidney, and thyroid. Cells are displaced into the cylinder of the needle by capillary action as the needle is incompletely retracted and redirected into the tissue three to six times. Personal preference is justified when deciding between aspiration and nonaspiration sampling for collection of the specimen. The operator may determine that each has value for sampling different tissues through trial and error.

KEY POINT: Acquisition of the cytology specimen is an art that can be honed only by practice. Selection of an appropriate indication enhances the probability of obtaining diagnostic information.

KEY POINT: Routinely dry-wipe the surface of the glass slide to remove "invisible" glass particles that cause spreading deficiencies. Never reuse washed glass slides.

MANAGING THE CYTOLOGIC SPECIMEN

Compression (Squash) Preparation

The compression (squash) technique is an important and adaptable procedure for the management of cytology specimens that are semisolid, mucus-like, or pelleted by centrifugation. A small amount of material is placed on a clean glass slide approximately ½ inch (1 cm) from the frosted end (Fig. 1–2A). A second clean glass slide is placed over the specimen at right angles. The specimen is gently but firmly compressed be-

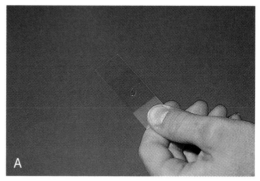

FIGURE 1-2. **A,** The application of only a small drop or portion of the specimen on the glass slide near the frosted end is an important initial step for making a quality cytologic preparation. Placing too much material on the slide results in a preparation that is too thick and/or spreads too close to the slide edges for diagnostic purposes.

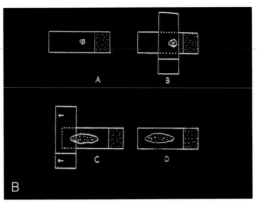

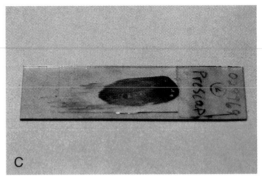

FIGURE 1–2. B, The specimen is gently but firmly compressed between the two glass slides (B) and in the same continuous motion (C) the top slide is glided along the surface of the slide with the material directed away from the frosted end, resulting in a featherlike spread of the specimen (D) referred to as the "sweet spot." (Reprinted with permission from Meyer DJ, Franks PT: Clinical cytology: Part I: Management of tissue specimens. Mod Vet Pract 1986; 67:255–259.)

FIGURE 1–2.   C, The location of the "sweet spot" is illustrated by this properly labeled and stained compression preparation of a lymph node specimen. (Reprinted with permission from Meyer DJ: The management of cytology specimens. Compend Contin Educ Pract Vet 1987; 9:10–17.)

tween the two glass slides and in the same continuous motion the top slide is glided along the surface of the slide with the material directed away from the frosted end (Fig. 1–2B). The objective is to distribute the material from a multicell-thick area to a monolayer spread for maximal flattening of individual cells and even stain penetration, thereby optimizing the microscopic examination of cell morphology. A properly prepared glass slide is characterized by a feather-shaped (oblong) area with a monolayer end referred to as the "sweet spot" (Fig. 1–2C). A common mistake is the initial placement of excess sample on the glass slide, resulting in a thick preparation that is not possible to adequately examine microscopically.

KEY POINT: Compression and spread of the specimen is a continuum; there should be no momentary pause as the upper slide contacts the specimen. Keep the flat surfaces of the two slides parallel. A common mistake is to slightly angle the upper slide near the end of the gliding motion by allowing a slight counterclockwise rotation of the wrist (clockwise if left handed) to occur, causing cell lysis or uneven spread of the specimen. A scraping sound of glass on glass can be heard when this occurs.

KEY POINT: The term *sweet spot* refers to that area around the center mass of a baseball bat, tennis racket, or golf club that is the most effective part with which to make a successful hit. The same concept applies to the location of the cytologic specimen if it is to make a successful diagnostic hit. Cellular material that is too close to the ends or edges of the slide cannot be properly examined. When slides go through an automated stainer, its guiding tracks can scrape off diagnostic material that is too close to the end of the slide (Fig. 1–3) or if placed too far from the end the specimen

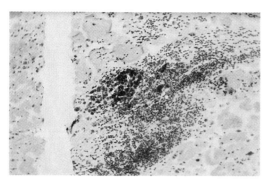

FIGURE 1–3. The clear area to the left of center represents the guide track of the automated stainer that has partially scraped off the only cytologic material present on the slide because it was located too close to the slide's end.

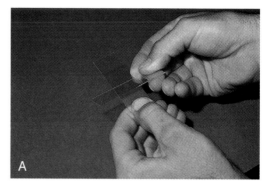

FIGURE 1–4. A, The procedure for making a cytologic preparation from a fluid specimen is illustrated. A *small* drop of the specimen is placed approximately ½ inch (1 cm) from the frosted end of the slide and the spreader slide is slowly backed into the drop. Just as the fluid begins to spread along its edge, the spreader slide is glided away from the frosted end.

may not be exposed adequately to the stain. The ends and longitudinal edges of the slide cannot be adequately examined because of the inability of the 40x dry and 50x and 100x oil objectives to properly focus at those extremes.

KEY POINT: If the compression preparation appears too thick, it probably is. Make another one. If the cytology specimen appears to be too close to the end or edge of the slide, it probably is. Make another one.

Management of Fluids

A fluid specimen should be immediately placed in an EDTA tube to prevent clot formation. Fluid with a plasmalike consistency can be handled similar to the preparation of a blood smear. A small drop of fluid is placed approximately ½ inch (1 cm) from the frosted end. The angled edge of a second glass slide, acute angle facing the operator, is backed into the specimen and drawn away from the frosted end as the fluid begins to spread along its edge (Fig.

1–4A). The speed at which the slide is moved depends on the viscosity of the sample—the thinner the specimen, the faster the slide is moved to distribute the specimen evenly and thinly. For a viscous fluid specimen such as synovial fluid, the spreader slide is moved with a slow and even movement.

All fluid initially applied to the slide must remain on the slide. It is tempting to go off the end of the slide with excess fluid, referred to as the "edge-of-the-cliff syndrome," resulting in potential loss of diagnostic material, i.e., it is thrown into the garbage with the spreader slide (Fig. 1–4B). The "edge-of-the-cliff syndrome" poses a notable threat to pleural and peritoneal fluids that contain clumps of neoplastic cells. These cellular clumps often follow the spreader slide, finally sticking to the surface when the fluid dissipates (Fig. 1–5A & B). To minimize this cytologic disaster when excess fluid remains, simply stop 1/2 inch from the end of the specimen slide and

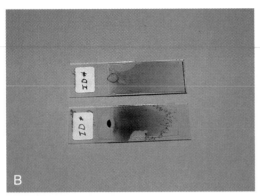

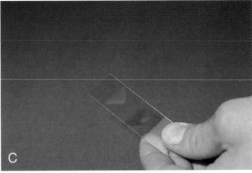

FIGURE 1–4. **B,** All of the original fluid drop should remain on the slide and the temptation to go off the end of the slide with excess fluid must be avoided. The lower slide illustrates a properly feathered fluid specimen with the entire specimen remaining on the slide. The upper slide demonstrates the "edge-of-the-cliff syndrome" in which the excess fluid was drawn off the slide's end.

FIGURE 1–4. **C,** Excess fluid that remains is allowed to partially flow back and air-dried as illustrated by the small opaque dried fluid triangle near the nonfrosted end of the slide. Alternatively, the edge of the spreader slide with the excess fluid adhering is transferred to another clean slide and another smear made.

apply the spreader slide to another clean glass slide and repeat the spreading procedure. A second option when minimal excess fluid remains is to permit it to slowly flow back on itself for a short distance. The thin part of the stained cytology slide preparation can be used to estimate cell numbers and the relatively thick concentrated part (where the excess fluid is dried) can be evaluated for types of cells and/or infectious agents (Fig. 1–4C). While not an optimal preparation, this "poor man's centrifuge" technique is useful in emergency settings for the initial, rapid triage of a fluid specimen.

The diagnostic yield of a predominantly bloody fluid specimen is enhanced with the buffy-coat concentration technique. A microhematocrit tube is prepared as if to measure a hematocrit. The tube is broken at the cell–plasma interface and the cellular concentrate (buffy coat) is applied to two or three slides and a direct smear technique is used to spread the specimen. The technique is valuable for hemorrhagic pericardial, peritoneal, and pleural samples (Fig. 1–6A & B). It is also useful for the examination of peripheral blood for neoplastic cells and cell-associated infectious organisms.

Transudates and cerebrospinal fluids are low in protein and cell numbers. The use of a cytocentrifuge (cytospin) is recommended for the capture all the cells (Fig. 1–7A & B). For cerebrospinal fluids, a cytologic preparation should be made ideally within 2 to 3 hours since the low specific gravity predisposes to cellular lysis. However, it appears that when inflammatory and neoplastic cells and infectious agents are present, their diagnostic cellular integrity is usually maintained for up to 12 hours with refrigeration.

KEY POINT: For the management of fluid samples, routinely make direct, centrifuged (or buffy coat), and cytospin (if pos-

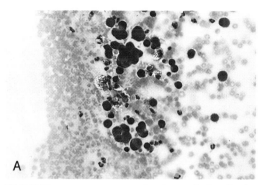

FIGURE 1–5. A, Examination of the feathered edge of the lower slide pictured in Figure 1–4B demonstrates clumps of cells located along the point where the fluid feathers out, emphasizing the need to leave excess fluid. The area to the right of the cell clumps consisted of only erythrocytes. (Wright; ×400.)

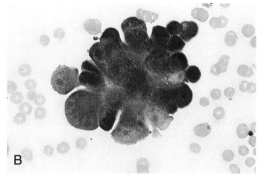

FIGURE 1–5. B, A diagnosis of a neoplastic effusion (adenocarcinoma) was made by examining the cell clumps. (Wright; ×1000.) The upper slide pictured in Figure 1–4B of the same specimen contained only erythrocytes and a few mesothelial cells but no cell clumps precluding a cytologic diagnosis.

sible) preparations and assess each for the best diagnostic yield.

KEY POINT: The refractometer-determined total solute (protein) concentration should be measured for all pleural and peritoneal fluids to facilitate classification as

transudate or modified transudate when that information has diagnostic importance (Meyer and Harvey, 1998).

KEY POINT: For low-protein fluids such as urinary sediments, cerebrospinal fluids, and transudates, the cells can be

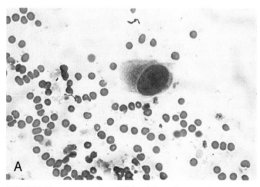

FIGURE 1–6. A, This bloody aspirate was obtained by pericardiocentesis. A rare large, atypical spindle-shaped cell suggestive of a sarcoma was observed among the many erythrocytes and a small number of reactive mesothelial cells. (Wright; ×1000.)

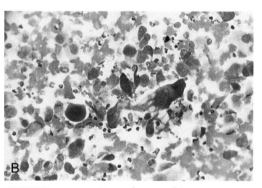

FIGURE 1–6. B, After making a smear from a buffy-coat preparation of the same bloody specimen, numerous spindle-shaped cells that show malignant characteristics are observed, affording a cytologic diagnosis of a neoplastic effusion consistent with a sarcoma. (Wright; ×600.)

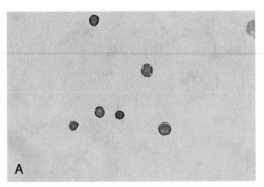

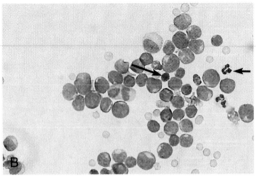

FIGURE 1–7. **A,** This is a direct smear of a pleural fluid specimen from a cat with a thoracic effusion. A small number of small, medium, and large lymphocytes were observed. (Wright; ×600.) The triglyceride concentration of the fluid approximated the serum value, making the diagnosis of a chylous effusion less likely. (Wright; ×1000.)

FIGURE 1–7. **B,** A cytospin preparation of the specimen easily demonstrates that most of the cells are medium to large immature lymphocytes indicative of malignant lymphoma. A normal small lymphocyte (long arrow) and a neutrophil (short arrow) are useful size comparators. (Wright; ×1000.) (Reprinted with permission from Meyer DJ, Franks PT: Effusion: Classification and cytologic examination. Compend Contin Educ Pract Vet 1987; 9:123–128.)

washed off during the staining process. The use of premade serum-coated slides facilitates the adhesion of the cells that can make a diagnostic world of difference. Several drops of the excess serum not used for clinical chemistries are applied to the entire surface of a glass slide and the film of serum is air-dried. Ten to 20 slide preparations are made. Once dry (not sticky to the touch), the slides can be stacked together in an empty slide box and placed in the freezer to prevent bacterial growth. Prior to use, several slides are brought to room temperature. It is critical that no condensation develops on the surface since it causes severe cell lysis.

HELPFUL HINT: A hair dryer set on low heat enhances the even drying of fluid specimens. It can also be used to remove condensation from the serum-covered slides taken from the freezer.

Touch Imprint

Cells will often exfoliate from excised tissue when the cut surface is touched to a glass slide. This type of cytologic preparation permits immediate evaluation of a biopsy, provides the pathologist with a second means of evaluating the tissue, and is a valuable instructional tool. The clinician's interpretation can be compared with the histopathologic findings. The cut surface of the excised tissue is aggressively blotted on a paper towel to remove blood and tissue fluid. The surface will have a dull, dry, tacky appearance. It is touched firmly to the surface of a clean glass slide in several places about the "sweet spot" (Fig. 1–8A). Properly prepared tissue is perceived to stick to the surface of the glass momentarily. If excess blood or tissue fluid is noted, the tissue is blotted again and a new touch imprint made. Imprint areas that appear too thick can be finessed to a monolayer by the gentle use of the compression technique. Touch imprints should be made of each area of tissue specimen that appears grossly different.

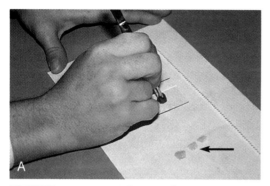

FIGURE 1–8. A, The touch imprint technique is illustrated. The cut surface of the specimen is firmly blotted on a paper towel (note wet spots arrow) until tacky and then firmly touched multiple times to the surface of a clean glass slide.

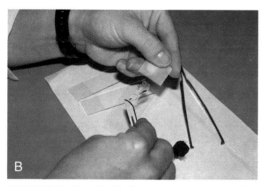

FIGURE 1–8. B, If the tissue does not adequately exfoliate, a scalpel blade is used to scrape or roughen up the surface of the tissue. The tissue can be touched to a glass surface and/or the material on the edge of the blade dragged along the surface of a slide, air-dried, and stained or, if thick, a compression preparation made. (Reprinted with permission from Meyer DJ: The management of cytology specimens. Compend Contin Educ Pract Vet 1987; 9:10–17.)

Tissues with a fibrous texture, such as, fibromas, fibrosarcomas, and cicatricial inflammation, may not exfoliate adequately with this technique. The surface of these firm, often pale-appearing tissues need to be roughened with a scalpel and then touched to the surface of a glass slide. In addition, the tissue on the edge of the scalpel can be used to make touch imprints and/or compression preparations (Fig. 1–8B). This technique works well on ulcerated cutaneous lesions when neoplasia or mycotic infection is suspected. Frequently, the surface is contaminated with debris, bacteria, and an attendant mixed inflammatory cell reaction composed of neutrophils, macrophages, and fibroplasia that can obscure the true etiology if a direct touch imprint is made. It is prudent to aggressively débride the area with moistened gauze and/or by aggressive, deep scraping of the area with a scalpel. The exfoliated material, including the tissue on the scalpel blade, is used to make touch imprints and compression preparations. In certain bullous skin diseases, touching a glass slide to a freshly ruptured bulla can be used to identify acantholytic epithelial cells along with nondegenerate neutrophils (Tzanck preparation), supporting a tentative diagnosis of an immune-mediated skin disorder.

STAINING THE SPECIMEN

Romanowsky, Romanowsky-type, and new methylene blue stains are used in veterinary medicine to identify nucleated cells.

Papanicolaou Stain

The Papanicolaou (Pap) stain is used routinely in the medical profession for cytologic specimens. The stain accentuates nuclear detail and is valuable in detecting early morphologic aberrations indicative of dysplasia and neoplasia. It is not used commonly in veterinary medicine because of the multistep staining procedure and its limitations in evaluating inflammatory reactions. A rapid Papanicolaou staining procedure has been recently described in veterinary medicine that may be advantageous for enhancing the nuclear abnormalities of cancer cells (Jorundsson et al., 1999).

New Methylene Blue Stain

New methylene blue (New Methylene Blue, Fisher Scientific) is a basic dye that stains nuclei, most infectious agents, platelets, and the granules of mast cells. Eosinophil granules do not stain nor do erythrocytes, which appear microscopically as translucent circular areas. Because there is no alcohol fixation, the lipids associated with lipomas and follicular infundibular cysts can be easily recognized. The cholesterol crystals associated with the latter are highlighted. The staining solution consists of 0.5 g of new methylene blue dissolved in 100 ml of 0.9% saline. Full-strength formalin (1 ml) is added as a preservative. The stock solution is kept refrigerated. For clinical use, a small stoppered bottle is replenished from the stock solution; the stain is passed through filter paper first, to remove all precipitate. A small drop of stain is applied directly to an air-dried cytology preparation. A dust-free coverslip (wipe it with a paper towel or a shirtsleeve) is placed on the drop of stain, which spreads by capillary movement. Larger coverslips, 20 mm $\times$ 40 or 50 mm, allow more of the specimen to be examined. The specimen should be immediately examined since the water-based stain will evaporate. A new methylene blue-stained cytologic specimen is useful for the detection of nucleated cells, bacteria (both gram-positive and gram-negative bacteria stain dark blue), fungi, and yeast. When applied to a blood smear, leukocyte and platelet numbers can be estimated and polychromatophils (as reticulocytes) recognized. This makes it a valuable triage stain for blood and fluid specimens examined on an emergency basis. When religiously filtered, it is an ideal stain to detect hemobartonellosis since the erythrocyte is essentially "invisible," accentuating the surface silhouette of the dark blue organism.

HELPFUL HINT: This is a valuable, cost-effective stain for the examination of cytologic preparations, blood smears, and urine sediments in veterinary practice. The added responsibility of replenishing the stain with filtered stock stain weekly is well worth the time invested.

Romanowsky-Type Stains

Romanowsky-type stains are often utilized in practice settings because of they are rapid and easy to use. They are combinations of basic and acidic dyes dissolved in methyl alcohol. These polychromatic stains impart the basophilic and eosinophilic tinctorial properties observed on blood films. Wright's stain (Wright's Stain Solution, Fisher Scientific) is used widely in most medical and veterinary laboratories because it results in well-stained blood films. Other Romanowsky-type stains used alone or in various combinations include Leishman's, May–Grunwald–Giemsa, and Diff-Quik® (Diff-Quik® Differential Stain Set, American Scientific Products). The latter is a polychromatic stain commonly used in veterinary practice because of its time-saving convenience. For certain specimens such as bone marrow samples, there may be tradeoff in the staining quality. Mast cell granules do not stain reliably with it. If a staining deficiency is suspected during the

TABLE 1–3	Causes of Abnormal Staining

Excessive blue (erythrocytes appear blue green)
   Prolonged contact time with the stain
   Inadequate wash
   Specimen too thick
   Stain or diluent too alkaline—ph > 7; check
   with pH paper
   Exposure of specimen to formalin or its
   fumes (e.g., open formalin container)
   Delayed fixation

Excessive pink
   Prolonged washing
   Insufficient contact time with the stain
   Stain or diluent too acid—ph < 7;
   erythrocytes can appear orange or bright
   red—formic acid can result from the
   oxidation of methyl alcohol with prolonged
   exposure to air; fresh methanol is
   recommended
   Mounting the coverslip before the specimen
   is dry

Inadequately stained nucleated cells and
erythrocytes
   Insufficient contact time with one or more of
   the staining solutions
   Surface of a second glass slide covers the
   specimen on the first slide (can occur when
   staining two slides back-to-back in Coplin
   jars)

Precipitate on the stained specimen
   Inadequate washing of the slide at the end of
   the staining period
   Inadequate filtration of the stain
   Unclear slides

examination of a discrete cell neoplasm, new methylene blue or Giemsa stain can be used to demonstrate the presence of mast cell granules.

Poorly stained specimens can result from improper staining times, weakened stain from overuse, and improperly managed cytologic preparations. One should become familiar with one kind of Romanowsky-type stain and not switch brands frequently. The composition of dyes in polychromatic stains has been demonstrated to vary considerably among suppliers and from batch to batch from the same supplier. Furthermore, prolonged storage at room temperature (25°C; 77°F) can impair staining intensity because of the formation of degradation products in the methanol. It is most convenient to purchase stains in liquid form. Table 1–3 lists the factors that can cause poorly stained specimens with Romanowsky-type stains.

Staining times vary depending on the thickness of the specimen and the freshness of the stain. The frequency with which the solutions are changed or refreshed depends on the number of slides processed. Dull-blue-appearing nuclei that lack sharp chromatin detail is one indication of a weak solution. Solutions should be changed completely whenever infectious agents or cellular elements inappropriately appear on specimens. The staining times for Diff-Quik® stain solutions need to be increased depending on the thickness of the cytologic preparation and the freshness of the stain. A pleural effusion with low cellularity may be stained adequately with three to five dips in each solution. A thick preparation from a lymph node or bone marrow specimen may require 60 to 120 seconds in each solution to obtain optimal staining (Fig. 1–9A & B). Table 1–4 lists staining time guidelines.

At the end of the staining process, the slide is washed with cold running water for 20 seconds to remove stain precipitate and allowed to dry in a nearly vertical position (also see KEY POINT regarding the use of a hair dryer). Any stain film on the back of the slide can be removed with an alcohol-moistened gauze sponge. The stained specimen is examined microscopically using the 10x or 20x objective for staining quality and uniformity. If acceptable, a coverslip is placed on the specimen if a 40x objective is to be used. A temporary mount is made by placing a drop of immersion oil on the specimen followed by a coverslip. A perma-

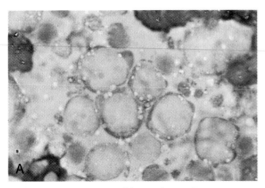

FIGURE 1–9. **A,** This aspirate from an enlarged lymph node was stained with approximately five dips in the fixative and each of the staining solutions. Cell outlines can be seen but the detailed cytomorphology can not be adequately examined. (Diff-Quik®; ×1000.)

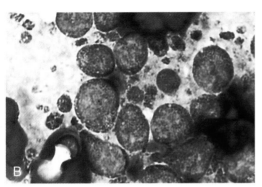

FIGURE 1–9. **B,** The same slide was replaced into the fixative and the staining solutions for approximately 60 seconds in each station while it was slowly moved up and down. A cytologic diagnosis of malignant lymphoma now can be made. A small lymphocyte near center is a helpful size comparator. (Diff-Quik®; ×1000.)

---

nent mount is made with a commercially available coverslip mounting glue (e.g., Eukitt®, Calibrated Instruments).

KEY POINT: A coverslip is always required for sharp focus when the 40x objective is used to examine hematologic and cytologic specimens. A second drop of oil can be placed on the coverslip for use of the oil objective.

TABLE 1–4	Suggested Procedure for Staining Cytologic Specimens Using Diff-Quik® Solutions*

Fixative: 60 to 120 seconds

Solution 1: 30 to 60 seconds

Solution 2: 5 to 60 seconds†

Rinse under cold tap water: 15 seconds

Examine staining adequacy using low power; eosinophilia or basophilia can be enhanced by returning to solution 1 or solution 2, respectively, followed by a rinse.

Air-dry and examine

---

* Suggested times are based on fresh stains; with time and use the stains weaken and longer times will be required. Consistently understained specimens are an indication for replenishing with fresh stain.

† The shortest times are suggested for hypocellular fluids that are low in protein such as transudates, cerebral spinal fluids, and urine sediments.

Modified from Henry MJ, Burton LG, Stanley MW, Horowitz CA: Application of a Diff-Quik® stain to fine needle aspiration smears: Rapid staining with improved cytologic detail. Acta Cytol 1987; 31:954–955.

KEY POINT: Two staining stations are routinely recommended. One is used for "clean" specimens such as blood films, effusions, and lymph nodes aspirates. The other is used for "dirty" specimens such as skin scrapings, fecal and intestinal cytology, and suspected abscesses.

SITE-SPECIFIC CONSIDERATIONS

Cutaneous Nodule and the Lymph Node

The cutaneous nodule and the enlarged lymph node are readily accessible tissues for exfoliative cytology. A minimum of two lymph nodes should be sampled if there is generalized lymphadenopathy. The center of an enlarged lymph node should be avoided to minimize the risk of obtaining necrotic debris and nondiagnostic cytologic material. The tissue is palpated for consistency and the margins are defined. Softer areas suggestive of fluid or necrotic tissue are identified and separate aspirates of these areas and firmer tissue are planned. The area of interest is clipped and scrubbed before aspiration. The tissue is immobilized firmly between the thumb and forefinger. The needle is inserted into the tissue, an aspiration or nonaspiration technique is used, and the needle is advanced into (but not through) the tissue of interest. The needle is redirected several times (Fig. 1–1). The plunger of the syringe is *gently* returned to the start position and the needle is withdrawn. Maintaining vacuum while removing the needle from the tissue causes splattering of the material in the syringe barrel and enhances the potential of blood contamination from a cutaneous vessel. When fluid is encountered it should be completely removed and handled as a fluid specimen. A separate sampling procedure is executed for the firmer tissue with a new needle and syringe combination.

KEY POINT: The exfoliation of cells occurs as a consequence of the needle's passage through the tissue. It is the repeated movement of the needle through the tissue that is the critical component of obtaining diagnostic material from nonfluid tissues.

KEY POINT: Not all solid tissues can be adequately sampled with exfoliation cytology. If diagnostic cells are not obtained with fine-needle aspiration biopsy (FNAB) after triaging the stained specimen, consider an excisional biopsy.

Liver, Spleen, Kidney

The use of exfoliative cytology for the investigation of organomegaly of the liver,
spleen, and kidney is the most rewarding indication. The cellular or cell-associated causation of the enlarged organ often exfoliates from these tissues. Ultrasonographic examination of these organs has increased the use of FNAB for the examination of focal lesions. The diagnostic efficiency of cytology is reduced in support of this indication. There is a greater possibility that the cell type may not exfoliate or the lesion will be missed and the surrounding tissue examined, resulting in an erroneous impression and misdiagnosis. In addition, greater expertise is required for the examination of FNAB specimens from these organs because nodular hyperplastic lesions of the spleen and canine liver become more prevalent in the geriatric patient (see Chapter 8).

KEY POINT: The nonaspiration sampling technique reduces blood contamination from vascular organs such as liver and spleen.

KEY POINT: Remember that the liver is a moving target due to its intimate association with the movement of the diaphragm. Consequently, a craniodorsad positioning of the needle reduces the risk of laceration (Fig. 1–10).

KEY POINT: Two actions should be taken if a bloody sample is obtained from the liver or spleen. First, place the sample immediately into an EDTA tube. A direct smear (similar to a peripheral blood film) and a buffy-coat preparation should be triaged for diagnostic material such as malignant mesenchymal cells (hemangiosarcoma). Do *not* attempt to "coat" an entire glass slide with the bloody specimen in hopes of a diagnostic specimen. The result will be a dismal diagnostic failure. Second, if no fluid-filled lesion is present upon ultrasound examination, repeat the FNAB with a clean needle and using a nonaspiration technique.

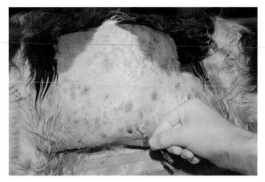

FIGURE 1–10. Fine-needle aspiration biopsy of the liver can be accomplished with the dog in left lateral recumbancy. In the picture, the head is to reader's left. The needle is inserted in a craniodorsad direction at the triangle formed by the left lateral edge of the xiphoid process and the union of the last rib with the sternum. Once the needle touches the surface of the liver, the hub of the needle will move in concert with the movement of the diaphram but in the opposite direction.

Nose and Lung

Evaluation of the nasal cavity is often compromised by the occult nature of the underlying pathology. Radiography always should precede an attempt to obtain a specimen for cytology or histopathology. They can define the area of the nasal cavity that is predominantly involved, thereby suggesting the side of the cavity to be sampled. In addition, manipulation within the nasal cavity often results in hemorrhage, which obscures radiographic detail. After radiography, the oropharynx is examined visually and by digital palpation. The dorsal area of the soft palate is examined with a dental mirror and by palpation. If no abnormal tissue is identified for aspiration and/or excisional biopsy, the recesses of the nasal cavity are sampled by a washing or aspiration technique. Examination of the nasal cavity with an otoscope can allow visualiza-

tion of abnormal tissue and can assist in procuring a tissue specimen.

Superficial lesions, such as eosinophilic or fungal rhinitis, can be occasionally identified by examination of nasal mucus or superficial mucosal scrapings. Most of the time, superficial swab-obtained specimens are nondiagnostic or yield only nonspecific inflammation and bacteria. More aggressive cytologic specimens from the nasal cavity can be obtained by flush or aspiration techniques. A soft, rubber urinary catheter is flexible enough for the retrograde flushing procedure. The saline flush is collected and squash preps made from mucoid globs and bits of tissue. The remaining saline is centrifuged in a conical-tip tube and preps (squash and/or direct smears) made from the pellet. A rigid, large-bore polyurethane urinary catheter or the plastic needle guard from a Sovereign® (Sherwood Medical) intravenous catheter is effective for obtaining a nasal specimen (Fig. 1–11A). The depth of the nasal cavity is approximated, and a corresponding length of catheter is cut at an angle. The catheter is attached to a sy-

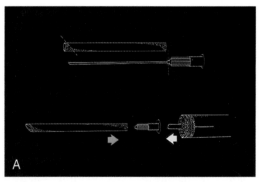

FIGURE 1–11. A, This schematic representation demonstrates a method of altering an intravenous catheter for use in obtaining nasal cytologic specimens by aspiration. One end of the outer plastic shield is cut at an angle and the needle is cut close to the plastic hub. The outer plastic shield is wedged firmly over the hub.

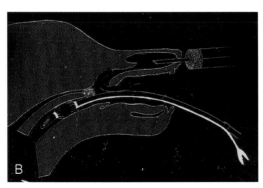

FIGURE 1–11. **B**, A sagittal schematic representation of a dog's head, demonstrating two possible techniques for obtaining a cytologic specimen from the nose. The altered intravenous catheter or a relatively rigid large-bore urinary catheter is aggressively inserted via the external nares and aspiration applied when resistance is encountered. Alternatively, a flexible rubber urinary catheter can be inserted above the soft palate and the nasal cavity flushed retrograde. The fluid and solid material are collected in a container. (Reprinted with permission from Meyer DJ: The management of cytology specimens. Compend Contin Educ Pract Vet 1987; 9:10–17.)

ringe and firmly advanced into the nasal cavity until moderate resistance is encountered. Aspiration is applied while the catheter is manipulated within the nasal cavity (Fig. 1–11B). For this procedure, aspiration and manipulation of the catheter can be more aggressive because of the mucus and cartilaginous nature of diseased tissue. Another deviation is the maintenance of negative pressure when withdrawing the catheter in an attempt to exteriorize bits of tissues. Fluid and bits of tissue can be used for cytologic preparations. Larger pieces of tissue fragments and clotted blood can be placed in 10% formalin for histopathologic examination to maximize the diagnostic yield.

FNBA of the lung parenchyma is rewarding when the interstitial infiltrative disease is diffuse or large focal lesions are identified radiographically. Unless the cellular infiltrate is radiographically or ultrasonographically notable, the diagnostic yield cannot be expected to be fruitful. Ultrasongraphic guidance of the needle is a more accurate way of ensuring that the desired lesion is sampled. Guessing the location of needle placement for small or ill-defined lesions from the radiograph is problematic.

Successful use of the transtracheal wash and brochoalveolar lavage for assessing pulmonary changes depends on the disease process involving the mucosa and/or the alveolar lumen, sampling the diseased region, and adequate collection of the saline lavage. There must be a relatively aggressive attempt to recover the wash or lavage that includes angulation of the patient's head downward to facilitate a diagnostic yield. Mucosal brushings/scrapings can enhance the cytologic yield of mucosal lesions.

KEY POINT: The lung is a dynamic organ prone to laceration by the needle. Momentary apnea can be achieved occasionally by touching or gently blowing on the patient's nose.

Joint

Lameness and swollen joints are the common indications for the examination of the synovial fluid. A review of the skeletal anatomy for the joint of interest is prudent prior to the sampling procedure. In general, an appropriate interosseous location is determined by digital palpation with the affected joint in a slightly flexed position. A 22- to 25-gauge needle attached to a 3-cc syringe is used. Normal synovial fluid is viscous and even inflamed synovial fluid may retain this quality. Consequently, gentle aspiration must be linked to patience as the thick fluid slowly rises up the smaller needle. Quantity is less important than quality of the specimen. One drop is adequate for a slide preparation and two or three drops in a sterile tube or applied to a culturette for potential culture will suffice. If nonlocalizing polyarticular disease is suspected, two or more joints, including at least one carpal joint, should be routinely sampled.

SUBMITTING CYTOLOGY SPECIMENS TO A REFERENCE LABORATORY

The busy practitioner often finds it more convenient to submit cytology specimens to a commercial veterinary laboratory for examination. Many of these facilities have personnel specifically trained to make buffy-coat and cytospin preparations of fluid specimens and experienced microscopists to examine cytologic specimens. Their expertise is effective only if the specimen is submitted properly.

Fluid specimens should be placed immediately in EDTA tubes to prevent clot formation. If the fluid will be in transit longer than 24 hours, a direct slide preparation should be made to accompany the tube. Experience indicates that the red-topped and purple-topped collection tubes are not reliably sterile. Bacterial growth can occur in a "sterile" specimen when transit is prolonged; therefore, an appropriate culture vehicle should be used when the specimen is being submitted for bacterial culture.

As previously indicated, touch imprints can be helpful adjuncts to the histologic examination of formalin-fixed tissues. Formalin vapors can alter the staining characteristics of touch imprints drastically (Fig.

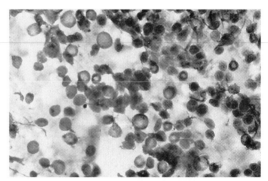

FIGURE 1–12. This lymph node specimen was inadvertently exposed to formalin fumes. Most of the elements present cannot be recognized as lymphocytes, precluding a cytologic interpretation. Formalin fumes alter the cytomorphology and staining characteristics of nucleated cells; this should be considered as a reason for a nondiagnostic specimen. (Wright; ×600.) A cytologic diagnosis of lymphoid hyperplasia was made from a second aspirate (not shown).

1–12). When touch imprints accompany formalin-fixed tissues, they should be placed in their own air-tight container. Breakage is a common problem when glass slides are mailed in cardboard containers. Rigid plastic or Styrofoam containers offer reliable protection. If there is a lack of familiarity with a particular sample submission procedure, the laboratory always should be contacted for advice before collection.

KEY POINT: Formalin fumes are pervasive and rapidly penetrating. They alter the staining and morphology of hematology and cytology specimens. Keep open formalin containers away from these specimens even if opened only momentarily.

References and Additional Reading

Clercx C, Wallon J, Gilbert S, et al: Imprint and brush cytology in the diagnosis of canine intranasal tumours. J Sm Anim Pract 1996; 37:423–437.

Eriksson O, Hagmar B, Ryo W: Effects of fine-needle aspiration and other biopsy procedures on tumor dissemination in mice. Cancer 1984; 54:74–78.

Farkas DH, Kaul KL, Wiedbrauk DL, et al: Specimen collection and storage for diagnostic molecular pathology investigation. Arch Pathol Lab Med 1996; 120:591–596.

Harvey JW: Canine bone marrow: Normal hematopoiesis, biopsy techniques, and cell identification. Compend Contin Educ Compan Anim Pract 1984; 6:909–925.

Henry MJ, Burton LG, Stanley MW, Horwitz CA: Application of a modified Diff-Quik stain to fine needle aspiration smears: Rapid staining with improved cytologic detail. Acta Cytol 1987; 31:954–955.

Jorundsson E, Lumsden JH, Jacobs RM: Rapid staining techniques in cytopathology: A review and comparison of modified protocols for hematoxylin and eosin, Papanicolaou and Romanowsky stains. Vet Clin Pathol 1999; 28:100–108.

Mair S, Dunbar F, Becker PJ, et al: Fine needle cytology—Is aspiration suction necessary? A study of 100 masses in various sites. Acta Cytol 1989; 33:809–813.

Meyer DJ: The management of cytology specimens. Compend Contin Educ Pract Vet 1987; 9:10–17.

Meyer DJ, Harvey JW: Effusions. In *Veterinary Laboratory Medicine: Interpretation and Diagnosis.* WB Saunders, Philadelphia, 1998, pp. 255–260.

Podell M: Epilepsy and seizure classification: A lesson from Leonardo. J Vet Intern Med 1999; 13:3–4.

Vos JH, van den Ingh TSGAM, van Mil FN: Non-exfoliative canine cytology: The value of fine needle aspiration and scraping cytology. Vet Q 1989; 11:222–231.

Willis M, Bounous DI, Hirsh S, et al: Conjunctival brush cytology: Evaluation of a new cytological collection technique in dogs and cats with a comparison to conjunctival scraping. Vet Comp Ophthalmol 1997; 7:74–81.

Yue X, Zheng S: Cytologic diagnosis by transthoracic fine needle sampling without aspiration. Acta Cytol 1989; 33:806–808.

CHAPTER 2

General Categories of Cytologic Interpretation

ROSE E. RASKIN

One use of cytology is to classify lesions so as to assist with the diagnosis, prognosis, and management of the case. Cytologic interpretations are generally classified into one of five cytodiagnostic groups (Table 2–1). A sixth category can be used for nondiagnostic interpretations. Nondiagnostic samples usually result from insufficient cellular material or excessive blood contamination.

KEY POINT: Interpretation of cytologic material may include more than one category, such as inflammation along with a response to tissue injury or neoplasia with inflammation.

NORMAL OR HYPERPLASTIC TISSUE

Normal and hyperplastic tissues are both composed primarily of mature cell types. Normal cells display uniformity in cellular, nuclear, and nucleolar size and shape. Cytoplasmic volume is usually high relative to the nucleus (Figs. 2–1 and 2–2). Hyperplasia is a non-neoplastic enlargement of tissue that can occur in response to hormonal disturbances or tissue injury. Hyperplastic tissue has a tendency to enlarge symmetrically in size in comparison to neoplasia. Cytologically, hyperplastic cells have a higher nuclear-to-cytoplasmic ratio than normal cells. Examples of hyperplastic responses include nodular proliferations within the parenchyma of the prostate (Fig. 2–3), liver, and pancreas (Fig. 2–4).

CYSTIC MASS

Cystic lesions contain liquid or semisolid material. The low-protein liquid usually contains a small number of cells. These benign lesions may result from proliferation of lining cells or tissue injury. Examples include seroma (Fig. 2–5), salivary mucocele, apocrine sweat gland cyst, epidermal/follicular cyst, and cysts associated with noncutaneous glands such as the mammary gland or prostate (Fig. 2–6).

TABLE 2–1.	General Categories of Cytologic Interpretation

Normal or hyperplastic tissue

Cystic mass

Inflammation or cellular infiltrate

Response to tissue injury

Neoplasia

Nondiagnostic sample

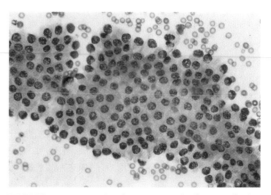

FIGURE 2–3. Canine prostatic hyperplasia. Tissue aspirate. Dog. The presenting clinical sign in this case involves blood dripping from the prepuce. Cytologically, the nuclear size is uniform, however, the nuclear-to-cytoplasmic ratio is increased as indicated by the close proximity of nuclei to each other. (Wright-Giemsa; ×125.)

FIGURE 2–1. Normal skeletal muscle. Tissue aspirate. Dog. Numerous threadlike myofibrils compose each cell whose nucleus is small, condensed, and oval. Cross-striations, characteristic of skeletal muscle, are barely visible against the dark blue cytoplasm. (Wright-Giemsa; ×125.)

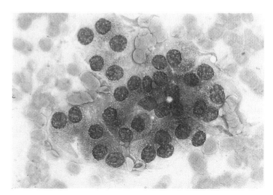

FIGURE 2–4. Nodular hyperplasia of the pancreas. Tissue aspirate. Dog. Ultrasound examination reveals a hypoechoic mass in the area of the pancreas. Cytologically, hyperplastic parenchymal organs commonly display binucleation. (Wright-Giemsa; ×250.)

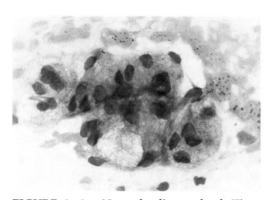

FIGURE 2–2. Normal salivary gland. Tissue aspirate. Dog. The gland has uniform features of nuclear size, nuclear-to-cytoplasmic ratio, and cytoplasmic content. (Wright-Giemsa; ×250.)

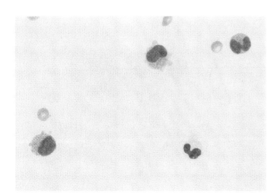

FIGURE 2–5. Seroma. Tissue aspirate. Dog. Blood-tinged fluid is removed from a swelling on the neck. Cytologically, low cellularity and low protein content is visible in the background. Large mononuclear cells with fine cytoplasmic granularity predominate along with low numbers of erythrocytes. (Wright-Giemsa; ×250.)

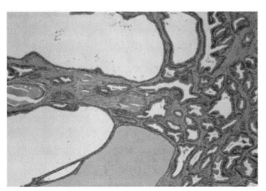

FIGURE 2–6. Prostatic cyst. Histopathology. Dog. Cuboidal epithelial cells line large cystic spaces that represent dilated ducts. (H & E; ×25.)

INFLAMMATION OR CELLULAR INFILTRATE

Inflammatory conditions are classified cytologically by the predominance of the cell type involved. Recognition of the inflammatory cell type often suggests an etiologic condition.

Purulent or suppurative lesions contain greater than 85% neutrophils; they are then classified by the presence or absence of degeneration affecting the neutrophil. Nondegenerate neutrophils are morphologically normal and predominate in relatively nontoxic environments such as immune-mediated conditions, neoplastic lesions (Fig. 2–7), and sterile lesions caused by irritants such as urine and bile. Degenerate neutrophils display nuclear swelling and decreased stain intensity termed *karyolysis* (Fig. 2–8),

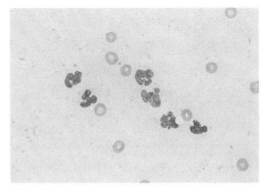

FIGURE 2–7. Nondegenerate neutrophils. Synovial fluid. Dog. Nonseptic inflammation with well-segmented neutrophils appears secondary to adjacent neoplasia of the bone. (Wright-Giemsa; ×250.)

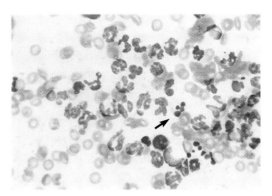

FIGURE 2–8. Karyolysis, karyorrhexis. Tissue aspirate. Dog. Mild to moderate karyolysis of neutrophils is evident by the decreased nuclear stain intensity and swollen nuclear lobes. Pyknosis of multiple nuclear segments appear as dark, dense, round structures, termed *karyorrhexis* (*arrow*), in this case of bacterial dermatitis. (Wright-Giemsa; ×250.)

indicating rapid cell death in a toxic environment (Perman et al., 1979b). Increased nuclear staining with coalescence of the nucleus into a single round mass and an intact cellular membrane characterizes *pyknosis* (Fig. 2–9), a slow progressive change often within a relatively nontoxic environment.

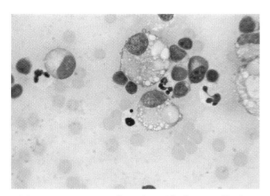

FIGURE 2–9. Pyknosis. Chylous effusion. Dog. Chronic inflammation of this fluid produces neutrophil nuclei that have condensed into a large, often single, dark, round structure related to the slow progression of cellular change in a nonseptic environment. The pyknotic cell in this case contains as well a second smaller round nuclear fragment. (Wright; ×250.)

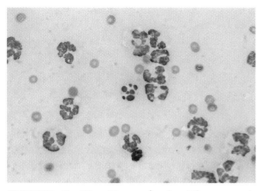

FIGURE 2–10. Karyorrhexis. Tissue aspirate. Inflammatory response with evidence of multiple pyknotic nuclear segments in the center cell. (Wright-Giemsa; ×250.)

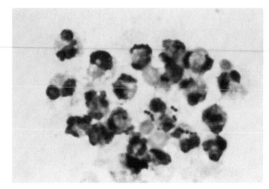

FIGURE 2–11. Bacterial sepsis. Tissue aspirate. Dog. Markedly karyolytic neutrophils are present with intracellular and extracellular coccoid bacteria. Karyolysis is so severe that the cells are barely recognizable as neutrophils. (Wright; ×500.)

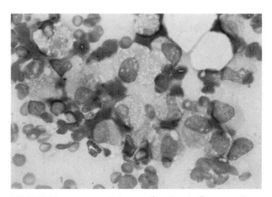

FIGURE 2–12. Macrophagic inflammation. Tissue imprint. Dog. Nodular lung disease with numerous large mononuclear cells having abundant gray cytoplasm and many cells with multiple cytoplasmic vacuoles. (Wright-Giemsa; ×250.)

An end stage of cell death, termed *karyorrhexis*, may be seen cytologically as the result of pyknosis of hypersegmented nuclei (Fig. 2–10). Degenerate neutrophils predominate in bacterial infections, particularly gram-negative types. Under septic conditions, bacteria may be found intracellularly (Fig. 2–11).

Histiocytic or macrophagic lesions contain a predominance of macrophages, suggesting chronic inflammation (Fig. 2–12). In granulomas, activated macrophages that morphologically resemble epithelial cells are termed *epithelioid macrophages*. These cells may merge to form giant multinucleated forms (Fig. 2–13). The granulomatous le-

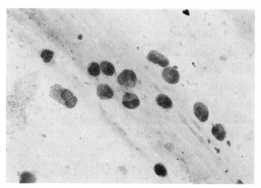

FIGURE 2–15. Eosinophilic inflammation. Transtracheal wash. Cat. Clinical presentation of a chronic cough in this cat with suspected pulmonary allergy. Fluid contains 95% eosinophils. Pictured are several eosinophils that stain pink to blue-green and adhere to pink mucus material. (Wright-Giemsa; ×250.)

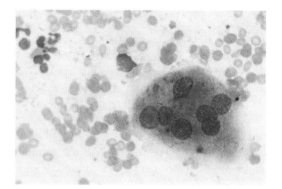

FIGURE 2–13. Multinucleate giant cell. Tissue aspirate. Cat. Skin lesion with pyogranulomatous inflammation, including many giant cells related to the presence of fungal hyphae. Pictured is a cell with seven distinct nuclei and abundant granular blue-gray cytoplasm. (Wright-Giemsa; ×250.)

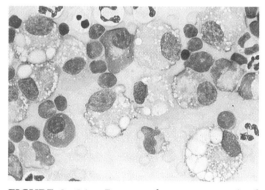

FIGURE 2–14. Pyogranulomatous or mixed cell inflammation. Chylous effusion. Dog. Chronic chylous effusion contains a variety of cell types; including nondegenerate neutrophils, vacuolated macrophages, small to medium lymphocytes, and two mature plasma cells. (Wright; ×250.)

sions are often associated with foreign body reactions and mycobacterial infection.

Pyogranulomatous or mixed cell inflammatory lesions contain a mixture of neutrophils and macrophages (Fig. 2–14) that may include increased numbers of lymphocytes or plasma cells. This type of inflammation is often associated with foreign body reactions, fungal infections, mycobacterial infections, panniculitis, lick granulomas, and other chronic tissue injuries.

Eosinophilic lesions contain greater than 10% eosinophils in addition to other inflammatory cell types (Fig. 2–15). It is seen with or without mast cell involvement. This inflammatory response is associated with eosinophilic granuloma, hypersensitivity or allergic conditions, parasitic migrations, fungal infections, mast cell tumors, and other neoplastic conditions that induce eosinophilopoiesis.

Lymphocytic or plasmacytic infiltration is often associated with allergic or immune reactions, early viral infections, and chronic inflammation. The lymphoid population is heterogeneous, with small or intermediate-sized lymphocytes and plasma cells mixed with other inflammatory cells (Fig. 2–14). A monomorphic population of lymphoid cells without other inflammatory cells present suggests lymphoid neoplasia.

RESPONSE TO TISSUE INJURY

Cytologic samples often contain evidence of tissue injury in addition to cyst formation, inflammation, or neoplasia. These changes include hemorrhage, proteinaceous debris, cholesterol crystals, necrosis, and fibrosis.

Hemorrhage that is pathologic can be distinguished from blood contamination encountered during the cytologic collection. Blood contamination is associated with the presence of numerous erythrocytes and platelets. Acute hemorrhage is associated with engulfment of erythrocytes by macrophages termed erythrophagocytosis (Fig. 2–16). Chronic hemorrhage is associated with active macrophages containing degraded blood pigment within their cytoplasm, for example, blue-green to black hemosiderin granules (Figs. 2–17 and 2–18) or yellow rhomboid hematoidin crystals (Fig. 2–18).

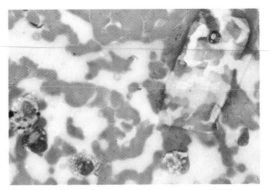

FIGURE 2–17.   Chronic hemorrhage. Tissue aspirate. Dog. Several activated macrophages are present in this follicular cyst lesion. The macrophage directly below the cholesterol crystal contains blue-green granular material in the cytoplasm consistent with hemosiderin, a breakdown product of erythrocytes. On the left edge is a macrophage with large black granules suggestive of hemosiderin. (Wright; ×250.)

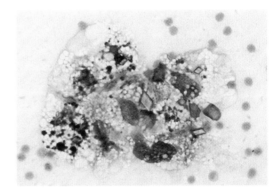

FIGURE 2–18.   Hematoidin crystals. Pericardial fluid. Dog. Activated macrophages with bright yellow rhomboid crystals of variable size appear in this hemorrhagic fluid related to hemoglobin breakdown in an anaerobic environment. Several macrophages also contain black granular material consistent with hemosiderin. (Wright-Giemsa; ×250.)

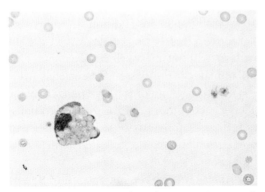

FIGURE 2–16.   Erythrophagocytosis. Cerebrospinal fluid. Cat. Many erythrocytes are in the background along with one large macrophage that engulfed numerous intact red cells. The cat had confirmed infection with feline coronavirus (feline infectious peritonitis). (Wright; ×250.)

Hemosiderin represents an excess aggregation of ferritin molecules or micelles. This form of iron storage now becomes visible by light microscopy and stains blue with the Prussian blue reaction. Hematoidin crystals do not contain iron although they are formed during anaerobic breakdown of hemoglobin such as may occur within tissues or cavities. Hematomas often contain phagocytized erythrocytes if the lesion is acute or hemosiderin-laden macrophages if the lesion is chronic.

Proteinaceous debris may be seen within the background of the preparation. Mucus stains lightly basophilic and appears amorphous (Fig. 2–19). Lymphoglandular bodies (Fig. 2–20) are cytoplasmic fragments from fragile cells, usually lymphocytes, which are discrete, round, lightly basophilic structures (Flanders et al., 1993). *Nuclear streaming* refers to linear pink to purple strands of nuclear remnants (Fig. 2–21) produced by excessive tissue handling during cytologic preparation or with necrotic material when sampled. Clear to light-pink amorphous strands representing collagen (Fig. 2–22) may be admixed with spindle cells and endothelium into a fibrovascular stroma. Amyloid is an uncommon pathologic protein

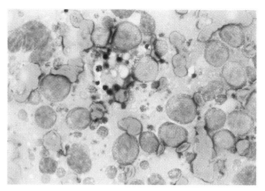

FIGURE 2–20. Lymphoglandular bodies. Tissue aspirate. Dog. The background of this lymph node preparation contains numerous small blue-gray cytoplasmic fragments called *lymphoglandular bodies* that are related to the rupture of the fragile neoplastic lymphocytes. An activated macrophage has phagocytized cellular debris appearing as large blue-black particles. (Wright; ×250.)

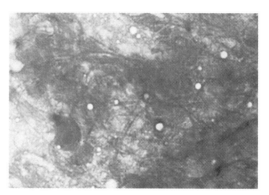

FIGURE 2–21. Nuclear streaming. Tissue aspirate. Purple strands of nuclear material are formed from ruptured cells either as an artifact of slide preparation or from fragile cells that are frequently neoplastic. (Wright-Giemsa; ×250.) (Courtesy of the University of Florida collection.)

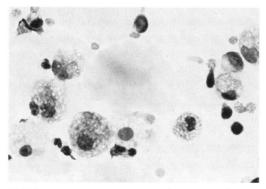

FIGURE 2–19. Mucus. Salivary mucocele. Dog. The background contains pale pink-blue amorphous material representative of mucus. Numerous activated macrophages or mucinophages compose the predominant population. (Wright; ×250.)

found between cells. It appears amorphous, eosinophilic, and hyaline and may be associated with chronic inflammation.

Cholesterol crystals represent evidence of cell membrane damage that is found in the background of some cytologic preparations. These rectangular plated crystals are transparent unless background staining is en-

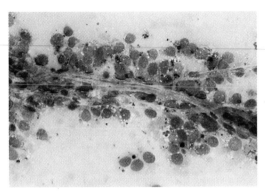

FIGURE 2–22. Collagenous fibers. Tissue aspirate. Dog. Clear to light pink strands of fibrous connective tissue may resemble fungal hyphae. Collagenous fibers will have poorly defined margins and a variable diameter, unlike hyphae, which have uniform width and distinct borders. Presumed neoplastic histiocytes are the predominant cell type. (Wright-Giemsa; ×125.)

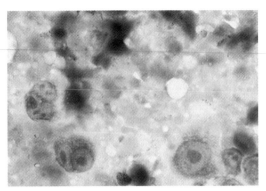

FIGURE 2–24. Necrosis. Tissue aspirate. Dog. Prominent nucleoli remain visible while other tissue has degenerated into dark blue-gray amorphous debris representative of necrotic material. The sample was taken from a case of prostatic carcinoma in which the necrotic site was focal. (Wright-Giemsa; ×250.)

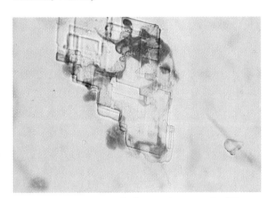

FIGURE 2–23. Cholesterol crystal. Tissue aspirate. Clear rectangular plates with notched corners are characteristic of cholesterol. This is often associated with degenerate squamous epithelium as in follicular cysts. Crystals may be highlighted with background cellular debris or stain. (New methylene blue; ×250.)

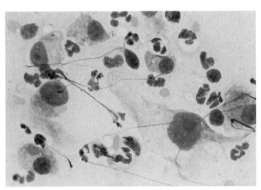

FIGURE 2–25. Reactive fibroplasia. Tissue scraping. Cat. Oral mass with associated septic inflammation. Pictured are several plump mesenchymal cells with a stellate to spindle appearance and prominent nucleoli along with suppurative inflammation. The severity of the inflammatory response warrants caution in suggesting a malignant mesenchymal mass or sarcoma. Note the nuclear streaming appear as purple strands. (Aqueous-based Wright; ×250.)

hanced as, for example, with new methylene blue stain (Fig. 2–23). The crystals are most often associated with epidermal/follicular cysts.

Necrosis and fibrosis may occur together or separately in some cytologic preparations. The death of cells is represented by fuzzy, indistinct cell outlines and definition

of cell type (Fig. 2–24). A reparative response accompanying tissue injury involves increased fibroblastic activity. It is common to see very reactive fibrocytes (Fig. 2–25) along with severe inflammation. One must be careful not to overinterpret this reactivity as a neoplastic condition.

NEOPLASIA

General Features

Neoplasia is initially diagnosed when a monomorphic cell population is present and significant inflammation is lacking. Further division into benign and malignant types is based on cytomorphologic characteristics. *Benign cells* display uniformity in size, nuclear-to-cytoplasmic ratio, and other nuclear features. *Malignant cells* often display three or more criteria (Table 2–2 and Figs. 2–26 to 2–32) of cellular immaturity or atypia, which should be identified before

TABLE 2–2.	Cytologic Criteria Used to Identify Malignant Cells

Pleomorphism of cell size, shape, or maturation state between cells of similar origin (Fig. 2–26)

High or variable nuclear-to-cytoplasmic ratio (Fig. 2–27)

Variation in nuclear size, termed *anisokaryosis* (Fig. 2–27)

Coarse nuclear chromatin clumping (Fig. 2–28)

Enlarged, multiple, or variably-shaped nucleoli (Fig. 2–29)

Nuclear molding related to the rapid growth of cells (Fig. 2–30)

Multinucleation (Fig. 2–31)

Abnormal mitotic figures evident as uneven divisions and isolated or lag chromatin (Fig. 2–32)

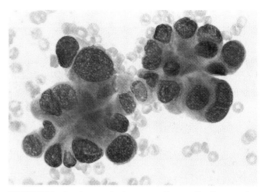

FIGURE 2–27. **Anisocytosis, anisokaryosis. Tissue aspirate. Dog.** Lung adenocarcinoma specimen has several features of malignancy. These features include high and variable nuclear-to-cytoplasmic ratio, anisokaryosis, binucleation, and coarse nuclear chromatin. (Wright-Giemsa; ×250.)

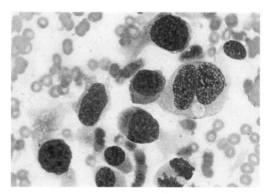

FIGURE 2–28. **Coarse chromatin. Tissue aspirate. Dog.** Same case as FIGURE 2–26. The nuclear material is mottled with light and dark spaces clearly evident. This appearance is often associated with neoplastic transitional epithelium but may be seen with other tissues. Binucleation is seen in one cell and a mitotic figure is present on the bottom edge. (Wright-Giemsa; ×250.)

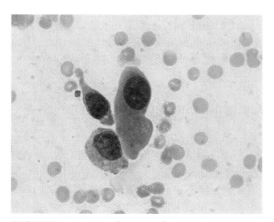

FIGURE 2–26. **Pleomorphism. Tissue aspirate. Dog.** Transitional cell carcinoma cells display variability in size and shape supportive of malignancy. (Wright-Giemsa; ×250.)

a diagnosis of malignancy is made. In cases of an equivocal diagnosis or severe inflammation, histopathologic examination is recommended.

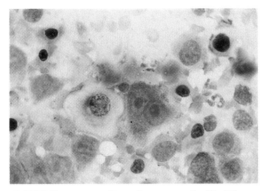

FIGURE 2–29. Prominent nucleoli. Tissue aspirate. Dog. Same case as FIGURE 2–24. A binucleate cell with very large single nucleoli in each nucleus is present. A prominent nucleolus is noted in the adjacent cell that also displays coarse chromatin or chromatin clumping. (Wright-Giemsa; ×250.)

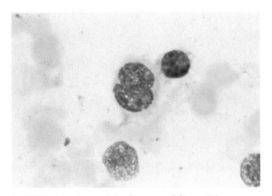

FIGURE 2–30. Nuclear molding. Tissue aspirate. Dog. Nasal chondrosarcoma pictured with a binucleate cell in which one nucleus is wrapped around the other. This feature is present in malignant tissues and is related to the lack of normal inhibition of cell growth. (Wright-Giemsa; ×500.)

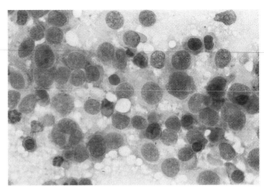

FIGURE 2–31. Multinucleation. Tissue imprint. Dog. Pheochromocytoma with two multinucleate cells, one in the lower left side with three nuclei and the other to the right of center with an irregularly shaped nuclear region. Multinucleation may be found also in epithelial, mesenchymal, and round cell neoplasms. (Wright-Giemsa; ×250.)

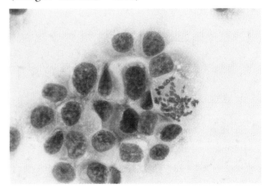

FIGURE 2–32. Abnormal mitosis. Tissue aspirate. Dog. Same case as FIGURE 2–26. Chromosomal fragments are dispersed irregularly with some isolated from the rest, termed *lag chromatin*. Increased mitotic activity may be suggestive of malignancy but abnormal division is diagnostic for malignancy. (Wright-Giemsa; ×250.)

Cytomorphologic Categories

Neoplasms may be divided into four general categories to assist in making the cytologic interpretation by restricting the list of differential diagnoses (Perman et al., 1979a, Alleman and Bain, 2000). The categories listed in Table 2–3 are based not on cell

TABLE 2–3.	Cytomorphologic Categories of Neoplasia	
Category	**General Features**	**Examples**
Epithelial	Clustered, tight arrangement of cells	Transitional cell carcinoma, lung tumors
Mesenchymal	Individualized, spindle to oval cells	Hemangiosarcoma, osteosarcoma
Round cell	Individualized, round, discrete cells	Lymphoma, transmissible venereal tumor
Naked nuclei	Loosely adherent cells with free round nuclei	Thyroid tumors, paragangliomas

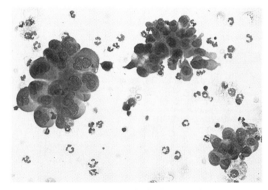

FIGURE 2–33. Epithelial neoplasm. Lung lavage. Dog. Large clusters of cohesive cells having distinct cell borders from a case of lung adenocarcinoma. (Wright-Giemsa; ×100.) (Courtesy of Dr. Robert King, Gainesville, FL.)

origin or function but rather on their general cytomorphologic characteristics. The first two terms are taken from embryology (Noden and de Lahunta, 1985).

Epithelial Neoplasms

This type of neoplasm is associated with a clustered arrangement of cells into ball shapes or monolayer sheets. Cell origin of these neoplasms often involves glandular or parenchymal tissue and lining surfaces. Examples of epithelial neoplasms include lung adenocarcinoma (Fig. 2–33), perianal adenoma (hepatoid tumor), basal cell tumor,

sebaceous adenoma, transitional cell carcinoma (Fig. 2–34), and mesothelioma. Specific cytologic features of epithelial neoplasms include the following characteristics:

■ Cells exfoliate in tight clumps or sheets

■ Cells are adherent to each other and may display distinct tight junctions, termed *desmosomes* (Fig. 2–35)

■ Cells are large and round to polygonal with distinct, intact cytoplasmic borders

■ Nuclei are round to oval

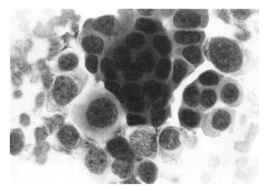

FIGURE 2–34. Epithelial neoplasm. Tissue aspirate. Dog. Same case as FIGURE 2–26. Cells are formed into tight balls or as sheets. Nuclei are round to oval and cells are large, round to polygonal with distinct cytoplasmic borders. (Wright-Giemsa; ×250.)

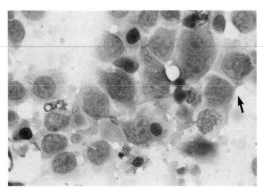

FIGURE 2–35. Desmosomes. Tissue aspirate. Dog. Same case as FIGURE 2–24. A sheet of carcinoma cells with prominent desmosomes. These clear lines (*arrow*) between adjacent cells represent tight junctions that are characteristic of epithelial cells. (Wright-Giemsa; ×250.)

Mesenchymal Neoplasms

Neoplasms with a mesenchymal appearance resemble the embryonic connective tissue, mesenchyme. This tissue is loosely arranged with usually abundant extracellular matrix (Noden and de Lahunta, 1985) and individualized spindle or stellate cells (Bacha and Wood, 1990). Benign and malignant mesenchymal neoplasms often originate from connective tissue elements, such as fibroblasts, osteoblasts, adipocytes, myocytes, and vascular lining cells. Examples of mesenchymal neoplasms include hemangiosarcoma (Fig. 2–36), osteosarcoma (Fig. 2–37), hemangiopericytoma, and amelanotic melanoma (Fig. 2–38). Specific cytologic features of mesenchymal neoplasms include the following:

- Cells usually exfoliate individually (however, clumps of cells are seen occasionally)
- Cells are oval, stellate, or fusiform with often indistinct cytoplasmic borders
- Samples are often poorly cellular
- Cells are usually smaller compared with epithelial cells
- Nuclei are round to elliptical

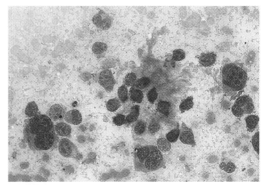

FIGURE 2–37. Mesenchymal neoplasm. Tissue aspirate. Dog. Individualized pleomorphic cells with abundant extracellular eosinophilic osteoid material is consistent with osteosarcoma. Binucleate and multinucleate forms are common and seen in this sample. (Wright-Giemsa; ×125.)

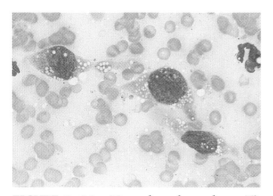

FIGURE 2–36. Mesenchymal neoplasm. Tissue imprint. Dog. Neoplastic cells exfoliate individually and appear oval, spindle, or fusiform. This bone lesion was confirmed as hemangiosarcoma on histologic examination. Characteristic of hemangiosarcoma cytology is a poorly cellular sample with plump mesenchymal cells that contain numerous small punctate cytoplasmic vacuoles. (Wright-Giemsa; ×250.)

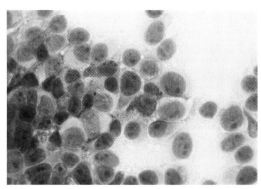

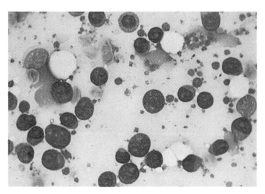

FIGURE 2–38. Mesenchymal neoplasm. Tissue imprint. Dog. Round to oval nuclei, anisokaryosis, high nuclear-to-cytoplasmic ratio, prominent and variably shaped nucleoli, and individualized cells with poorly distinct cytoplasmic borders suggest a malignant mesenchymal neoplasm. This lesion is from a gum mass with a histologically confirmed diagnosis of amelanotic melanoma. One cell in the center contains small amounts of melanin pigment granules. (Aqueous-based Wright; ×250.)

FIGURE 2–39. Round (discrete) cell neoplasm. Tissue aspirate. Dog. Discrete cells with a round shape, distinct cytoplasmic borders and a very high nuclear-to-cytoplasmic ratio are characteristic of lymphoid cells. This sample is taken from a lymph node effaced by lymphoma cells. (Wright-Giemsa; ×250.)

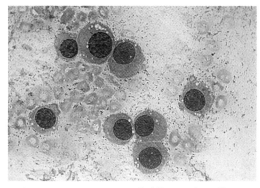

FIGURE 2–40. Round (discrete) cell neoplasm. Tissue aspirate. Dog. This fleshy vulvar mass is composed of round cells bearing a single prominent nucleolus and moderately abundant cytoplasm with frequent punctate cytoplasmic vacuolation. The cytologic diagnosis is transmissible venereal tumor. (Wright-Giemsa; ×250.)

Round Cell Neoplasms

These neoplasms have discrete, round cellular shapes and are often associated with hematopoietic cells. Examples of round cell neoplasms include mast cell tumor, histiocytoma, lymphoma (Fig. 2–39), plasmacytoma, and transmissible venereal tumor (Fig. 2–40). Specific cytologic characteristics of round cell neoplasms include the following:

- Cells exfoliate individually, having distinct cytoplasmic borders
- Cell shape is generally round
- Samples are moderately cellular
- Cells are usually smaller compared with epithelial cells
- Nuclei are round to indented

Naked Nuclei Neoplasms

Naked nuclei neoplasms have a loosely adherent cellular arrangement with free nuclei. This cytologic appearance is an artifact related to the fragile nature of these cells. These neoplasms are usually associated with endocrine and neuroendocrine tumors. Ex-

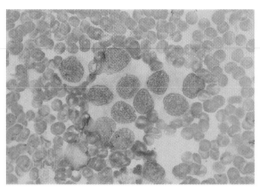

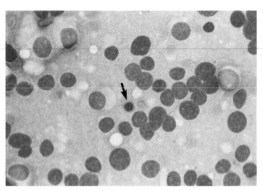

FIGURE 2–41. Naked nuclei neoplasm. Tissue aspirate. Dog. Cervical mass in the area of the thyroid from an animal with a honking cough. Cytologically the sample presents as a syncytium of round nuclei with relatively uniform features. This is characteristic of an endocrine mass. Typically the distinction between hyperplasia, adenoma, and carcinoma is difficult cytologically and sometimes histologically. (Wright-Giemsa; ×250.)

FIGURE 2–42. Naked nuclei neoplasm. Tissue imprint. Dog. Clinical signs include a head tilt and temporal muscle atrophy. Magnetic resonance imaging suggested a mass involving the osseous bulla. Surgery found a mass at the bifurcation of the common carotid artery. Cytologically, the preparation contains mostly loose or free round nuclei against a finely granular eosinophilic background. Few intact cells remain with pale cytoplasm at the edges and center. Adjacent to the center intact cell is a nucleated red cell (*arrow*) suggestive of extramedullary hematopoiesis. The histologic diagnosis is paraganglioma, specifically a malignant chemodectoma in this case, since it metastasized and was thought to involve the chemoreceptor organ in that site. (Wright-Giemsa; ×250.)

amples include thyroid tumors (Fig. 2–41), islet cell tumors, and paragangliomas (Fig. 2–42). Specific cytologic features of naked nuclei neoplasms include the following:

- Cells exfoliate in loosely attached sheets with many free nuclei present, having often indistinct cytoplasmic borders
- Occasional cell clusters may be present with distinct cell outlines
- Cell shape is generally round to polygonal
- Samples are highly cellular
- Nuclei are round to indented

The use of these four cytomorphologic categories may help to classify neoplastic lesions by their general cellular appearance and suggest specific tumor types. Remember that these categories may not fit well for some neoplasms, especially for poorly differentiated tumors. It is recommended that biopsy specimens for histopathologic examination be taken to determine the specific tumor type and extent of the lesion.

References

Alleman AR, Bain PJ: Diagnosing neoplasia: The cytologic criteria for malignancy. Vet Med 2000; 95:204–223.

Bacha WJ, Wood LM: *Color Atlas of Veterinary Histology.* Lea & Febiger, Philadelphia, 1990, pp. 14–15.

Flanders E, Kornstein MJ, Wakely PE, et al: Lymphoglandular bodies in fine-needle aspiration cytology smears. Am J Clin Pathol 1993; 99: 566–569.

Noden DM, de Lahunta A: *The Embryology of Domestic Animals.* Williams & Wilkins, Baltimore, 1985, pp. 10–11.

Perman V, Alsaker RD, Riis RC: *Cytology of the*

Dog and Cat. American Animal Hospital Association, South Bend, IN, 1979a, pp. 4–5.

Perman V, Alsaker RD, Riis RC: *Cytology of the Dog and Cat.* American Animal Hospital Association, South Bend, IN, 1979b, pp. 5–7.

CHAPTER 3

Skin and Subcutaneous Tissues

Rose E. Raskin

NORMAL HISTOLOGY AND CYTOLOGY

There are regional differences in histology of the skin of the dog and cat related to the thickness of the epidermis and dermis (Fig. 3–1A). In general, the epidermis is composed of several layers of squamous epithelium, including a keratinized layer, a granular layer, a spinous layer, and a basal layer. The adnexal structures of the epidermis include hair follicles, sweat glands, and sebaceous glands (Fig. 3–1B). The dermis present below the epidermal layer contains the adnexal structures, smooth muscle bands, blood and lymphatic vessels, nerves, and variably sized collagen and elastic fibers. Located beneath the dermis lies the subcutis, composed of loose adipose tissue and collagen bundles. Normal cytology of the dermis and subcutis contains a mixture of epidermal squamous epithelium and well-differentiated glandular elements as well as mature adipose and collagen tissue.

Basal epithelial cells are round and deeply basophilic with a high nuclear-to-cytoplasmic ratio. Cells of the other epidermal layers are known as *keratinocytes* because of their composition of keratin. Polygonal cells of the granular layer are evident cytologically by the presence of basophilic to magenta keratohyaline granules within an abundant lightly basophilic cytoplasm having a small contracted nucleus. The most superficial keratinized layer consists of flattened, sharply demarcated, blue-green hyalinized squames that lack a nucleus. Elongated dark-blue to purple squames are termed *keratin bars,* which represent rolled or coiled cells. Melanocytes from neural crest origin are located within the basal layer of the epidermis or hair matrix. Their brownish-black to greenish-black fine granules may be seen in some keratinocytes. Also present may be a low number of mast cells from perivascular and perifollicular sites.

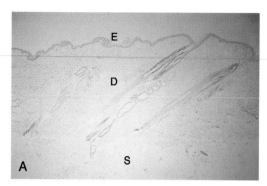

FIGURE 3–1. A, Normal skin histology.
Section of thin-haired skin from the abdomen
of a dog showing the epidermis (E), dermis
(D), and subcutis (S). (H & E; ×10.)

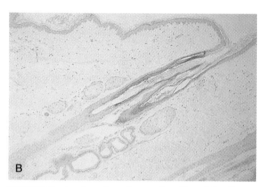

FIGURE 3–1. B, Normal skin histology.
Same case as in Figure 3–1A. The dermis contains the adnexal structures of hair follicles,
sebaceous glands, and ducts of the sweat
glands. In addition, loose and dense collagen
bundles are present superficially and deep, respectively, within the dermis. (H & E; ×25.)

NORMAL-APPEARING EPITHELIUM

KEY POINT: Presence of only mature
epithelium in a skin mass most often indicates a non-neoplastic condition.

Non-neoplastic noninflammatory tumorlike
lesions account for approximately 10% of
skin lesions removed from dogs and cats

(Goldschmidt and Shofer, 1992). These include cysts and glandular hyperplasia.

Epidermal Cyst or Follicular Cyst

Also termed *epidermal inclusion cysts* or *epidermoid cysts,* these cysts are found in one
third to one half of the non-neoplastic noninflammatory tumorlike lesions removed in
dogs and cats, respectively (Goldschmidt
and Shofer, 1992). They occur most frequently in middle- to older-aged dogs (Yager and Wilcock, 1994). Cysts may be single
or multiple, firm to fluctuant, with a
smooth, round, well-circumscribed appearance. These are often located on the dorsum and extremities (Goldschmidt and
Shofer, 1992). The cyst lining arises from
well-differentiated stratified squamous epithelium (Fig. 3–2A). By definition, the lack
of adnexal differentiation without a connec-
tion to the skin surface seen histologically is
termed an *epidermal inclusion cyst.* The
more common follicular cyst is characterized by a distended hair follicle infundibu-
lum that opens to the surface via a pore

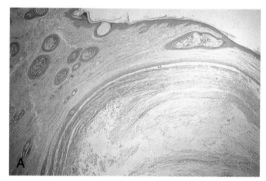

FIGURE 3–2. A, Follicular cyst. Dog. The
large cystic structure is composed of laminated
keratin surrounded by a thin rim of stratified
squamous epithelium. Note the nearby smaller
cysts with pores that open to the surface, suggesting these are of follicular origin. (H & E;
×10.)

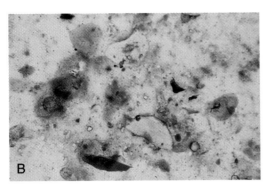

FIGURE 3–2. B, Follicular cyst. Tissue aspirate. Amorphous cellular debris with anuclear squamous epithelium and keratin bars. (Wright; ×125.)

(Fig. 3–2A). The distinction cannot be made cytologically. Keratin bars, squames, or other keratinocytes predominate on cytology (Fig. 3–2B). Degradation of cells within the cyst may lead to the formation of cholesterol crystals, which appear as negative-stained, irregularly notched, rectangular plates best seen against the amorphous basophilic cellular debris of the background (Fig. 3–2C). The behavior of these masses is benign, but rupture of the cyst wall can induce a localized pyogranulomatous cellulitis. When this occurs, neutrophils and mac-

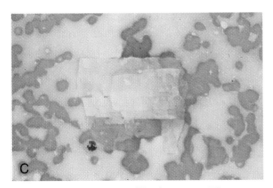

FIGURE 3–2. C, Follicular cyst. Tissue aspirate. Cholesterol crystals appear as clear, rectangular plates visible against the proteinaceous background. (Wright; ×125.)

rophages may be frequent. To prevent this inflammatory response, surgery is frequently suggested and the prognosis is excellent.

Cytologic differential diagnosis: **intracutaneous cornifying epithelioma (keratoacanthoma), dermoid cyst, follicular tumors.**

Apocrine Cyst

This is a common lesion in dogs and cats that is formed from occlusion of the apocrine or sweat gland duct. Grossly, it appears as a fluctuant swelling filled with light-brown to colorless fluid. On cytology, this fluid is usually acellular, having a clear background. Treatment involves surgical excision and the prognosis is excellent.

Cytologic differential diagnosis: **apocrine gland hyperplasia, apocrine gland adenoma.**

Sebaceous Hyperplasia

Grossly, these masses are single to multiple and often resemble a wart. Most are less than 1 cm in diameter. They are firm, elevated, with a hairless, cauliflower or papilliferous surface. Sebaceous hyperplasia is more prevalent than sebaceous adenoma (Yager and Wilcock, 1994). They are very common in old dogs and less common in cats. Distinction cannot be made cytologically and may even be difficult histologically when distinguishing between sebaceous hyperplasia and sebaceous adenoma. Symmetrical proliferation of mature sebaceous lobules around a central squamous-lined duct is the histopathologic basis used to classify the condition as hyperplasia. Mature sebaceous epithelial cells are seen cytologically, sometimes in clusters, or as individual pale foamy cells with a small dense centrally placed nucleus, often mistaken for phagocytic macrophages. These are benign proliferations that have an excellent prognosis following surgical excision.

Cytologic differential diagnosis: sebaceous adenoma.

NONINFECTIOUS INFLAMMATION

Acral Lick Dermatitis/Lick Granuloma

This is a chronic inflammatory response to persistent licking or chewing of a limb, producing a thickened, firm, raised plaque lesion that often becomes ulcerated (Fig. 3–3A). Causes include infectious agents, hypersensitivity reactions, trauma, and psychogenesis. Cytologically, there is a mixed population of mononuclear inflammatory cells, including plasma cells, along with intermediate squamous epithelium (Fig. 3–3B) related to acanthosis, i.e., hyperplasia of the epidermal stratum spinosum layer. The healing response to surface erosion may produce fibroblastic cells, which appear in the cytologic specimens as plump fusiform cells along with numerous erythrocytes re-

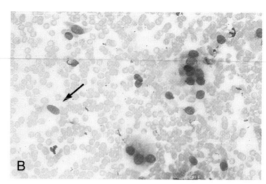

FIGURE 3–3. B, Lick dermatitis. Tissue aspirate. Dog. Sheets of intermediate squamous epithelium predominate related to the thickened epidermis found in these cases. Adjacent to the neutrophil in the lower left is a fibroblastic cell present in response to stromal reaction. (Wright-Giemsa; ×125.)

lated to increased vascularization. Lesions may also involve a secondary bacterial infection with suppuration. Treatment will be determined by the underlying cause, and frequently involves control of pyoderma.

Cytologic differential diagnosis: foreign body reaction, parasitic bite reaction.

Foreign Body Reaction

These reactions caused by penetration of plant, animal, or inorganic material into the skin, producing an erythematous wound that progresses to a nodular response that often drains fluid. Cytologically, a mixed inflammatory response is present, composed mostly of macrophages and lymphocytes with smaller numbers of neutrophils and possibly eosinophils (Fig. 3–4). Multinucleated giant cells are frequently present. A fibroblastic response is common. A secondary bacterial infection may occur. Treatment includes surgical exploration or excision with histologic biopsy and culture if warranted.

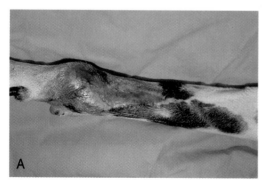

FIGURE 3–3. A, Lick dermatitis. Dog. Thickened, ulcerated, hairless lesion on the limb. (Courtesy of Rosanna Marsella, Gainesville, FL.)

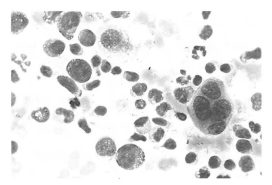

FIGURE 3–4. Foreign body reaction. Tissue fluid sediment smear. Dog. Small lymphocytes and macrophages predominate, with occasional neutrophils found. Note the giant cell, suggesting granulomatous inflammation. The inflammatory reaction was secondary to calcinosis circumscripta that was diagnosed on histopathology. (Aqueous-based Wright; ×250.)

Cytologic differential diagnosis: **fungal, bacterial, noninfectious, or parasitic inflammatory lesions.**

Parasitic Bite Reaction

Insects, ticks, and spiders, for example, may induce a mild to severe reaction characterized usually by erythema and swelling (Rakich et al., 1993). Cytology reveals a mixed inflammatory infiltrate composed of neutrophils, macrophages, and usually increased numbers of eosinophils related to a hypersensitivity reaction (Fig. 3–5). These lesions often regress spontaneously, but some may require additional wound care.

Cytologic differential diagnosis: **bacterial, fungal, noninfectious, or foreign body reactions.**

Nodular Panniculitis/Steatitis

Causes of noninfectious panniculitis include trauma, foreign bodies, vaccination reac-

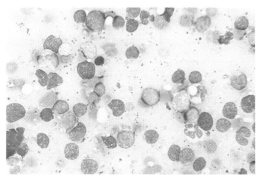

FIGURE 3–5. Insect bite reaction. Tissue aspirate. Dog. Small and intermediate-sized lymphocytes infiltrated this mass on the ventral neck in addition to low numbers of eosinophils and neutrophils. (Wright-Giemsa; ×250.)

tions, immune-mediated conditions, drug reactions, pancreatic conditions, nutritional deficiencies, and idiopathy. The condition appears in the cat and dog as solitary or multiple, firm to fluctuant, raised, well-demarcated lesions. These may ooze an oily yellow-brown fluid (Fig. 3–6A). Sites of prevalence include the dorsal trunk, neck, and proximal limbs. Cytologically, nondegenerate neutrophils and macrophages predominate against a vacuolated background composed of adipose tissue (Fig. 3–6B). Small lymphocytes and plasma cells may be

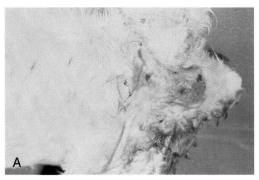

FIGURE 3–6. A, Sterile nodular panniculitis. Dog. Wet, draining nodule from the leg. (Courtesy of Leslie Fox, Gainesville, FL.)

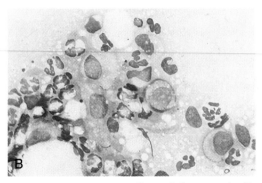

FIGURE 3–6. **B, Sterile nodular panniculitis. Tissue discharge. Dog.** Tracts drained in the lumbar region of this poodle for one year. Infectious agents were not found. Present are numerous degenerate neutrophils, several epithelioid macrophages, and occasional lymphocytes. (Wright-Giemsa; ×250.)

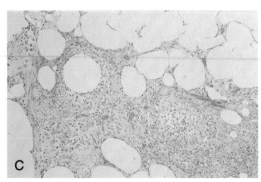

FIGURE 3–6. **C, Sterile nodular panniculitis. Dog.** Focal collections of neutrophils and macrophages appear within the subcutis of this animal, which was presented with multiple subcutaneous nodules. No evidence was found for an infectious agent. (H & E; ×5.)

numerous, especially in lesions induced by vaccination reactions. Frequently, macrophages present with abundant foamy cytoplasm or as giant multinucleated forms. When chronic, evidence of fibrosis is indicated by the presence of plump fusiform cells with nuclear immaturity. The fibrosis may be so extensive as to suggest a mesenchymal neoplasm. Prognosis is usually best for solitary lesions, which respond to surgical excision. Histologically, sterile panniculitis may demonstrate inflammatory cells within the subcutis (Fig. 3–6C) that extend into the dermis. Multiple lesions are often associated with systemic disease in young dogs, and treatment revolves glucocorticoid administration. Dachshunds and poodles may be predisposed to this form of the disease. Culture and histopathologic examination are recommended to rule out infectious causes. Fungal stains should be applied to cytologic specimens.

Cytologic differential diagnosis: **infectious panniculitis.**

Eosinophilic Plaque/Granuloma

Feline eosinophilic plaque presents initially as alopecic focal areas of intense pruritus that progress to ulceration with exudation. It has been associated with flea-bite allergy, food allergy, and atopy. Sites affected include the face, neck, abdomen, and medial thighs. Lesions may become secondarily infected with bacteria. Cytologically, eosinophils and mast cells predominate, with few lymphocytes. When lesions become secondarily infected, neutrophils are prominent. Treatment includes glucocorticoid administration and antibiotics, if necessary.

Eosinophilic granuloma occurs in dogs and young cats in response to a hypersensitivity reaction, similar to plaque formation. Grossly, lesions may appear as raised linear bands of yellow to erythematous tissue along the posterior legs or as papules and nodules on the nose, ears, and feet. Lesions have been seen in the oral cavity. Cytologically, a mixed inflammatory response is seen, with macrophages, lymphocytes, plasma

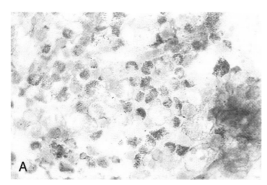

FIGURE 3–7. A, Eosinophilic granuloma. Tissue aspirate. Cat. Note the dense collections of eosinophils, many of which have degranulated. (Wright-Giemsa; ×250.)

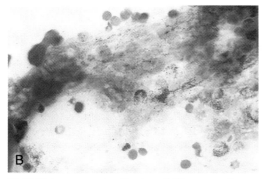

FIGURE 3–7. B, Eosinophilic granuloma. Same case as in Figure 3–7A. Collagenolysis appears as amorphous basophilic material associated with degranulated eosinophils. (Wright-Giemsa; ×250.)

cells, neutrophils, and increased numbers of eosinophils and mast cells (Fig. 3–7A). Rare multinucleated giant cells may be present. Collagen necrosis may occur as a result of eosinophil granule release giving rise to the occasional appearance of amorphous basophilic material in the background (Fig. 3–7B). Eosinophil numbers are usually less than are seen in eosinophilic plaque. Surgical excision is recommended for solitary nodular lesions.

Cytologic differential diagnosis: arthropod bite reactions, foreign body reactions.

Pemphigus Foliaceus

This is the most common autoimmune skin disease in dogs and cats. Drugs, chronic disease, and spontaneous causes have been associated with their occurrence. Grossly, lesions appear as erythematous macules that progress to white or yellow pustules and finally to crusts (Fig. 3–8A). The head and feet are preferred sites although the ears, trunk, and neck are also commonly affected in the cat. Direct imprint of the underside of a crust or aspiration of a pustule reveals nondegenerate neutrophils and acantholytic cells appearing as intensely stained individualized oval keratinocytes (Fig. 3–8B). Eosinophils may be present as well, but bacterial infection is usually lacking. Treatment includes antibiotics and immunotherapy. Excisional biopsy of early lesions is recommended. Histologic examination along with direct immunofluorescent antibody tests or direct immunoperoxidase staining tests are necessary to distinguish the different pem-

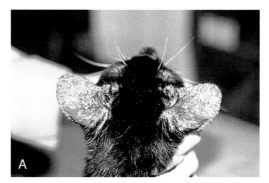

FIGURE 3–8. A, Pemphigus foliaceous. Cat. Crusty and erythematous lesions on the ear pinnae. (Courtesy of Janet Wojciechowski.)

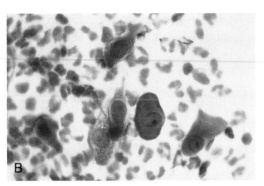

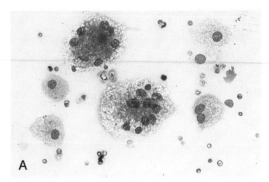

FIGURE 3–8. B, Acantholytic cells. Pustule aspirate. Cat. Densely stained individualized keratinocytes from a skin pustule on an animal with pemphigus foliaceous. These cells are often associated with immune-mediated skin diseases. Numerous neutrophils, mostly nondegenerate, are present in large numbers. (Wright-Giemsa; ×250.)

FIGURE 3–9. A, Cutaneous xanthomatosis. Tissue aspirate. Cat. Multinucleated giant cells and mononuclear foamy macrophages predominate in this specimen. This 1-year-old Siamese presented with multiple skin masses. (Wright-Giemsa; ×125.)

phigus subtypes. Antinuclear antibody tests also may be helpful.

Cytologic differential diagnosis: **pyoderma.**

Xanthomatosis

This is an uncommon granulomatous inflammation in cats, birds, and amphibians related to primary or secondary diabetes mellitus, high-fat diets, and hereditary hyperchylomicronemia (Grieshaber et al., 1991). The deposition of cholesterol and triglycerides in tissues results in lipid-laden macrophages. Grossly, the lesions are single or multiple, white to yellow plaques or nodules, which may ulcerate or drain caseous material. Sites preferred are the face, trunk, and foot pads. Cytologically, aspirates contain numerous foamy macrophages (Fig. 3–9A) that stain positive with lipid stains (Fig. 3–9B). Lymphocytes and occasional eosinophils or neutrophils are present as

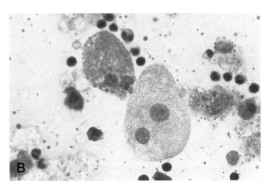

FIGURE 3–9. B, Cutaneous xanthomatosis. Same case as in Figure 3–9A. This stain demonstrates the lipid content within the cytoplasm of variably sized macrophages. (Oil red O/new methylene blue; ×250.)

well. Histologically, cholesterol clefts and giant cells may be prominent (Fig. 3–9C). Treatment is aimed at identifying and controlling the underlying cause.

Cytologic differential diagnosis: **sterile granuloma, e.g., foreign body reaction.**

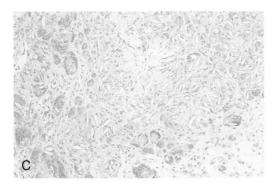

FIGURE 3–9. C, Cutaneous xanthomatosis. Same case as in Figure 3–9A. Aggregates of giant cells surround clusters of cholesterol clefts within the dermis. (H & E; ×50.)

INFECTIOUS INFLAMMATION

Acute Bacterial Abscess

The abscess is a common subcutaneous lesion in cats and dogs, often related to bites or other penetrating wounds. This may be localized to the skin or associated with systemic signs. The area is firm to fluctuant, swollen, erythematous, warm, and painful. A creamy white exudate may be aspirated, which is characterized cytologically by numerous degenerate neutrophils displaying karyolysis, karyorrhexis, and pyknosis (see Chapter 2). Bacteria may be found in association with the swollen, round nuclei. Case management includes culture and sensitivity tests, with treatment aimed at surgical incision and antibiotics.

Clostridial Cellulitis

The infection is usually associated with penetrating wounds. The swollen skin may be crepitant with a serosanguineous wound exudate. Cytologically, tissue aspirates may reveal large rods measuring 1×4 μm, some with a clear, oval, subterminal endospore, occurring singly or in short chains (Fig. 3–10A). This anaerobic organism is gram positive (Fig. 3–10B), but may be variably staining as a result of a chronic infection or following antibiotic therapy. The specimen background often contains cellular debris and lipid with few inflammatory cells, if present. Neutrophils, when present, are often degenerate. Anaerobic culture is necessary for diagnosis. Treatment includes surgical management and appropriate antibiotic administration.

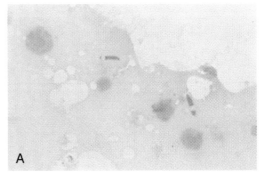

FIGURE 3–10. A, Clostridial cellulitis. Tissue aspirate. Dog. Bacilli with terminal spore formation in the subcutis in an animal with subcutaneous emphysema and adjacent bone lysis. (Wright-Giemsa; ×500.)

FIGURE 3–10. B, Clostridial cellulitis. Same case as in Figure 3–10A. Gram-positive rods on aerobic culture were confirmed as *Clostridium* sp. (Gram; ×500.)

Actinomycosis/Nocardiosis

The infection presents as subcutaneous swellings that progress to ulceration with exudation of red-brown fluid. The cause is often related to penetrating wounds. The infections may be associated with systemic signs that often include pyothorax. Cytologically, degenerate neutrophils predominate, with macrophages and small lymphocytes also present. Bacteria may be intracellular or extracellular, the latter often found as dense clusters of organisms (Fig. 3–11A–C).

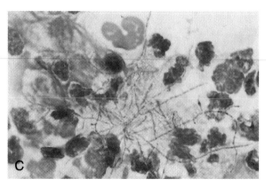

FIGURE 3–11. C, Nocardiosis. Same case as in Figure 3–11B. Branching, beaded slender bacterial filaments are demonstrated in this fluid pocket from a dog with a swollen hind leg. (Wright-Giemsa; ×500.)

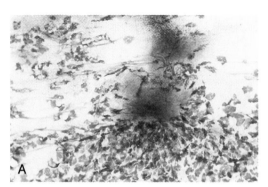

FIGURE 3–11. A, Actinomycosis. Tissue aspirate. Dog. Note the basophilic clusters of filamentous organisms that resemble amorphous debris. (Wright-Giemsa; ×125.)

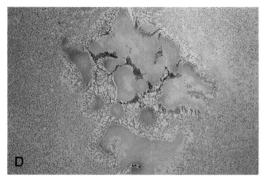

FIGURE 3–11. D, Actinomycosis. Dog. Pyogranulomatous cellulitis surrounding irregular islands of filamentous organisms that are gram positive and acid-fast negative. The periphery of these foci contain densely eosinophilic hyalinized material thought to represent antigen-antibody complexes. This reaction has been termed the *Splendore–Hoeppli phenomenon.* (H & E; ×25.)

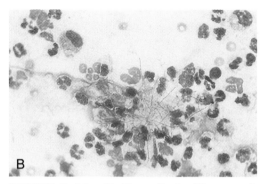

FIGURE 3–11. B, Nocardiosis. Tissue aspirate. Dog. Cluster of organisms surrounded by many degenerate neutrophils and few macrophages. Culture confirmed presence of *Nocardia* sp. (Wright-Giemsa; ×250.)

These bacteria are slender, filamentous, branching, lightly basophilic rods with red spotted or beaded areas. Histologically, inflammatory cells group around dense mats of organisms (Fig. 3–11D). *Actinomyces* sp. are gram positive and acid-fast negative, whereas *Nocardia* sp. are gram positive but variably positive for acid-fast stain. Culture is necessary for diagnosis of the specific type and samples should be obtained anaerobically. Treatment includes surgical drainage and appropriate antibiotics.

KEY POINT: Look at the dense areas of the specimen for basophilic mats of bacteria.

Dermatophilosis

This is a rare infection that has been reported in cats and dogs, usually as the result of penetrating wounds contaminated with infected soil or water. The lesion presents as a firm, alopecic, subcutaneous draining mass. The thick gray exudate below the crusted surface is purulent, with numerous degenerate neutrophils but few eosinophils and macrophages. The organism appears as gram-positive branching filaments that segment horizontally and longitudinally into coccoid forms (Carakostas et al., 1984; Tyler et al., 1999). Diagnosis is made by morphologic identification of the organism on biopsy or through culture. Treatment involves appropriate antibiotics and appropriate wound management.

Mycobacteriosis

Three clinical forms of mycobacteriosis in dogs and cats are recognized, which include internal tuberculous, localized cutaneous nodules (lepromatous), and spreading subcutaneous forms (Greene and Gunn-Moore, 1998). Diagnosis is best performed by tissue culture and histopathology. Definitive identification may be made by polymerase chain reaction (PCR) of tissue specimens. Treatment may include surgical excision and appropriate antibiotics. The tuberculous form is related to *Mycobacterium tuberculosis, Mycobacterium bovis,* or the opportunistic *Mycobacterium avium-intracellulare* complex. Contact with infected people, cattle, birds,

or soil may be documented. The disease may be also associated with immunosuppressed animals. This form is characterized by a systemic disease with weight loss, fever, and lymphadenopathy. While internal organs are most affected, skin nodules can appear on the head, neck, and legs of dogs and cats (Miller et al, 1995). These are slow-growing organisms normally requiring 4 to 6 weeks to culture. Detection may be hastened to 2 weeks and may require PCR and other molecular techniques for identification. Cytologically, macrophages contain few to many beaded bacilli, and some organisms may be extracellular (Fig. 3–12A). Acid-fast staining is helpful in the recognition of the organisms (Fig. 3–12B). Lymphocytes and neutrophils are more abundant than in lepromatous forms.

The lepromatous form is caused by *Mycobacterium lepraemurium* and is common in wet, cooler climates with exposure to infected rodents. Nonpainful raised nodules are found on the head and distal limbs without systemic signs in cats. Nodules are soft to firm, fleshy, and often localized, with occasional ulceration and little exudation.

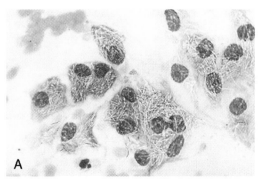

FIGURE 3–12. A, Mycobacteriosis. Tissue aspirate. Cat. A swollen area over the nose was confirmed positive for *M. avium-intracellulare* complex. Note the abundance of negative-staining rods with the cytoplasm of macrophages. (Wright-Giemsa; ×250.)

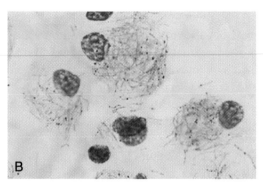

FIGURE 3–12. B, Mycobacteriosis. Same case as in Figure 3–12A. Acid-fast stain is positive for the beaded linear bacteria. (Ziehl-Neelsen; ×500.)

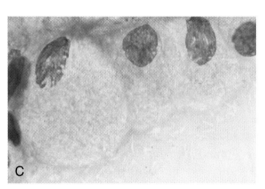

FIGURE 3–12. C, Feline leprosy. Tissue imprint. Cat. Negative-stained linear bacteria fill the cytoplasm and appear extracellular, visible against the proteinaceous background. (Giemsa; ×500.) (Glass slide material courtesy of John Kramer, Washington State University; presented at the 1988 ASVCP case review session.)

Cultivation of the organism is difficult. Spontaneous remission has been reported in a cat (Roccabianca et al., 1996). Cytologically, macrophages containing numerous intracellular organisms predominate (Fig. 3–12C). Other cells seen include lymphocytes, plasma cells, neutrophils, and occasional multinucleated giant cells.

The more common presentation of cutaneous mycobacteriosis in dogs and cats involves those fast-growing species having an atypical growth pattern or culture characteristic, such as *Mycobacterium fortuitum, Mycobacterium chelonei,* and *Mycobacterium smegmatis.* These are the result of inoculation with contaminated soil or standing water. Lesions are characterized by a spreading subcutaneous pyogranulomatous inflammation having frequent draining tracts. This

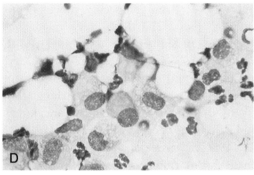

FIGURE 3–12. D, Atypical mycobacteriosis. Tissue aspirate. Dog. Frequent neutrophils and macrophages appear without obvious evidence of sepsis. Neutrophils are mildly degenerate in this 2-cm mass located on the back. (Wright-Giemsa; ×250.)

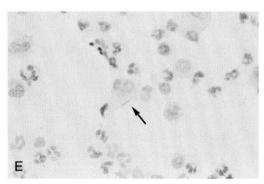

FIGURE 3–12. E, Atypical mycobacteriosis. Same case as in Figure 3–12D. Single positive filamentous bacterium found within macrophage (*arrow*). (Fite's acid-fast; ×250.)

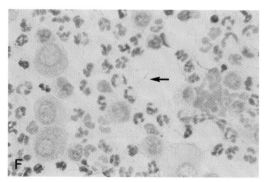

FIGURE 3–12. F, Atypical mycobacteriosis. Same case as in Figure 3–12D. Tissue aspirate. Single positive filamentous bacterium found within a lipocyst (*arrow*). (Fite's acid-fast; ×250.)

form also lacks systemic signs. Bacterial culture of deep tissue sites is required and growth may occur within 3 to 5 days. Cytologically, a mixed population of neutrophils and macrophages predominates, with occasional lymphocytes, plasma cells, multinucleated giant cells, or reactive fibroblasts (Fig. 3–12D). Organisms are occasionally found on cytology with the aid of acid-fast staining (Fig. 3–12E & F). On histopathology, lesions appear diffuse and organisms may be found within lipocysts surrounded by inflammatory cells. Prognosis for this form is guarded, as response to antibiotics is often unrewarding.

KEY POINT: Mycobacterial organisms are gram positive and acid-fast positive. They appear on cytology as nonstaining, long, thin rods due to the high lipid content of their cell wall.

Localized Opportunistic Fungal Infections

Cutaneous or subcutaneous lesions occur as the result of penetrating wounds contaminated with infected soil or water, commonly in tropical or subtropical climates. One

common type is phaeohyphomycosis, caused by a group of dematiaceous (pigmented) fungi such as *Alternaria, Curvularia,* or *Bipolaris (Drechslera)* spp. (Fig. 3–13A–C). A rare type is hyalohypomycosis, produced by nonpigmented fungi such as *Paecilomyces* spp. (Fig. 3–13D) (Elliott et al., 1984). Nodules develop slowly, usually on extremi-

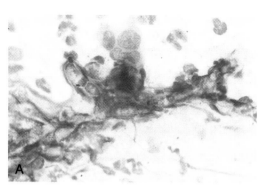

FIGURE 3–13. A, Phaeohyphomycosis (pigmented fungi). Tissue aspirate. Dog. Small mass on plantar surface of the foot was positive for *Curvularia* sp. on culture. Degenerate neutrophils and macrophages surround the fungal hyphae with yeastlike swellings. (Aqueous-based Wright; ×250.)

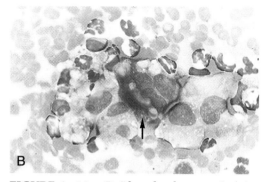

FIGURE 3–13. B, Phaeohyphomycosis (pigmented fungi). Tissue aspirate. Dog. Mixed inflammation with macrophages, degenerate neutrophils, and lymphocytes surround a hyphal structure (*arrow*) with yeastlike swellings. (Wright-Giemsa; ×250.)

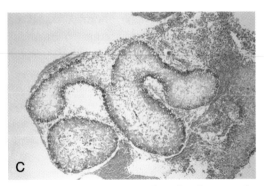

FIGURE 3–13. C, Phaeohyphomycosis. Same case as in Figure 3–13B. Large colonies of brown fungi confirm the diagnosis of dematiaceous or pigmented fungi. (H & E; ×25.)

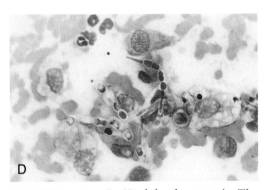

FIGURE 3–13. D, Hyalohyphomycosis. Tissue aspirate. Cat. This swollen digit contained hyphal structures with yeastlike swellings suspected to be caused by *Paecilomyces* sp. Numerous macrophages are noted along with few neutrophils. (Wright-Giemsa; ×250.)

ties, later becoming ulcerated with draining tracts. Cytologically, these produce a pyogranulomatous inflammation with degenerate neutrophils, macrophages, multinucleated giant cells, lymphocytes, plasma cells, and mature fibroblasts. Hyphal structures are septate and periodic constrictions may be seen producing globose dilations. Yeast forms rarely occur. Diagnosis involves histopathologic biopsy and tissue culture.

Treatment involves surgical excision but prognosis is often poor to guarded.

Cutaneous Lesions from Systemic Fungal Infections

Lesions usually present as single or multiple nodules that ulcerate and drain a serosanguineous exudate. Regional lymphadenopathy is common along with affected organ systems. Examination of the exudate is diagnostic but surgical excision with histopathologic biopsy is recommended. Serum titers and tissue culture are helpful in difficult cases. In general, treatment is aimed at systemic antifungal therapy. Prognosis is guarded.

Blastomycosis

Blastomycosis is a pyogranulomatous or granulomatous inflammation of dogs and rarely cats that is related to yeast and rare hyphal forms of *Blastomyces dermatitidis*. The disease is endemic in areas around the Mississippi and Ohio River basins and into Canada. Lesions appear often on the extremities and nose. Cytologically, degenerate neutrophils, macrophages, multinucleated giant cells, and lymphocytes are present. Yeast forms measure 7 to 15 μm in diameter and have a refractile deeply basophilic thick cell wall (Fig. 3–14A). Organisms may be phagocytized by macrophages or found extracellularly. Cell division occurs by budding that is broad based compared with the narrow-based budding of *Cryptococcus* sp. Structures stain positive with periodic acid-Schiff (PAS) (Fig. 3–14B) and methenamine silver. Definitive diagnosis involves immunostaining of tissue sections and tissue culture. Serum tests involve agar immunodiffusion and enzyme-linked immunosorbent assay (ELISA) methods.

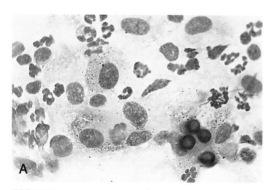

FIGURE 3–14. A, Blastomycosis. Tissue imprint. Dog. A mass on the digit revealed several deeply basophilic thick-walled budding yeast forms along with a mixture of macrophages and degenerate neutrophils. (Aqueous-based Wright; ×250.)

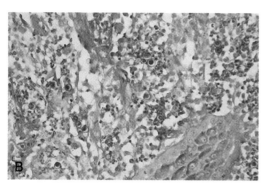

FIGURE 3–14. B, Blastomycosis. Dense accumulation of inflammatory cells surround densely stained yeast forms that collapse on fixation away from the thick cell wall. (PAS ×50.)

Coccidioidomycosis

This disease, caused by *Coccidioides immitis,* produces a pyogranulomatous response similar to that of blastomycosis in dogs and occasionally cats. It is endemic in the southwestern United States. Cytologically, the organism appears as thick-walled spherules measuring 20 to 200 μm diameter (Fig. 3–15A). Within the basophilic spherule (Fig. 3–15B) are uninucleate round endo-

spores measuring 2 to 5 μm in diameter. The free endospores (Fig. 3–15C) may be confused with yeast forms of *Histoplasma.* Empty small spherules resemble *Blastomyces.* Both cell wall and endospores stain positive with methenamine silver, while PAS stains the cell wall purple and the endospores red. Intact spherules are poorly chemotactic for neutrophils compared with free

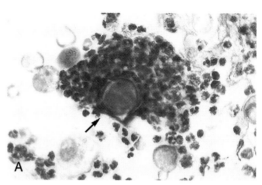

FIGURE 3–15. A, Coccidioidomycosis. Tissue aspirate. Dog. Presented with several semi-firm skin masses and no systemic signs. Purple thick-walled spherule (*arrow*) measuring approximately 60 μm in diameter is surrounded by numerous degenerate neutrophils. (Wright; ×250.)

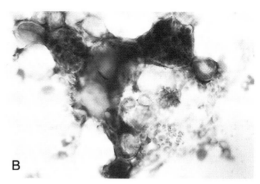

FIGURE 3–15. B, Coccidioidomycosis. Tissue aspirate. Dog. Several variably sized spherules containing numerous small endospores are noted in this animal with systemic involvement. (Romanowsky; ×250.)

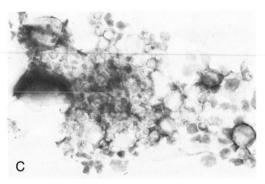

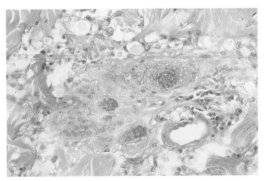

FIGURE 3–15. C, Coccidioidomycosis. Same case as in Figure 3–15B. Numerous small round endospores are released from adjacent spherules in the presence of a mixed inflammatory response. (Romanowsky; ×250.)

FIGURE 3–16. Cryptococcosis. Cat skin. Perifollicular inflammation related to the presence of numerous clear-walled yeast forms. (H & E; ×100.)

endospores, which attract many neutrophils (Fig. 3–15A). Serologic tests used include tube precipitin, latex agglutination, complement fixation, agar immunodiffusion, and ELISA. Fluorescent antibody methods may be used for tissue biopsy. Tissue culture is not recommended because of the public health risk.

Cryptococcosis

Cryptococcosis is found in several geographic areas, but frequently in tropical or subtropical climates or with soil infected by pigeon droppings. Lesions in dogs and cats may present as crusts or erosions on the nose in addition to nodules. The cellular response is granulomatous with macrophages predominant (Fig. 3–16). Other cells present include lymphocytes and multinucleated giant cells. There is minimal inflammation in immunocompromised patients and when organisms retain their thick outer capsule. The causative agent, *Cryptococcus neoformans,* is found in cytologic specimens as a round to oval yeast form measuring 4 to 10 μm in diameter. Cell sizes may be variable, ranging from 2 to 20

μm. When present, the thick lipid capsule remains unstained with Romanowsky-type stains (see Figure 5–10A). As a result, the biopsy background appears vacuolated, often with many dense, round cell bodies. Stains such as new methylene blue and India ink are used to enhance visibility of the capsule on unstained specimens (see Figure 5–10B). The internal cell body stains positive with methenamine silver and PAS, while the cell wall requires mucicarmine stain. Cell division involves narrow-based budding compared with the broad-based budding of *Blastomyces.* Definitive diagnosis involves immunostaining in tissue biopsies, latex agglutination test, complement fixation, or fungal culture.

Histoplasmosis

This disease produces a pyogranulomatous response by the agent *Histoplasma capsulatum,* and is similar in geographic distribution to blastomycosis. Bird and bat droppings provide an ideal growth medium for the organisms. Cutaneous lesions (Fig. 3–17) are uncommon compared with those in gastrointestinal and hematopoietic

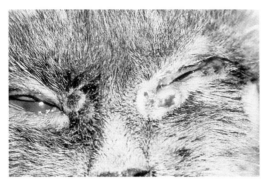

FIGURE 3–17. Histoplasmosis. Skin lesions as well as ocular lesions were present in this cat. (Courtesy of Heidi Ward.)

organs. Cytologically, macrophages predominate, but lymphocytes, plasma cells, and occasional multinucleated giant cells may be present. Numerous intracellular and extracellular oval yeast forms measuring 2 to 4 μm are frequently found in specimens. They stain positive with PAS and methenamine silver. The yeast structures resemble the protozoan *Leishmania* except *Histoplasma* has a clear halo due to cell shrinkage and the cell body lacks a kinetoplast. Definitive diagnosis of histoplasmosis requires identification by cytology, immunostaining in tissue biopsy, or fungal culture. There are no reliable serologic tests.

Other systemic infections may involve *Aspergillus* sp., *Candida* sp., or *Paecilomyces* sp. These often occur in immunosuppressed patients.

Dermatophytosis

The lesions vary from alopecia, broken hair shafts, crusts, scales, and erythema to raised nodules on the head, feet, and tail of dogs and cats. Cytologic specimens reveal a pyogranulomatous inflammation with degenerate neutrophils and large epithelioid macrophages (Tyler et al., 1999). Arthrospores and nonstaining hyphae are associated with

hair shafts, which are best visualized using clearing agents with plucked hairs (Fig. 3–18A & B) or methenamine silver staining (Fig. 3–18C). Fungal culture is necessary for identification.

An uncommon presentation is a pseudomycetoma in Persian cats, usually caused by *Microsporum canis,* that presents as a nodular granuloma with fistulous tracts deep into subcutaneous tissues. Cytologically, this involves macrophages with abundant foamy

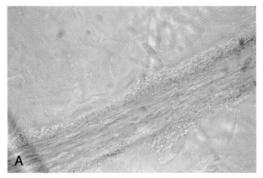

FIGURE 3–18. A, Dermatophytosis. Low-magnification view of unstained, keratin-cleared hair shaft with attached arthrospores. (Courtesy of the University of Florida Dermatology Section.)

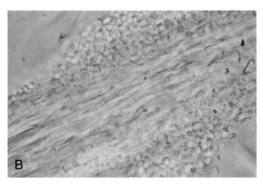

FIGURE 3–18. B, Dermatophytosis. High-magnification view of unstained, keratin-cleared hair shaft demonstrating arthrospores outside and fungal hyphae within the hair. (Courtesy of the University of Florida Dermatology Section.)

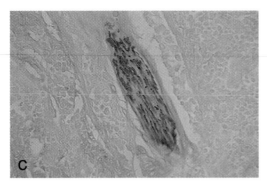

FIGURE 3–18. C, Dermatophytosis. Dog. Note the black stained hyphae within the hair shaft from this tissue section of skin. Diagnosis confined as *M. canis* by culture. (Gomori's methenamine silver; ×100.)

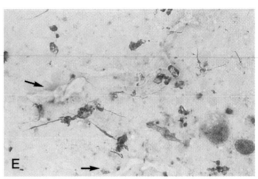

FIGURE 3–18. E, Feline dermatophytic pseudomycetoma. Same case as in Figure 3–18D. Fungal hyphae are variably visible with Romanowsky staining (*arrows*). Culture confirmed infection by *M. canis*. (Wright-Giemsa; ×250.)

cytoplasm and numerous multinucleated giant cells (Fig. 3–18D). Fungal hyphae have an irregular shape and size and may stain variably with Romanowsky-type stains (Fig. 3–18E). Positive staining occurs with PAS and methenamine silver (Fig. 3–18F). Treatment of the nodules involves surgical excision and antifungal drugs.

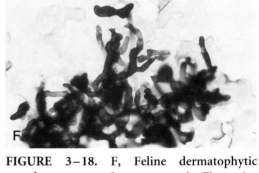

FIGURE 3–18. F, Feline dermatophytic pseudomycetoma. Same case as in Figure 3–18D. Hyphal elements are clearly visible with silver staining. (Gomori's methenamine silver; ×250.)

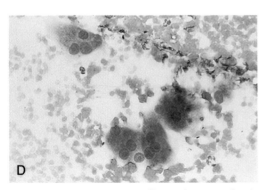

FIGURE 3–18. D, Feline dermatophytic pseudomycetoma. Tissue aspirate. Cat. Several multinucleated giant cells are present in this 3-cm superficial mass on the lateral abdomen of a Persian cat. (Wright-Giemsa; ×125.)

Malassezia

The causative agent, *Malassezia pachydermatis*, is an opportunistic invader of the skin and ear canal. It is associated with widespread seborrheic dermatitis as well as otitis externa in dogs. Organisms are found in surface scabs or crusts of exudative lesions. Sites of predilection include the face, ventral

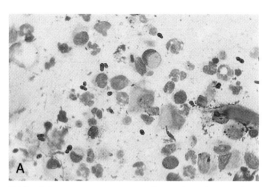

FIGURE 3–19. A, *Malassezia* dermatitis. Pustule imprint. Dog. Abundant budding yeast forms with a mixed-cell inflammatory response were noted in an animal with pustular dermatitis. Mildly degenerate neutrophils are present along with lymphocytes and macrophages. (Wright-Giemsa; ×250.)

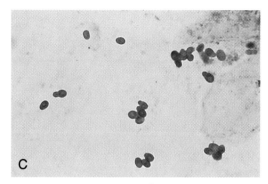

FIGURE 3–19. C, *Malassezia* otitis. Same case as in Figure 3–19B. Characteristic shoe print morphology of the broad-based budding yeast form associated with chronic otitis externa. (Aqueous-based Wright; ×500.)

Romanowsky stains reveal purple broad-based budding organisms characterized by a bottle or shoe shape (Fig. 3–19C). Treatment includes surface cleaning and appropriate antifungal agents.

Pythiosis

The causative agent, *Pythium insidiosum,* is a water mold of the oomycete class in the Protista kingdom. It differs from true fungi in producing motile, flagellate zoospores, having cell walls without chitin, and having differences in nuclear division and cytoplasmic organelles (Foil, 1998). This disease is common in dogs from tropical or subtropical climates, such as the southeastern United States. Animals are infected by standing in or drinking contaminated water. Systemic signs result from gastrointestinal involvement, and are more common than the cutaneous presentation. Dermal ulcerative nodules develop into draining tracts and serosanguineous exudation from sites that include the extremities, tail head, and perineum (Fig. 3–20A). Cytologically, specimens consist of a pyogranulomatous inflammation with increased eosinophils and

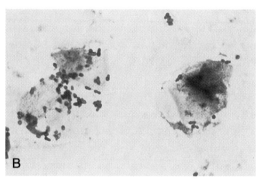

FIGURE 3–19. B, *Malassezia* otitis. Ear swab. Dog. *Malassezia* sp. organisms adhere to keratinized squamous epithelium without evidence of inflammation. (Aqueous-based Wright; ×250.)

neck, dorsum of paws, ventral abdomen, and caudal thighs. Cytologically, the skin infection involves primarily a mononuclear inflammation, with lymphocytes and macrophages, but secondary pyoderma may occur with the presence of focal neutrophils (Fig. 3–19A). Typically, the ear infection is minimally inflamed with organisms adhered to squamous epithelium (Fig. 3–19B).

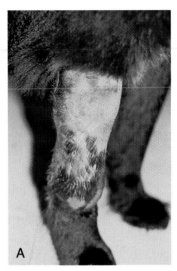

FIGURE 3–20. A, Pythiosis. Dog. This draining lesion present on the leg of a long-haired dog was confirmed as pythiosis. (Courtesy of Diane Lewis, Gainesville, FL.)

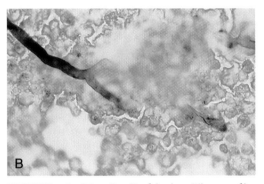

FIGURE 3–20. B, Pythiosis. Tissue discharge. Dog. Hyphal elements appear as broad, poorly septate branched structures surrounded by inflammatory cells. (Gomori's methenamine silver; ×250.)

the presence of broad, poorly septate and branching hyphal elements. Methenamine silver stain is preferred over PAS stain to demonstrate the organisms (Fig. 3–20B). Fluorescent antibody testing can be performed for diagnosis in tissue biopsies. Pos-

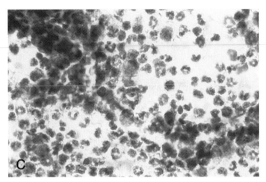

FIGURE 3–20. C, Pythiosis. Same case as in Figure 3–20B. Clear-staining linear pattern with degenerate neutrophils closely adherent are noted in this draining lesion on the limb and perianal area. Eosinophils are present in significant numbers but are difficult to see in this field. (Aqueous-based Wright; ×250.)

sible treatment involves wide surgical excision or amputation of affected limbs. Prognosis is guarded to poor.

KEY POINT: Organisms stain poorly with Romanowsky stains and are best seen within dense clumps of inflammatory cells at low magnification. The presence of clear, uniformly sized, linear strands suggest hyphal elements (Fig. 3–20C), but these must be distinguished from collagen debris, which may also appear as unstained strands.

Protothecosis

This is a rare disease in dogs and cats related to an achloric algae, *Prototheca wickerhamii*, that is found in sewage-contaminated food and water. It is frequently associated with immunosuppression or concurrent disease. Cats usually develop a cutaneous disease, while dogs may develop both cutaneous and systemic forms. Systemic involvement primarily includes the gastrointestinal tract, eye, and nervous system. Cutaneous lesions in dogs are chronic, nodular, exudative, and ulcerative, occurring on the trunk and extremities. Large, firm nodules on limbs, feet, head, and tail base have been reported in cats. Cytologically, the inflammation is granulomatous or pyogranulomatous. Epithelioid macrophages predominate, but lymphocytes, plasma cells, and occasional multinucleated giant cells may also be found. Organisms, present outside or within macrophages, measure 5 to 20 μm in diameter. They are round to oval with internal septation producing 2 to 20 endospores within the cell wall. The endospores are basophilic and granular with a single nucleus, and have a clear halo around them. Both PAS and methenamine silver stains demonstrate the cell wall. Definitive diagnosis requires culture or tissue biopsy using immunofluorescence or immunoperoxidase techniques. Treatment involves surgical excision for cutaneous lesions. Antimicrobial drugs have been used with limited success in systemic forms. Prognosis is guarded to poor.

Sporotrichosis

This disease is associated with immunosuppression, such as occurs with glucocorticoid administration or concurrent disease. It presents in several clinical forms—cutaneous, systemic, and the most frequent, cutaneolymphatic—usually as the result of penetrating wounds (Werner and Werner, 1993). Grossly, a dermal to subcutaneous nodule progresses into an ulcerated lesion that drains a serosanguineous exudate. In dogs, the skin of the trunk and extremities is preferred, while in cats the large firm nodules appear on the limbs, feet, head, and tail base. The etiologic agent, *Sporothrix schenckii,* is a saprophytic fungus that appears classically as cigar-shaped yeast forms measuring 3 to 5 μm in diameter with a thin, clear halo around the pale-blue cyto-

plasm (Fig. 3–21A). The shape of the yeast is pleomorphic, with round to oval shapes also observed (Fig. 3–21B). Cytologically, the yeast is located intracellularly or extracellularly, being abundant in cats and few in number in dogs. In dogs, pyogranuloma-

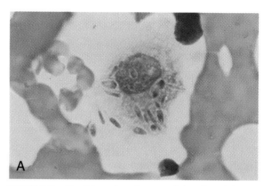

FIGURE 3–21. A, Sporotrichosis. Tissue imprint. Cat. This 2-cm granulomatous lesion on one digit contains a macrophage with numerous oval to cigar-shaped yeast forms having a thin clear halo around the basophilic center. These structures measure 2 × 5 μm, approximately the width of an erythrocyte. (Wright; ×500.)

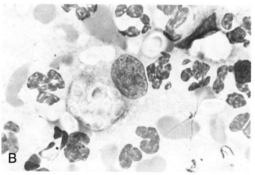

FIGURE 3–21. B, Sporotrichosis. Tissue imprint. Cat. Pyogranulomatous inflammation with engulfed yeast within a macrophage. These forms have a round to oval shape and are difficult to distinguish from *Histoplasma* sp. on the basis of morphology. Culture-confirmed *Sporothrix* sp. (Romanowsky; ×500.) (Courtesy of Peter Fernandes.)

tous inflammation with degenerative neutrophils is common, while macrophages and lymphocytes predominate in the cat. The diagnosis may be made from the characteristic cytologic appearance. Definitive diagnosis requires fungal culture of the exudate or tissue biopsy using immunofluorescence or immunoperoxidase techniques. The organism stains positive with both methenamine silver and PAS. There are no reliable serologic tests available for dogs and cats. Surgical excision may be performed on single cutaneous lesions. Treatment of the systemic form involves a variety of antimicrobial drugs, which have been used with variable success. Prognosis is poor to guarded. Good response has been obtained with itraconazole (Peaston, 1993).

KEY POINT: Organisms resemble those of histoplasmosis, which may be round or oval, but only sporotrichosis has cigar-shaped or slender yeast forms.

KEY POINT: The disease may spread to people, usually transmitted by cats.

Cytologic differential diagnosis: **histoplasmosis, toxoplasmosis, cryptococcosis.**

Leishmaniasis

This is an uncommon multisystemic disease with cutaneous presentation and regional lymphadenopathy. It is caused by the protozoan *Leishmania* spp, which is transmitted by sand flies. The disease is often associated with Mediterranean travel although endemic areas such as Oklahoma and Ohio are found in the United States. It is more likely to occur in dogs than in cats. The condition may begin in the skin, then spread internally. Periorbital alopecia and scaling or ulcerative and erosive lesions of the nose are common signs that may progress to poorly

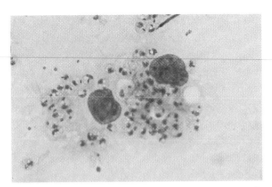

FIGURE 3–22. Leishmaniasis. Tissue aspirate. Cat. Ear nodule consists of macrophages with intracellular and extracellular organisms having a characteristic appearance of *Leishmania* sp. (Aqueous-based Wright; ×500.) (Glass slide material courtesy of Ruanna Gossett et al., Texas A & M University; presented at the 1991 ASVCP case review session.)

defined cutaneous and mucocutaneous nodules. *Leishmania mexicana* has been associated with a nonsystemic, cutaneous form of the disease in cats from Texas and Mexico (Barnes et al., 1993). On cytology, macrophages predominate but other cells present include lymphocytes, plasma cells, and occasional multinucleated giant cells. The intracellular organisms, termed *amastigotes,* measure 1.5 to 2.0 × 2.5 to 5 μm and possess a red nucleus and characteristic bar-shaped kinetoplasts (Fig. 3–22). In addition to the skin, the bone marrow and lymphoid organs are common sites of involvement. Other laboratory abnormalities include polyclonal or monoclonal gammopathy and nonregenerative anemia. The characteristic cytology or culture is used to obtain a definitive diagnosis. Also immunoperoxidase staining may be performed on tissue biopsies. An indirect fluorescent antibody test is available for *Leishmania donovani* but this only indicates previous exposure. Treatment involves pentavalent antimony compounds, itraconazole, or allopurinol (Lester and Kenyon, 1996) for systemic disease and surgical excision for focal skin lesions. Prognosis is good to guarded, however, this is a zoonotic disease and euthanasia may need to be considered.

PARASITIC INFESTATION

Dracunculiasis

An uncommon parasitic condition in dogs and potentially in cats causes pruritic, painful erythematous subcutaneous swellings (Giovengo, 1993) that can be diagnosed by cytologic evaluation of aspirated tissue fluid (Panciera and Stockham, 1988) or imprints from a lesion discharge. First-stage larvae from *Dracunculus insignis* measuring approximately 25 μm wide $\times$ 500 μm long appear pale blue when stained (Baker and Lumsden, 2000) or granulated (Fig. 3–23) and have a long tapered tail. The life cycle involves ingestion of infected water fleas or frogs containing larvae, which leave the digestive tract and migrate, usually to the limbs. Surgical excision is used to remove the adult nematode, which often measures 20 cm long (Beyer et al., 1999) but may

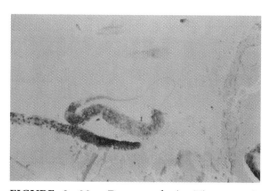

FIGURE 3–23. Dracunculosis. Tissue aspirate. Dog. A wormlike subcutaneous mass on the thorax contained these large larvae with long tapered tails. (Romanowsky; ×100.) (Courtesy of Judy Radin et al., The Ohio State University; presented at the 1990 ASVCP case review session.)

reach lengths up to 120 cm. Antihelmintics appear ineffective in killing adults.

NEOPLASIA

Epithelial

Squamous Papilloma

These warts are usually solitary lesions, most often affecting older dogs. They are rare in cats. It usually presents as a raised growth with keratin-covered finger-like projections appearing on the head or limbs. On cytology, squamous epithelium in all stages of development is present, but mature forms with benign-appearing nuclei predominate. In younger dogs, papillomas occurring at mucocutaneous sites may be induced by another papovavirus, and these can regress spontaneously. If necessary, surgical excision results in a good to excellent prognosis.

> *Cytologic differential diagnosis:* squamous cell carcinoma, intracutaneous cornifying epithelioma.

Squamous Cell Carcinoma

This is a common tumor in the dog and cat occurring as solitary or multiple proliferative or ulcerative masses (Fig. 3–24A). It accounts for 15% of skin tumors in cats but only 2% in dogs (Yager and Wilcock, 1994). It is most common on the limbs of dogs and thinly haired areas of the pinnae or face of cats. Tumors are usually locally invasive and may metastasize to regional lymph nodes. Those on the digit are considered to be highly malignant with a greater chance for metastasis. Cytologically, purulent inflammation often accompanies immature or dysplastic squamous epithelium (Fig. 3–24B). Bacterial sepsis may occur if the surface has eroded. A tadpole

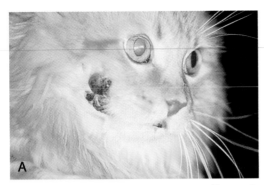

FIGURE 3–24. A, Squamous cell carcinoma. Ulcerative lesion on the face. Cat. (Courtesy of Jamie Bellah.)

plasm of another, termed *emperipolesis,* may be noted in well-differentiated squamous cell carcinomas (Fig. 3–24E). Moderately differentiated tumors have few angular cells and greater than 50% round or oval dysplastic cells (Fig. 3–24F). Round individualized cells having a high nuclear-to-cytoplasmic ratio predominate in the poorly differentiated tumors. Cellular and nuclear pleomorphism are marked in the poorly differentiated squamous cell carcinomas.

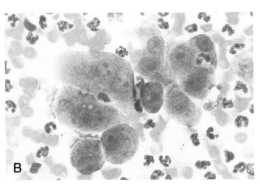

FIGURE 3–24. B, Squamous cell carcinoma. Nose planum mass aspirate. Dog. Dysplastic epithelium with purulent inflammation. (Wright-Giemsa; ×250.)

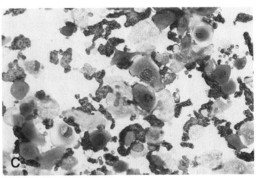

FIGURE 3–24. C, Squamous cell carcinoma. Cheek mass aspirate. Cat. Note the intermediate, superficial, and anucleated squame forms often with angular cell borders and keratinized cytoplasm seen in the well-differentiated type of neoplasm. (Aqueous-based Wright; ×125.)

shape with a tail-like projection and keratinized blue-green hyalinized cytoplasm may be helpful criteria in determining the cell of origin (Garma-Avina, 1994). The neoplastic epithelium may appear as individual cells or as sheets of adherent cells. Squames and highly keratinized nucleated angular squamous epithelium with nuclear atypia predominate in well-differentiated tumors (Fig. 3–24C). When these cells are concentrically arranged, they correspond to the keratin pearls seen histologically (Fig. 3–24D). The presence of one cell type within the cyto-

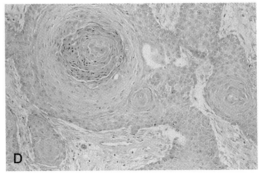

FIGURE 3–24. D, Squamous cell carcinoma. Dog. Keratin pearl in the center of a lobule of neoplastic squamous epithelium. (H & E; ×50.)

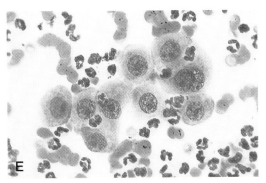

FIGURE 3–24. E, Squamous cell carcinoma. Same case as in Figure 3–24B. Emperipolesis noted by neutrophils migrating through epithelium. (Wright-Giemsa; ×250.)

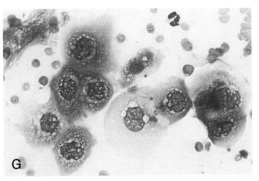

FIGURE 3–24. G, Squamous cell carcinoma. Thigh mass aspirate. Cat. Small sheets of epithelium with marked anisokaryosis and anisocytosis are present. The keratinized cytoplasm displays prominent perinuclear vacuolation. (Aqueous-based Wright; ×250.)

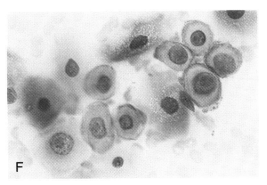

FIGURE 3–24. F, Dysplastic squamous epithelium. Foot mass aspirate. Dog. Rounded cells and keratinized intermediate squamous epithelium similar to cells found in squamous cell carcinoma. (Aqueous-based Wright; ×250.)

KEY POINT: It is often difficult to determine if dysplastic changes are the result of the reaction to chronic inflammation or an indication of malignancy.

Cytologic differential diagnosis: **intracutaneous cornifying epithelioma, squamous papilloma, basosquamous carcinoma.**

Basal Cell Tumor

This tumor is found commonly in dogs and cats and typically presents as a single, firm, elevated, well-demarcated round intradermal mass that may be ulcerated or cystic (Fig. 3–25A). Many tumors appear pigmented because of their abundant melanin. Tumors in cats may be cystic. Basal cell tumors are the most common cutaneous neoplasm in cats as indicated by one study that reported a prevalence of 22% (Yager and Wilcock, 1994). They are less common in dogs, accounting for 6% of skin tumors (Yager and Wilcock, 1994). They are located mostly about the head with frequent occurrence on the neck and limbs. Cytolog-

Perinuclear vacuolation is thought to represent colorless keratohyalin granules and may be present most frequently in well and moderately differentiated tumor types (Fig. 3–24G). Treatment considerations include surgical excision, cryosurgery, radiotherapy, intralesional chemotherapy, and photodynamic therapy. Prognosis is guarded as recurrence is common, especially in white-faced cats.

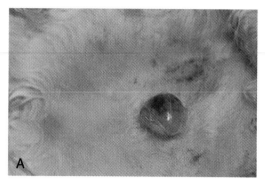

FIGURE 3–25. A, Basal cell tumor. Cat.
Note the single, firm, raised, alopecic, well-demarcated round intradermal mass. (Courtesy of the University of Florida Dermatology Section.)

baceous differentiation, or basal tumors with follicular differentiation (Fig. 3–25F), respectively. Histologically, several patterns of basal cell tumors exist, including solid, ribbon, medusoid (Fig. 3–25G), and cystic (Fig. 3–25H). Basal cell tumors in general are benign, but rare reports of metastasis exist (Day et al., 1994). Basosquamous carcinoma may recur locally at the site of excision. Treatment considerations include

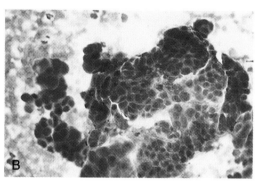

FIGURE 3–25. B, Basal cell tumor. Lip mass imprint. Dog. Large clusters of tightly adherent epithelial cells with intensely basophilic cytoplasm are present. (Aqueous-based Wright; ×125.)

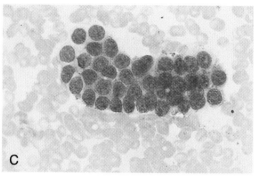

FIGURE 3–25. C, Basal cell tumor. Mass aspirate. Dog. Tight cluster of uniform cells having a high nuclear-to-cytoplasmic ratio. The cytoplasm is scant and basophilic. (Wright-Giemsa; ×250.)

ically, basal cells are small cells characterized by high nuclear-to-cytoplasmic ratios, monomorphic nuclei, and deeply basophilic cytoplasm that may be pigmented (Fig. 3–25B–D). They may be arranged as clusters or in row formation. Basal cells may predominate in a tumor but foci of atypical squamous differentiation, individual sebocytes, or scattered keratinocytes (Fig. 3–25E) should suggest the presence of basosquamous carcinoma, basal cell tumors with se-

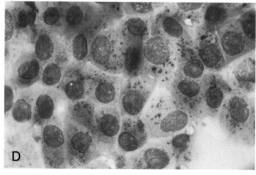

FIGURE 3–25. D, Basal cell tumor. Neck mass aspirate. Dog. Sheet of basal epithelium with prominent cytoplasmic granulation and pigmentation, consistent with keratohyalin and melanin. (Wright-Giemsa; ×250.)

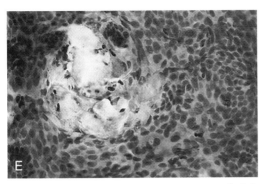

FIGURE 3–25.   E, Basal cell tumor with fol-licular differentiation. Shoulder mass aspi-rate. Dog. Dense clusters of basal epithelium with foci of keratinocytes. (Aqueous-based Wright; ×125.)

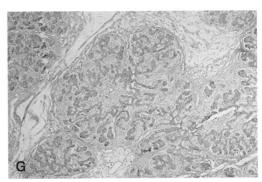

FIGURE 3–25.   G, Basal cell tumor. Dog. Note the medusoid pattern with cords of basal epithelium radiating out from the center. (H & E; ×25.)

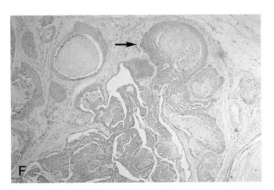

FIGURE 3–25.   F, Basal cell tumor with fol-licular differentiation. Same case as in Figure 3–25E. Note the gradual process of keratiniza-tion within the thickened basal epithelium (*ar-row*). This tumor also may be termed *baso-squamous epithelioma*, similar to a tricho-epithelioma. (H & E; ×25.)

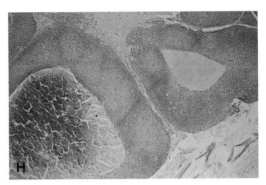

FIGURE 3–25.   H, Cystic basal cell tumor. Cat. Head mass with basal epithelium prolifer-ation surrounding centers containing choles-terol, calcium deposits, or liquefactive material. (H & E; ×25.)

surgical excision, cryosurgery, and radio-therapy. Prognosis is fair to good.

KEY POINT: There is considerable over-lap cytologically between basal cell tumors and adnexal or follicular tumors, related to their common origin.

Cytologic differential diagnosis: **sebaceous carcinoma, sebaceous epithelioma, follic-ular tumors, squamous cell carcinoma.**

Hair Follicle Tumors

These infrequent benign tumors are usually solitary but may be multiple. They are most often found in older dogs. These are firm, raised, hairless, well-circumscribed masses that may ulcerate. Most often considered are trichoepithelioma (Fig. 3–26) and pi-lomatrixoma. Cytologically, keratinaceous debris, keratinocytes, and low numbers of germinal epithelium resembling basal cells

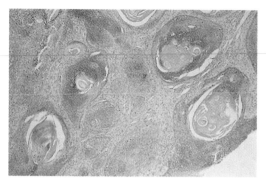

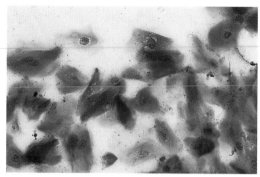

FIGURE 3–26. Trichoepithelioma. Note the abrupt keratinization in the center surrounded by thickened basal epithelium, suggesting rudimentary hair formation. (H & E; ×25.)

FIGURE 3–27. Keratoacanthoma. Digit mass aspirate. Dog. Keratinocytes predominate in this lesion, which is cytologically indistinguishable from a follicular cyst or follicular neoplasm. (Wright-Giemsa; ×125.)

are present. Histologically, the abrupt keratinization from the basal epithelium forming horn cysts helps to distinguish this tumor from the basal cell tumor showing early differentiation. Treatment consists of surgical excision or cryosurgery. Prognosis is excellent.

Cytologic differential diagnosis: intracutaneous cornifying epithelioma, epidermal cyst or follicular cyst, basosquamous tumors.

Intracutaneous Cornifying Epithelioma (Keratoacanthoma)

This tumor represents a proliferation of the epithelium containing adnexal and follicular structures with a pore to the outside. It may be predisposed in some breeds (Norwegian elkhound, keeshond). Pore contents are similar to that of epidermal cyst or follicular cyst. Cytologically, keratinous debris, keratinocytes, and cholesterol crystals characterize this tumor (Fig. 3–27). Low numbers of basal cell epithelium may be found. Treatment consists of surgical excision, cryosurgery, and retinoids, particularly for

multiple tumor presentation. Prognosis is good.

Cytologic differential diagnosis: epidermal cyst or follicular cyst, hair follicle tumors.

Sebaceous Adenoma

This appears as a single, smooth, raised, hairless cauliflower lesion or as an intradermal multilobulated mass that usually measures less than 1 cm in diameter (Fig. 3–28A). The overlying skin is alopecic and sometimes ulcerated. These are common in dogs, accounting for approximately 6% of all canine skin and subcutaneous tumors in one survey (Gross et al., 1992). Fifty percent of these tumors in older dogs occur on the head (Goldschmidt and Shofer, 1992). Multiple tumors occur infrequently. Although uncommon in the cat, these tumors are most often found on the head and back. Cystic degeneration and lipogranulomatous inflammation may occur in the center of lobules. Cytologically, mature sebocytes arranged in lobules or clusters predominate and are characterized by pale foamy cyto-

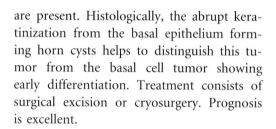

plasm having a small dense centrally placed nucleus (Fig. 3–28B & C). A variable number of germinal epithelial cells having basophilic cytoplasm and a higher nuclear-to-cytoplasmic ratio may accompany the secretory cells. Necrotic centers containing amorphous basophilic with remnants of foamy cells may be found (Fig. 3–28D). Treatment consists of surgical excision or cryosurgery. Prognosis is excellent.

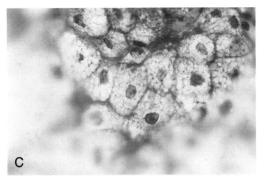

FIGURE 3–28. C, Sebaceous adenoma. Same case as in Figure 3–28B. Note the low nuclear-to-cytoplasmic ratio and the foamy cytoplasm with delicate streaks. (Aqueous-based Wright; ×250.)

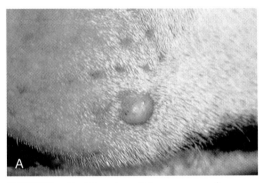

FIGURE 3–28. A, Sebaceous adenoma. Dog. Raised, alopecic, lobulated lesion present on the lip. (Courtesy of the Dermatology Section, University of Florida.)

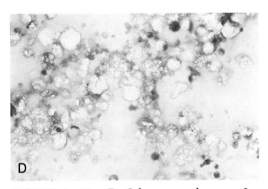

FIGURE 3–28. D, Sebaceous adenoma. Interdigital mass aspirate. Dog. Large amount of globular material is present, with occasional degenerated sebocytes. Necrotic centers of tumors produce this cellular debris. (Wright-Giemsa; ×125.)

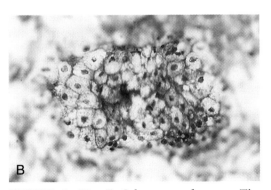

FIGURE 3–28. B, Sebaceous adenoma. Tissue aspirate. Dog. The monomorphic population of vacuolated epithelial cells having a small centrally placed nucleus is consistent with mature sebocytes. (Aqueous-based Wright; ×125.)

KEY POINT: Histologic examination is necessary to distinguish between hyperplastic and adenomatous sebaceous tumors.

Cytologic differential diagnosis: **sebaceous hyperplasia.**

Sebaceous Epithelioma

This is similar in gross appearance to sebaceous adenoma. When present on the eyelid, it is termed *meibomian adenoma*. Pathologists may classify sebaceous epithelioma in the same category as sebaceous adenoma or basal cell tumor. Histologically, germinal epithelium predominates and small lobules

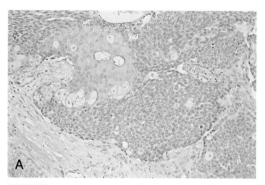

FIGURE 3–29. A, Sebaceous epithelioma. Ear mass. Dog. Dermal mass composed of lobules and islands of neoplastic basal epithelium with occasional foci of sebocytes and keratinocytes. (H & E; ×50.)

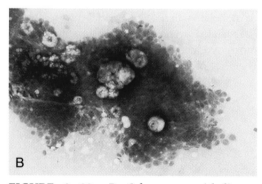

FIGURE 3–29. B, Sebaceous epithelioma. Shoulder mass aspirate. Dog. Clusters of basal epithelium with scattered sebocytes. Six months later, this mass was diagnosed as basal cell carcinoma related to progressive infiltration into subcutaneous tissues. (Wright-Giemsa; ×100.)

of mature sebaceous epithelium are intermixed (Fig. 3–29A). Cytologically, the tumor resembles a basal cell tumor with small basophilic epithelial clusters along with scattered groups of mature sebocytes (Fig. 3–29B) and low numbers of individualized well-differentiated squamous epithelial cells. Clinical behavior is benign but they may rarely recur locally. Prognosis is usually excellent following surgical excision.

> *Cytologic differential diagnosis:* sebaceous adenoma, basal cell tumor.

Sebaceous Carcinoma

This is an uncommon tumor found most frequently on the head of dogs. Cocker spaniels appear predisposed. It presents as a rapid growing, large, ulcerated, poorly circumscribed mass. Cytologically, pleomorphic glandular epithelium displays malignant nuclear features such as anisokaryosis,

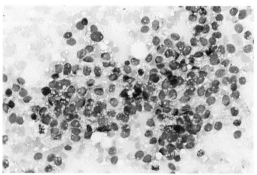

FIGURE 3–30. Sebaceous carcinoma. Shoulder mass aspirate. Dog. A monomorphic population of cohesive cells in sheets and clumps. Malignant features include a high nuclear-to-cytoplasmic ratio, anisokaryosis, multinucleation, clumped chromatin, and prominent, variable nucleoli. The cytoplasm is basophilic, with frequent clear, punctate vacuoles suggestive of sebaceous differentiation. Histopathology confirmed the diagnosis. (Wright-Giemsa; ×125.)

prominent nucleoli, and frequent atypical mitotic figures. The finely vacuolated cytoplasm suggests sebaceous differentiation (Fig. 3–30). This malignant tumor is usually locally invasive, but may occasionally metastasize to regional lymph nodes. Treatment consists of wide surgical excision. Prognosis is good.

Cytologic differential diagnosis: basal cell tumor.

Perianal Gland Adenoma

This is a common tumor mostly associated with intact male dogs, suggesting androgen dependency. Goldschmidt and Shofer (1992) reported this tumor involving 9% of skin tumors. Perianal gland tumors are rarely found in the cat. The tumor may be single or multiple, occurring generally near the anus (Fig. 3–31A), but may also be found on the tail, perineum, prepuce, and thigh, and along the dorsal or ventral midline. Initially they grossly appear as smooth, raised round lesions that lobulate and ulcerate as they enlarge. The tumor arises from modified sebaceous gland epithelium within the dermis that is lined by small basophilic re-

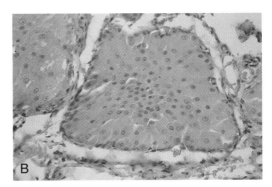

FIGURE 3–31. B, Normal perianal gland tissue. Dog. The hepatoid cells are packets of modified sebaceous epithelium having a low nuclear-to-cytoplasmic ratio that are lined by small basophilic reserve cells. (H & E; ×100.)

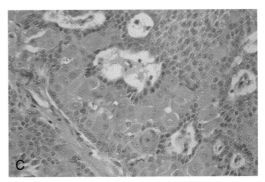

FIGURE 3–31. C, Perianal gland adenoma. Perianal mass. Dog. The lesion is well circumscribed, consisting of islands of polygonal hepatoid cells and a dense proliferation of basal reserve cells in the upper right area. (H & E; ×100.)

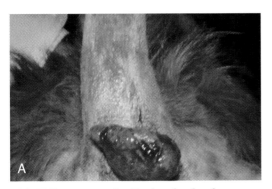

FIGURE 3–31. A, Perianal gland tumor. Anal mass. Dog. (Courtesy of Colin Burrows, Gainesville, FL.)

serve cells (Fig. 3–31B & C). Cytologically, sheets of mature round hepatoid cells predominate characterized by abundant finely granular pinkish-blue cytoplasm (Fig. 3–31D). Nuclei resemble those of normal hepatocytes appearing round with an often single or multiple, prominent, nucleolus. A low number of smaller basophilic reserve cells having a high nuclear-to-cytoplasmic

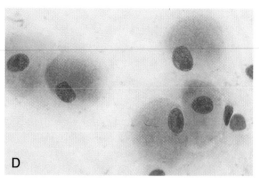

FIGURE 3–31. D, Perianal gland adenoma. Mass aspirate. Dog. Individual hepatoid cells display a small round nucleus and abundant pink-blue finely granular cytoplasm. (Aqueous-based Wright; ×250.)

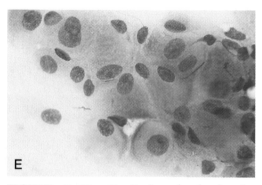

FIGURE 3–31. E, Perinanal gland adenoma. Same case as in Figure 3–31C. Smaller basophilic reserve cells are interspersed between hepatoid cells. (Aqueous-based Wright; ×250.)

ratio may also be present, but these lack features of cellular pleomorphism (Fig. 3–31E). Perianal gland adenomas are benign tumors, which respond to surgical excision or cryosurgery, coupled with castration. Prognosis is good to excellent. The malignant counterpart of this tumor is infrequently encountered. Nuclear pleomorphism is generally marked in those cases.

Cytologic differential diagnosis: perianal gland hyperplasia, well-differentiated perianal gland carcinoma.

Apocrine Gland Adenocarcinoma of Anal Sac (Anal Sac Adenocarcinoma)

There is an increased incidence of the disease in older spayed female dogs but a sex predilection has not been confirmed (Goldschmidt and Shofer, 1992). The majority of cases involve dogs, but occasional cases have been reported in the cat. Grossly, this is a subcutaneous mass, firmly fixed around the anal sacs that arises from the glands in the wall of these sacs. A paraneoplastic syndrome of hypercalcemia is associated with 50% to 90% of cases, which may result in renal disease (Ross et al., 1991). Cytologically, dense cell clusters with a papillary shape have poorly defined cell borders in the solid and anaplastic forms of carcinoma (Fig. 3–32A). Malignant characteristics are easily detected in glandular epithelium, which displays cellular and nuclear pleomorphism, a high nuclear-to-cytoplasmic ratio, and in some cases multiple small cytoplasmic vacuoles (Fig. 3–32B). An acinar

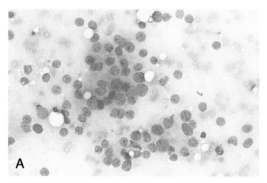

FIGURE 3–32. A, Anal sac apocrine gland adenocarcinoma. Tissue aspirate. Dog. Loosely cohesive cell clusters with indistinct cell borders. (Wright-Giemsa; ×125.)

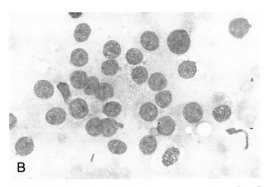

FIGURE 3–32. B, Anal sac apocrine gland adenocarcinoma. Same case as in Figure 3–32A. Malignant features include high and variable nuclear-to-cytoplasmic ratios, aniso-karyosis, coarse chromatin, and prominent nucleoli. (Wright-Giemsa; ×250.)

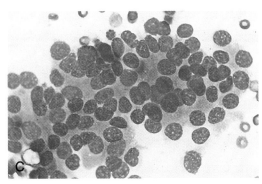

FIGURE 3–32. C, Anal sac apocrine gland adenocarcinoma. Anal mass. Dog. An acinar arrangement with nuclei peripheralized within a cluster of cells helps to diagnose a tumor of glandular origin. (Wright-Giemsa; ×250.)

arrangement may be detected to aid in the diagnosis and distinguish it from perianal (hepatoid) carcinoma (Fig. 3–32C). Treatment consists of wide surgical excision with postoperative radiation therapy. These malignant tumors commonly metastasize initially to regional lymph nodes. Prognosis is poor to fair.

Cytologic differential diagnosis: **perianal gland carcinoma.**

Ceruminous Gland Adenoma/ Adenocarcinoma

These tumors arise from specialized apocrine sweat glands in the external ear. They are more frequently encountered in cats than dogs, especially in aged cats, and involve approximately 1% of all feline tumors submitted to a diagnostic laboratory (Moisan and Watson, 1996) and 6% of all feline skin tumors (Goldschmidt and Shofer, 1992). The adenoma grossly resembles ceruminous cystic hyperplasia, a non-neoplastic growth also common in the cat that is associated with chronic otitis externa. Both adenoma and hyperplasia present as smooth nodular or pedunculated masses that rarely ulcerate. Brown to black oily fluid collects within the enlarged gland ducts. Cytologically, amorphous debris along with low numbers of inflammatory cells and ductal epithelium may be found. Treatment consists of conservative surgical excision. Prognosis is good. Ceruminous gland adenocarcinoma is found in two thirds of the ceruminous gland tumors in cats (Fig. 3–33A & B). It is invasive locally and frequently metastasizes to regional lymph nodes. Nuclear pleomorphism is expected

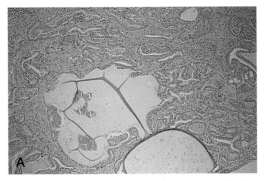

FIGURE 3–33. A, Ceruminous gland adenocarcinoma. Ear canal mass. Cat. Neoplastic proliferation of ductular epithelium with large cysts formed that contain brown sebum. (H & E; ×25.)

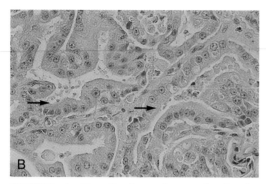

FIGURE 3–33. B, Ceruminous gland adenocarcinoma. Same case as in Figure 3–33A. Malignant changes noted by anisokaryosis, vesicular nuclei, prominent nucleoli, and marked anisocytosis of ductular epithelium. Note the apocrine function of these cells is demonstrated by eosinophilic droplets at the apical surface (*arrows*). (H & E; ×125.)

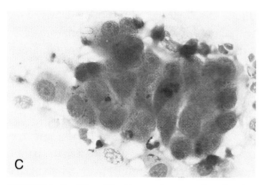

FIGURE 3–33. C, Ceruminous gland adenocarcinoma. Tissue imprint. Same case as in Figure 3–33A. Tight clusters of epithelium demonstrate increased nuclear-to-cytoplasmic ratio, prominent single nucleoli, coarse chromatin, anisokaryosis, and anisocytosis. Note the intracytoplasmic presence of black globular secretory material in some cells, which when finely dispersed in other cells resembles melanin pigment. (Aqueous-based Wright; ×250.)

on cytology and cells in some cases contain fine to coarse black granular material that mimics melanin pigment (Fig. 3–33C). Radical surgical excision is recommended and some suggest postoperative radiotherapy to limit recurrence.

Cytologic differential diagnosis: ceruminous gland hyperplasia (for adenoma).

Sweat Gland Adenocarcinoma

This is an uncommon tumor, accounting for up to 2% to 3% of skin tumors of dogs and cats, respectively (Bevier and Goldschmidt, 1981a; Miller et al., 1991). They are often located on the back, flanks, and feet of dogs and present as solitary, raised, well-circumscribed, and solid masses, many of which ulcerate. In older cats, most occur on the head and limbs, appearing as a solid nodular mass. An alternate form observed in the dog and cat is an ulcerative, hemorrhagic, and frequently inflamed lesion that resembles acute dermatitis. Cytologically, ductular epithelium is present as clusters of basophilic cells that display numerous criteria of malignancy. In some cases, significant fibroplasia occurs so aspirates may yield fibroblasts along with epithelium. Treatment consists of wide surgical excision. Prognosis is fair to guarded as local recurrence and metastasis has been reported.

Cytologic differential diagnosis: mammary gland adenocarcinoma, anal sac adenocarcinoma, other adenocarcinomas, basal cell tumor.

Mesenchymal

Fibroma

This is an uncommon tumor of adult dogs and cats, accounting for approximately 1% of cutaneous neoplasms in dogs (Yager and Wilcock, 1994). It presents as a solitary lesion on the extremities, head, flanks, and groin. Grossly, it is firm to soft, well circumscribed, hairless, and dome shaped or pedunculated. Cytologically, variable numbers of spindle or fusiform cells with small, uniform, dense oval nuclei occur individually or occasionally in small bundles. Generally, few cells exfoliate into cytologic preparations. Cytoplasm is lightly basophilic and cell borders are poorly defined as they form cytoplasmic tails on opposite sides of the nucleus (Fig. 3–34A). Amorphous eosinophilic material representing intercellular collagen protein may be associated with the neoplastic cells. Histologically, spindle cells may be arranged loosely (Fig. 3–34B) or as dense collagen bundles that are found rarely on cytology (Fig. 3–34C). These tumors are

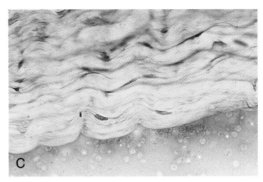

FIGURE 3–34. C, Fibroma. Same case as in Figure 3–34A. Dense bundles of collagen stained lightly pink with basophilic oval nuclei enmeshed in the connective tissue. (Aqueous-based Wright; ×125.)

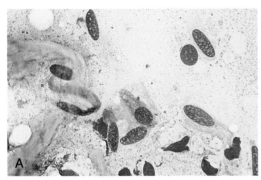

FIGURE 3–34. A, Fibroma. Metatarsal mass imprint. Dog. Spindle cells are present, with indistinct lightly basophilic cytoplasm that extends from both ends of the oval nucleus. Note the amorphous eosinophilic material interspersed between cells. (Aqueous-based Wright; ×250.)

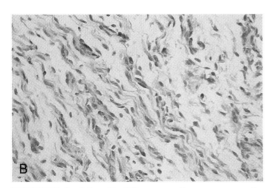

FIGURE 3–34. B, Fibroma. Same case as in Figure 3–34A. Loose proliferation of benign fibrocytes into wavy strands of collagen. (H & E; ×100.)

benign and treatment consists of surgical excision. Prognosis is generally good except for occasional local recurrence following removal of large tumors.

Cytologic differential diagnosis: **myxoma, well-differentiated fibrosarcoma, neural sheath tumors.**

Fibrosarcoma

This common tumor of dogs and cats accounts for 15% to 17% of skin neoplasms in the cat and is the fourth most common skin tumor in that species (Miller et al., 1991; Goldschmidt and Shofer, 1992). Those in young cats may be caused by the feline sarcoma virus and may be multiple. In older dogs and cats, tumors are solitary with a predilection for the limbs, trunk, and head. They are poorly circumscribed and sometimes ulcerated (Fig. 3–35A). These malignant tumors are invasive and approximately 25% will metastasize via hematogenous routes. Vaccine-induced fibrosarcomas, possibly related to subcutaneous administered killed vaccines in cats (Hendrick and Brooks, 1994), are locally invasive and slow to metastasize. Cytologically, fi-

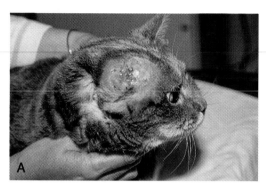

FIGURE 3–35. A, Fibrosarcoma. Cat. Recurrence of tumor in the site of previous surgery to remove the ear and surrounding tissue. (Courtesy of Jamie Bellah.)

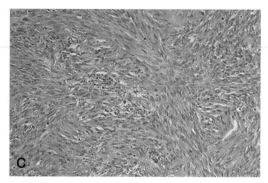

FIGURE 3–35. C, Fibrosarcoma. Skin mass aspirate. Dog. Broad interlacing bundles of spindle cells with malignant features are present. (H & E; ×50.)

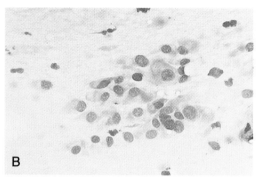

FIGURE 3–35. B, Fibrosarcoma. Leg mass aspirate. Cat. Individualized plump oval cells with wispy cytoplasmic tails. Rare multinucleated cell noted as shown in lower right. (Aqueous-based Wright; ×125.)

brosarcomas consist of abundant numbers of large plump cells (Fig. 3–35B) occurring individually or in aggregates often associated with pink collagenous material. Multinucleated giant cells may be present occasionally. Nuclear pleomorphism may be marked compared with the benign counterpart. Cells are less uniform and generally have high nuclear-to-cytoplasmic ratios. Treatment consists of wide surgical excision and/or amputation. Recurrence involves 30% of canine cases. Alternately, radiotherapy with or without hyperthermia may be

helpful postsurgery. Immunostimulants in combination with surgery and radiotherapy have also shown promising results. Chemotherapy alone has not proven effective in treatment of fibrosarcoma but may be helpful used with other modalities. Prognosis is good to poor depending on the site and degree of anaplasia.

KEY POINT: Histologic examination is necessary to distinguish between fibrosarcoma and other spindle cell mesenchymal malignancies or granulation tissue (Fig. 3–35C). Immunohistochemistry may be similarly useful in distinguishing tissue origin.

Cytologic differential diagnosis: **granulation tissue, malignant neural sheath tumors, malignant fibrous histiocytoma, hemangiopericytoma, myxosarcoma.**

Myxoma/Myxosarcoma

Myxomas are rare tumors in dogs and cats, accounting for less than 1% of skin tumors (Goldschmidt and Shofer, 1992). Myxomas are infiltrative growths with a soft, fluctuant feel that present as slightly raised masses.

Common sites in the dog and cat include the limbs, thorax, and abdomen. Cytologically, an intercellular matrix is often present in the background as granular eosinophilic amorphous material (Fig. 3–36A & B). Well-differentiated fusiform and stellate cells are found in low numbers in the benign lesion, which increase in the degree of cellular and nuclear pleomorphism with the malignant form (Fig. 3–36C). Multinucle-

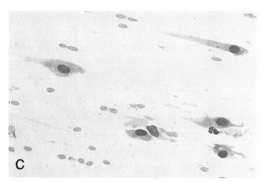

FIGURE 3–36. C, Myxosarcoma. Same case as in Figure 3–36B. Pleomorphic spindle cells with vesicular oval nuclei characterize the malignant form of myxomatous tumor. (Aqueous-based Wright; ×125.)

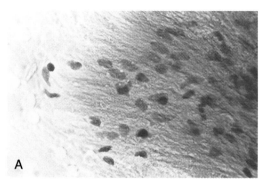

FIGURE 3–36. A, Myxoma. Carpal mass aspirate. Dog. Dense granular eosinophilic intercellular matrix is present with small dense nuclei, suggesting a benign proliferation. (Aqueous-based Wright; ×250.)

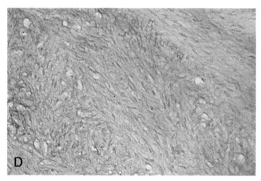

FIGURE 3–36. D, Myxoma. Same case as in Figure 3–36A. The ground substance stains blue or positive for mucin shown between nuclei staining red. (Alcian blue; ×100.)

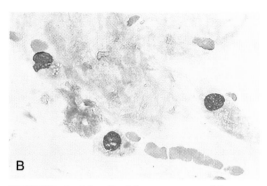

FIGURE 3–36. B, Myxosarcoma. Metacarpal mass aspirate. Dog. An intracellular and extracellular granular eosinophilic matrix is shown with plump individualized mesenchymal cells. (Aqueous-based Wright; ×250.)

ated cells are occasionally present in myxosarcomas. Alcian blue staining of the ground substance for mucin is diagnostic (Grindem et al., 1990) (Fig. 3–36D). Treatment consists of surgical excision. Prognosis is good to fair since recurrence is common, but it rarely metastasizes.

Cytologic differential diagnosis: **fibroma, fibrosarcoma, neural sheath tumors, hemangiopericytoma.**

Canine Hemangiopericytoma

This is a common tumor generally considered to affect dogs only. It may be present in 7% of skin neoplasms (Goldschmidt and Shofer, 1992). The origin of the neoplastic cells is still unproven, but association with the periphery of blood vessels may be observed. These are often solitary tumors with a predilection for the joints of the limbs, but are found commonly on the thorax and abdomen. They are firm to soft, multilobu-

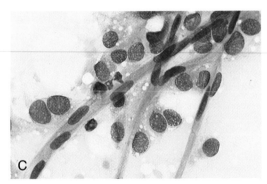

FIGURE 3–37. C, Hemangiopericytoma. Same case as in Figure 3–37A. Plump spindle cells are shown adherent to the surface of capillaries. (Aqueous-based Wright; ×250.)

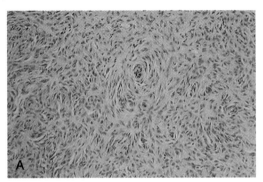

FIGURE 3–37. A, Hemangiopericytoma. Thigh mass. Dog. Classic fingerprint whorls of plump spindle cells around blood vessels. (H & E; ×50.)

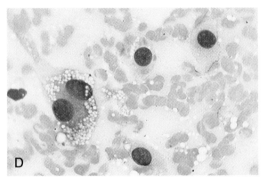

FIGURE 3–37. D, Hemangiopericytoma. Same case as in Figure 3–37A. The cytoplasm is basophilic with numerous small discrete vacuoles, and one cell contains eosinophilic globules. (Aqueous-based Wright; ×250.)

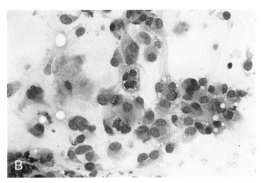

FIGURE 3–37. B, Hemangiopericytoma. Sternal subcutaneous mass aspirate. Dog. Slide preparation is highly cellular, with aggregates of plump mononuclear or multinucleated mesenchymal cells. (Wright-Giemsa; ×125.)

lated, and often well circumscribed. Histologically, it belongs to a broad group of spindle cell tumors with the classic appearance of fingerprint whorls of plump spindle cells and a low mitotic index (Fig. 3–37A). Cytologically, preparations are moderately to highly cellular (Fig. 3–37B). Plump spindle cells may be individualized or arranged in bundles, sometimes found adherent to the surface of capillaries (Fig. 3–37C). Nuclei are ovoid, with one or more prominent central nucleoli. Multinucleated cells are occasionally seen. Associated with cells may be a pink amorphous collagenous stroma. The cytoplasm is basophilic with often numerous small discrete vacuoles and occasional eosinophilic globules (Fig. 3–37D). Lymphoid cells have been found in approximately 10% of cases. Treatment consists of wide surgical excision or amputation, and radiotherapy with or without hyperthermia. Prognosis is fair as 20% to 60% will recur locally, especially with conservative excision. Metastasis is rare.

Cytologic differential diagnosis: **neural sheath tumors, well-differentiated fibrosarcoma, myxomatous tumors, malignant fibrous histiocytoma.**

Malignant Fibrous Histiocytoma

This is an uncommon tumor in dogs, comprising 0.34% of all canine tumors (Waters et al., 1994), and involves up to 3% of skin tumors in cats (Miller et al., 1991). It is a pleomorphic spindle cell tumor (Fig. 3–38A), the origin of which likely involves a primitive dermal pluripotent precursor cell since immunocytochemistry does not support a histiocytic origin (Pace et al., 1994). A subtype of it is known as giant cell tumor of soft parts, in which multinucleated cells are frequent. These tumors may be solitary or multiple, occurring mostly on the limbs of older dogs and cats, but may occur in abdominal organs, lungs, and lymph nodes. The subcutis and skeletal muscle of the shoulder and regional lymph node were diagnosed with malignant fibrous histiocytoma in a report of a dog (Desnoyers and St-Germain, 1994). Tumors are firm and poorly circumscribed. Cytologically, preparations contain a mixed population of multinucleated cells and plump spindle cells (Gibson et al., 1989; Desnoyers and St-Germain, 1994) (Fig. 3–38B & C). Treatment involves radical excisional surgery with or without radiotherapy, and chemotherapy. Prognosis is guarded as these tumors are locally invasive with frequent recurrence and rarely may metasta-

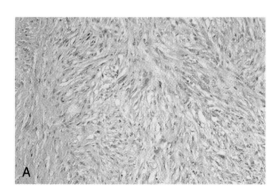

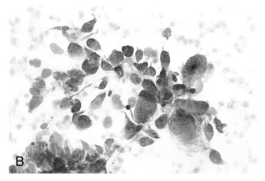

FIGURE 3–38. A, Malignant fibrous histiocytoma. Thoracic skin mass aspirate. Cat. Pleomorphic spindle cells form tightly swirling or interlacing (storiform) bundles. Note frequent multinucleated cells scattered throughout the mass. This tumor recurred 3 months after previous surgical excision. (H & E; ×50.)

FIGURE 3–38. B, Malignant fibrous histiocytoma. Flank mass aspirate. Dog. A mixed population of plump spindle cells is present, with multiple criteria for malignancy, including increased and variable nuclear-to-cytoplasmic ratios, prominent nucleoli, anisokaryosis, and multinucleation. (Wright-Giemsa; ×100.)

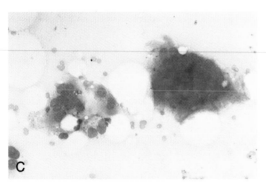

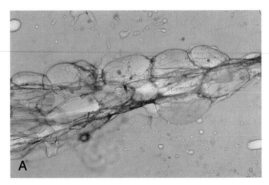

FIGURE 3–38.   C, Malignant fibrous histio-cytoma. Same case as in Figure 3–38A. Several variably sized giant cells are present. The cytoplasm contains fine eosinophilic granulation. (Wright-Giemsa; ×125.)

FIGURE 3–39.   A, Lipoma. Skin mass aspirate. Dog. Adipocytes are not dissolved in the water-soluble stain and are more visible. Note the pyknotic basophilic nucleus in relation to the massive cytoplasmic volume. (New methylene blue; ×50.)

size, especially in those cases containing higher percentages of giant cells.

Cytologic differential diagnosis: fibrosarcoma, hemangiopericytoma, granulation tissue.

Lipoma

This is a very common mesenchymal tumor in dogs, accounting for 8% of skin tumors (Goldschmidt and Shofer, 1992). It is a benign growth affecting generally older obese female dogs. It is present in 6% of cats (Goldschmidt and Shofer, 1992). The tumor may be single or multiple, occurring mostly on the trunk and proximal limbs. These are dome shaped, well circumscribed, soft, often freely moveable masses within the subcutis that can grow slowly, becoming quite large. Some may infiltrate between muscles. Cytologically, unstained slides appear wet with glistening droplets that do not dry completely. Lipid may be best demonstrated with a water-soluble stain such as new methylene blue (Fig. 3–39A) or the fat stain oil red O. When alcohol fixatives are used with Romanowsky stains, lipid is dis-

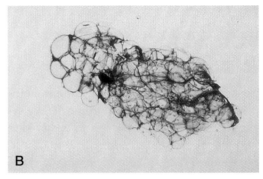

FIGURE 3–39.   B, Lipoma. Skin mass aspirate. Dog. Large aggregate of adipocytes. (Romanowsky; ×25.)

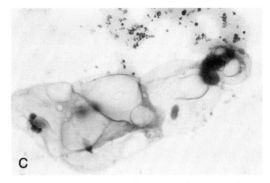

FIGURE 3–39.   C, Lipoma. Tissue aspirate. Cat. Adipocytes with small dense nucleus. The pale-blue background material is an artifact likely resulting from incomplete washing of the slide of stain. (Wright-Giemsa; ×125.)

solved, leaving slides often void of cells. When present, intact adipocytes have abundant clear cytoplasm with a small compressed nucleus to one side of the cell (Fig. 3–39B & C). Treatment involves surgical excision. Prognosis is excellent, however, some infiltrative lipomas may be difficult to completely excise.

Cytologic differential diagnosis: normal subcutaneous fat.

Liposarcoma

Rare tumors of dogs and cats composing less than 0.5% of skin tumors (Goldschmidt and Shofer, 1992a), liposarcomas are usually solitary masses occurring anywhere but most often on the ventral abdomen. An association with a foreign body was documented in one report (McCarthy et al., 1996). They are firm, poorly circumscribed and adherent to underlying tissues (Fig. 3–40A). Ulceration of the epidermis may occur. Cytologically, dense aggregates of mesenchymal cells contain variable amounts of lipid vacuoles (Fig. 3–40B). Cells appear plump, have a spindle shape with large ve-

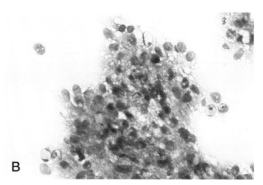

FIGURE 3–40. B, Liposarcoma. Leg mass aspirate. Dog. Large aggregates of mesenchymal cells with scattered lipid vacuoles that appear shrunken and well defined in this sample. (Aqueous-based Wright; ×125.)

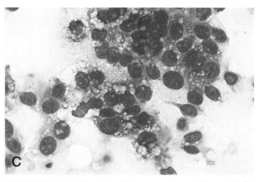

FIGURE 3–40. C, Liposarcoma. Dog. Cells appear plump and spindle shaped, with large vesicular nuclei and prominent nucleoli with variably sized intracytoplasmic fat vacuoles. (Aqueous-based Wright; ×250.) (Case material courtesy of Peter Fernandes.)

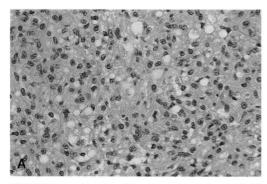

FIGURE 3–40. A, Liposarcoma. Dog. Lipid vacuoles are scattered between dense sheets of mesenchymal cells with vesicular nuclei. (H & E; ×100.)

sicular nuclei and prominent nucleoli, and may contain variably sized intracytoplasmic fat vacuoles (Fig. 3–40C). Multinucleated cells may be present. These are malignant tumors that have moderate metastatic potential. Treatment involves wide surgical excision, but may be coupled with radiation and hyperthermia to control recurrence.

Prognosis is guarded as they are likely to recur and may metastasize.

> *Cytologic differential diagnosis:* fibrosarcoma, undifferentiated sarcoma, anaplastic carcinoma.

Hemangioma

These benign tumors are common in dogs but less common in cats, representing about 5% and 2% of skin masses, respectively (Goldschmidt and Shofer, 1992; Miller et al., 1991). They may be solitary or multiple. Hemangiomas are discrete nodules present on the head, trunk, or limbs that appear dark red to purple and may feel spongy (Fig. 3–41). Cytologically, aspirates appear bloody, resembling blood contamination. Small basophilic endothelial cells are infrequent. Evidence for acute or chronic hemorrhage is often noted, resulting in erythrophagocytosis or hemosiderin-laden macrophages. Platelets are not commonly seen. Treatment involves surgical excision or cryosurgery. Prognosis is excellent.

> *Cytologic differential diagnosis:* hematoma, blood contamination.

Hemangiosarcoma

This is a malignant infiltrative mass of the dermis or subcutis. It is an infrequent tumor of older dogs and cats, occurring in about 1% and 3% of skin tumors, respectively (Goldschmidt and Shofer, 1992). Studies show an association between dermal vascular tumors and solar radiation (Hargis et al., 1992). Tumors are found more frequently in thin-haired areas such as the ventral abdomen of dogs and the ear pinnae of cats (Hargis et al., 1992; Miller et al., 1992). Lesions are raised, poorly circumscribed, ulcerated, and hemorrhagic. Cytologically, slide preparations often have low cellularity with numerous blood cells within the background. Solid, anaplastic cases of hemangiosarcoma may contain large dense aggregates of markedly pleomorphic mesenchymal cells (Fig. 3–42A). Evidence of acute erythrophagia or chronic hemorrhage with hemosiderin-laden macrophages is expected (Fig. 3–42B). Neoplastic cells are pleomorphic, ranging from large spindle to stellate. Cytoplasm is basophilic, having indistinct cell borders and occasional punctate vacuolation. Cells have high nuclear-to-cytoplasmic ratios, oval nuclei with coarse

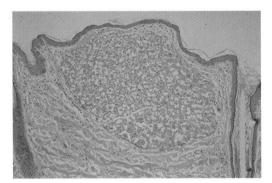

FIGURE 3–41. Hemangioma. Dog. Well-defined dermal nodule with endothelial proliferation and cavernous spaces filled with blood cells. (H & E; ×10.)

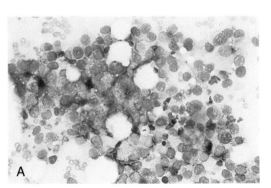

FIGURE 3–42. A, Hemangiosarcoma. Skin mass aspirate. Dog. Large dense aggregates of markedly pleomorphic mesenchymal cells. (Wright-Giemsa; ×125.)

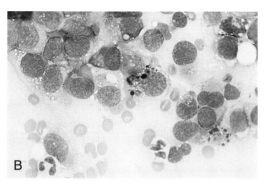

FIGURE 3–42. B, Hemangiosarcoma. Same case as in Figure 3–42A. Note the blue-black granules related to chronic hemorrhage. A mitotic figure is shown in the upper right corner. (Wright-Giemsa; ×250.)

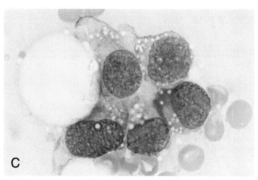

FIGURE 3–42. C, Hemangiosarcoma. Same case as in Figure 3–42A. Cells have high nuclear-to-cytoplasmic ratios, oval nuclei with coarse chromatin, and prominent multiple nucleoli. Note the punctate vacuoles in the cytoplasm seen commonly in this tumor. (Wright-Giemsa; ×500.)

chromatin, and prominent multiple nucleoli (Fig. 3–42C). Diagnosis may be assisted through immunohistochemistry using von Willebrand's factor (factor VIII-related antigen) and vimentin (Miller et al., 1992). Treatment consists of radical surgical excision and in the case of possible metastatic lesions, combination chemotherapy. Prognosis is guarded because of regional inva-

sion and local recurrence. Metastasis is uncommon but those occurring within the subcutis are more likely to spread.

Cytologic differential diagnosis: **fibrosarcoma, undifferentiated sarcoma, hemangiopericytoma, lymphangiosarcoma.**

Melanoma

Benign and malignant forms are common, accounting for 5% of canine skin tumors and 3% of feline skin tumors (Yager and Wilcock, 1994). Older animals are usually affected, as are those with dark skin pigmentation. Gross features differ for benign and malignant forms. About 70% of the melanocytic tumors are benign, appearing as mostly dark-brown to black, circumscribed, raised, dome-shaped masses covered by smooth hairless skin (Fig. 3–43A & B). Malignant tumors are variably pigmented, infiltrative, frequently ulcerated, and inflamed. Cytologically, cells from benign and malignant forms are pleomorphic, ranging from epithelioid (Fig. 3–43C) to fusiform (Fig. 3–43D), or occasionally are discrete and round, resembling those found in cutaneous plasmacytoma (Fig. 3–43E).

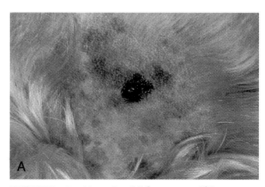

FIGURE 3–43. A, Melanoma. Skin mass. Dog. Note the dark-brown to black, circumscribed, raised, dome-shaped mass typical of most well-differentiated melanocytic tumors. (Courtesy of Leslie Fox, Gainesville, FL.)

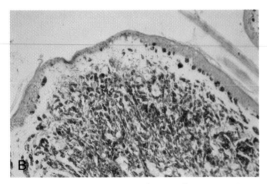

FIGURE 3–43.   B, Benign melanoma. Dorsum mass imprint. Dog. Melanocytes are present in the basal layer of the epidermis and within the superficial dermis arranged in clusters and diffusely. Cells are heavily pigmented. (H & E; ×50.)

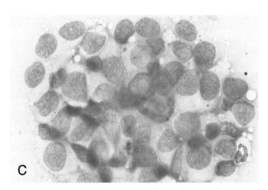

FIGURE 3–43.   C, Amelanotic melanoma. Gum mass imprint. Dog. Cells lacking pigment are clustered, giving a cohesive epithelial appearance. Abundant clear cytoplasm is present in the poorly differentiated type of melanoma. (Wright-Giemsa; ×250.)

In well-differentiated tumors, numerous fine black-green cytoplasmic granules may mask nuclei (Fig. 3–43D, F). Nuclei in benign forms are small and uniform compared with characteristics of anisocytosis, anisokaryosis, coarse chromatin, and prominent nucleoli seen in the malignant melanomas (Fig. 3–43G). Poorly differentiated tumors may contain few or no cytoplasmic

granules (Fig. 3–43C). A gray dustlike appearance in a few cells may help determine that the tumor is melanocytic (Fig. 3–43H). Treatment usually involves wide surgical excision. Prognosis depends on tumor site of origin and histologic characteristics. Benign skin tumors have a low mitotic rate and frequently have a good prognosis. Malig-

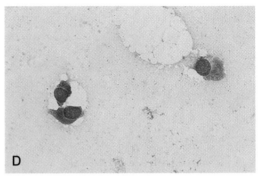

FIGURE 3–43.   D, Benign melanoma. Same case as in Figure 3–43B. Individual fusiform cells with abundant melanin pigment. (Aqueous-based Wright; ×250.)

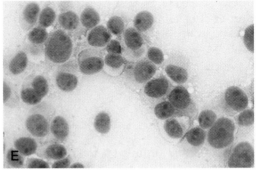

FIGURE 3–43.   E, Amelanotic melanoma. Same case as in Figure 3–43C. In other parts of the slide, individualized cells with a plasmacytoid appearance are evident. Note the prominent and multiple nucleoli, anisokaryosis, coarse chromatin, and oval to round nuclei in the poorly differentiated melanoma. (Aqueous-based Wright; ×250.)

nant forms arise more often from the nail bed, lip, and other oral mucocutaneous junctions in dogs. The latter forms carry a guarded or poor prognosis related to frequent recurrence and metastasis.

KEY POINT: The number of melanin granules will vary within a tumor, with deeper regions composed of fusiform cells

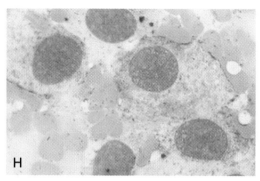

FIGURE 3–43. H, Melanoma. Skin mass aspirate. Dog. The uniform fine, gray-black melanin granules help determine the diagnosis in poorly differentiated melanocytic tumors. (Wright-Giemsa; ×500.)

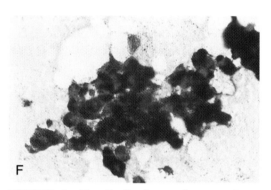

FIGURE 3–43. F, Benign melanoma. Same case as in Figure 3–43B. Large aggregates of darkly pigmented cells are found that mask nuclear details. (Aqueous-based Wright; ×250.)

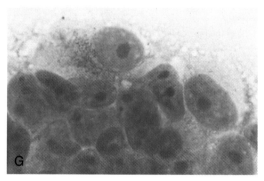

FIGURE 3–43. G, Amelanotic melanoma. Oral lesion imprint. Dog. Malignant features seen include large and multiple nucleoli, anisokaryosis, coarse chromatin, and variable nuclear-to-cytoplasmic ratios. Note the cell with few dustlike dark granules. (Aqueous-based Wright; ×500.)

having fewer granules compared with superficial areas composed of epithelioid cells. Special stains such as the Fontana stain may be used on cytology preparations to detect poorly visible melanin granules, especially useful for amelanotic melanomas. Prussian blue stain will help identify hemosiderin granules, which appear dark green and may resemble melanocytes. Additionally, the immunohistochemical stain S-100 may help distinguish amelanotic melanoma from plasmacytoma.

Cytologic differential diagnosis for benign melanoma: normal skin melanocytes, normal pigmented basal cells, melanophages, hemosiderin-laden macrophages.

Cytologic differential diagnosis for malignant melanoma: plasmacytoma, fibrosarcoma, undifferentiated sarcoma, other cutaneous spindle cell tumors.

Round or Discrete Cell

Canine Histiocytoma

This is a very common benign, rapidly growing tumor of mostly young dogs, composing about 12% to 14% of skin masses (Goldschmidt and Shofer, 1992; Yager and Wilcock, 1994). Its origin is the Langerhans cell of the epidermis. The tumor appears as a small solitary, well-circumscribed, dome-shaped, red ulcerated, hairless mass, the so-called button tumor (Goldschmidt and Beaver, 1981). It occurs commonly on the head, especially the ear pinnae, as well as on the hindlimbs, feet, and trunk. Histologically, a nonencapsulated dense dermal infiltrate of round cells is closely associated with hyperplastic epithelium (Fig. 3–44A). Mitotic figures are frequently found (Fig. 3–44B). Cytologically, cells have variably distinct cytoplasmic borders (Fig. 3–44C). Nuclei are round, oval, or indented with fine chromatin and indistinct nucleoli (Fig. 3–44D). Cells exhibit minimal anisocytosis and anisokaryosis. The cytoplasm is abundant and clear to lightly basophilic (Fig. 3–44E). A variable number of small well-differentiated lymphocytes, likely cytotoxic T-cells, are common in regressing lesions (Fig. 3–44F). Cytochemical staining and immunostaining of these tumor cells may be positive for histiocytic markers, including nonspecific esterases (Fig. 3–44G) and

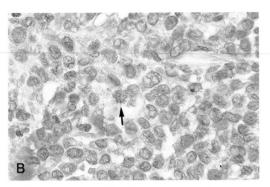

FIGURE 3–44.   B, Histiocytoma. Same case as in Figure 3–44A. Mitotic figures are frequently found among the pleomorphic histiocytic cells. One mitotic figure is shown in the center (*arrow*). (H & E; ×250.)

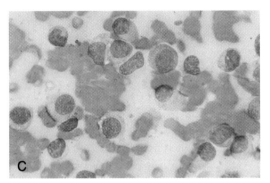

FIGURE 3–44.   C, Histiocytoma. Dorsum mass aspirate. Dog. Cells have variably distinct cytoplasmic borders. (Wright-Giemsa; ×250.)

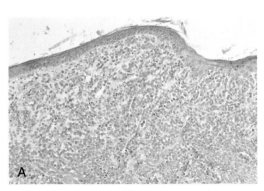

FIGURE 3–44.   A, Histiocytoma. Skin mass. Dog. The dermis contains a diffuse nodular and dense infiltrate of round cells that is closely associated with hyperplastic epithelium. (H & E; ×50.)

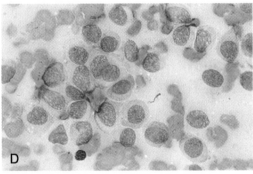

FIGURE 3–44.   D, Histiocytoma. Same case as in Figure 3–44C. Nuclei are round, oval, or indented with fine chromatin and indistinct nucleoli. Anisocytosis and anisokaryosis are mild. One small lymphocyte is present at the bottom, left of center. (Wright-Giemsa; ×250.)

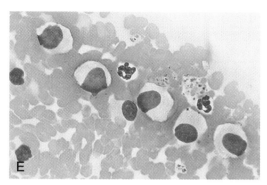

FIGURE 3–44. E, Histiocytoma. Lip mass aspirate. Dog. The cytoplasm is abundant and clear to lightly basophilic and cells appear discrete. (Wright-Giemsa; ×250.)

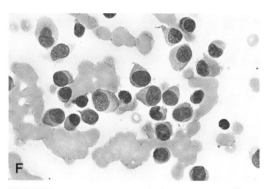

FIGURE 3–44. F, Histiocytoma. Elbow mass aspirate. Dog. Several lymphocytes are present, suggesting regression of the lesion. (Aqueous-based Wright; ×250.)

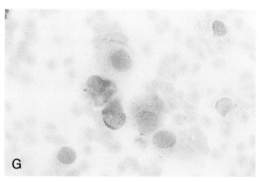

FIGURE 3–44. G, Histiocytoma. Same case as in Figure 3–44E. Red cytoplasmic staining indicates positive reaction to this histiocytic cytochemical marker. (Alpha naphthyl butyrate esterase; ×250.)

lysozyme (Moore, 1986). Treatment involves surgical excision if necessary. Prognosis is excellent to good as the tumor frequently regresses spontaneously within 3 months and recurrence is rare.

Cytologic differential diagnosis: lymphoma, plasmacytoma, benign cutaneous histiocytosis, systemic histiocytosis, nodular granulomatous dermatitis.

Mast Cell Tumor

This tumor in dogs accounts for about 10% of skin tumors, with higher prevalence in certain breeds such as the boxer, pug, and Boston terrier (Yager and Wilcock, 1994). Tumors in dogs are generally solitary, nonencapsulated, and highly infiltrative into dermis and subcutis (Fig. 3–45A–C). They may occasionally occur in puppies. Tumors are most common on the trunk and limbs in the dog. Cytologically, canine tumor cells vary in the degree of granularity and nuclear atypia. Canine mast cells having numerous distinct metachromatic stained granules with uniform small nuclei are considered grade I (well differentiated). Grade II (intermediate) mast cells have fewer

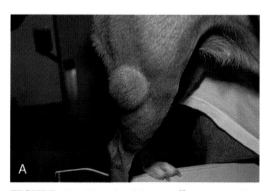

FIGURE 3–45. A, Mast cell tumor. Leg mass. Dog. Note the large raised haired nodule on the lateral stifle area that resembles grossly a lipoma. (Courtesy of Leslie Fox, Gainesville, FL.)

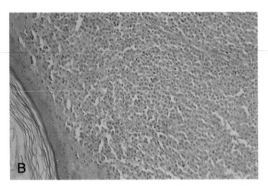

FIGURE 3–45. B, Mast cell tumor. Cat. Diffuse dense dermal infiltration of round cells. (H & E; ×50.)

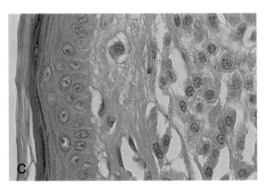

FIGURE 3–45. C, Mast cell tumor. Same case as in Figure 3–45B. Some granulation is present within the round cells. Nuclear size is uniform in this well-differentiated tumor. (H & E; ×250.)

associated with hemorrhage, vascular necrosis, edema, and collagenolysis (Fig. 3–45F). Treatment involves wide surgical excision, cryosurgery, radiotherapy, and chemotherapy. Prognosis for dogs varies with stage and histologic grade. Another prognostic tool involves the frequency of argyrophilic nucleolar organizer regions, which was shown to correlate well with the histologic grade of the tumor in dogs (Kravis et al., 1996). Grade III tumors have a high chance

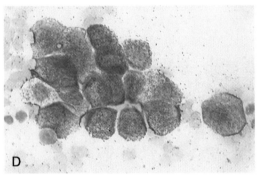

FIGURE 3–45. D, Mast cell tumor. Mammary area mass aspirate. Dog. Variable staining of granules and anisokaryosis suggest a moderately differentiated tumor. (Wright-Giemsa; ×250.)

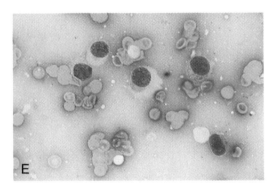

FIGURE 3–45. E, Mast cell tumor. Submandibular area mass imprint. Dog. Few scattered fine metachromatic granules are present in cells of this poorly differentiated tumor. Malignant nuclear changes include coarse chromatin, anisokaryosis, high and variable nuclear-to-cytoplasmic ratios, and prominent nucleoli. (Wright-Giemsa; ×250.)

granules and nuclei may vary in size and shape (Fig. 3–45D). Grade III (poorly differentiated) mast cells have few to no cytoplasmic granules and nuclei display marked atypia with mitotic figures (Fig. 3–45E). This involves anisokaryosis, coarse chromatin, and multiple and prominent nucleoli. Cytoplasmic borders in grade III mast cells are often indistinct. Giant binucleated cells are more commonly found in grade III forms. Eosinophils are more numerous in canine tumors than feline tumors. The background is usually filled with granules from ruptured cells. Degranulation may be of local recurrence and metastasis to lymph nodes. Less than 10% survive more than 1 year with grade III tumors (Yager and Wilcock, 1994). Those tumors occurring on the perineum, digits, or prepuce in dogs appear to be more aggressive (Moriello and Mason, 1995).

Mast cell tumors in cats represent the second most common skin tumor type, accounting for 12% to 20% of skin tumors (Goldschmidt and Shofer, 1992; Miller et

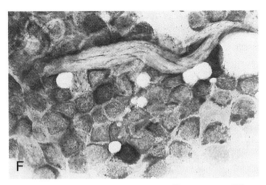

FIGURE 3–45. F, Mast cell tumor. Thoracic skin mass aspirate. Dog. This moderately differentiated tumor contains pale pink collagen strands as a result of collagenolysis. (Wright-Giemsa; ×250.)

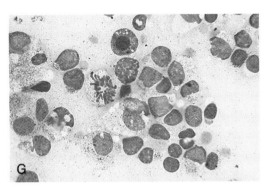

FIGURE 3–45. G, Mast cell tumor. Digit mass imprint. Cat. Note the granular background from released cytoplasmic granules. Cells are pleomorphic with a "histiocytic" appearance and contain a variable number of cytoplasmic granules. This 8-year-old cat had multiple digits on two feet affected by the same tumor. (Wright-Giemsa; ×250.)

al., 1991). These are usually solitary, well-circumscribed, dermal masses that occur on the head, neck, and limbs. Multiple masses are common in young Siamese cats (Wilcock et al., 1986). Small well-differentiated lymphocytes may be associated with the feline tumors. Tumor cells that resemble poorly granulated histiocytes are associated with the multiple form of mast cell tumor (Fig. 3–45G). For cats, the solitary form of the disease is generally considered benign with some exceptions of recurrence and invasion. Tumor histopathological grade involving nuclear pleomorphism, mitotic rate, and deep dermal invasion has no prognostic significance in cats with solitary mast cell tumors (Molander-McCrary et al., 1998). A significant number of young cats with multiple masses respond with spontaneous regression within months.

KEY POINT: Giemsa or toluidine blue staining should be used to reveal cytoplasmic granules in poorly differentiated forms. It should be noted that aqueous-based Wright stains, such as Diff-Quik®, often show a lack of granulation, especially in less differentiated forms of mast cell tumor. This is related to the water-soluble nature of the granule contents (Fig. 3–45H & I).

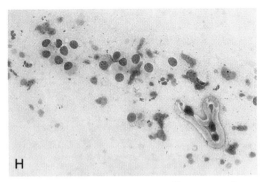

FIGURE 3–45. H, Mast cell tumor. Same case as in Figure 3–45D. Note the *Dirofilaria immitis* microfilaria in the lower right area among the poorly granulated mast cells. (Aqueous-based Wright; ×125.)

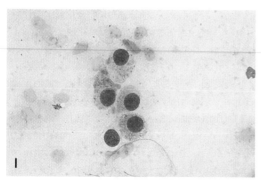

FIGURE 3–45. I, Mast cell tumor. Same case as in Figure 3–45D. Note the poorly granulated mast cells related to the use of a water-soluble stain. (Aqueous-based Wright; ×250.)

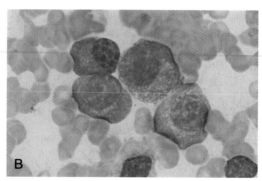

FIGURE 3–46. B, Plasmacytoma. Same case as in Figure 3–46A. Note the plasmacytoid appearance with eccentrically placed nuclei and variably coarse chromatin. This case had a monoclonal production of gamma globulins. (Wright-Giemsa; ×500.)

Cytologic differential diagnosis: **normal mast cells, chronic allergic dermatitis, lymphoma.**

Plasmacytoma

This tumor is present in about 2% of canine skin tumors and is rare in cats (Yager and Wilcock, 1994). They present as mostly solitary, well-circumscribed masses often on

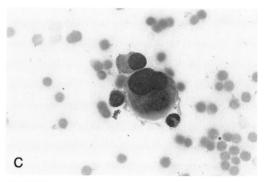

FIGURE 3–46. C, Plasmacytoma. Digit mass imprint. Dog. Multinucleated cells are often present, as shown in this case. (Wright-Giemsa; ×250.)

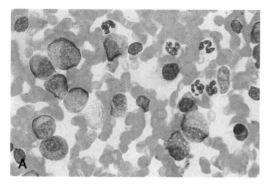

FIGURE 3–46. A, Plasmacytoma. Nasal planum mass aspirate. Cat. Cellular specimen with cells that have variable amounts of basophilic cytoplasm in which borders are discrete. (Wright-Giemsa; ×250.)

the digits, ears, and mouth. Cytologically, aspirates are moderately to markedly cellular. Individual cells have variable amounts of basophilic cytoplasm in which borders are discrete (Fig. 3–46A & B). Anisocytosis and anisokaryosis are prominent features. Nuclei are round to oval with fine to moderately coarse chromatin and indistinct nucleoli. The nuclei are often eccentrically placed and frequently binucleated. Multinucleated cells may be present (Fig. 3–46C &

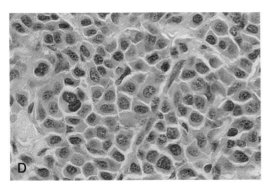

FIGURE 3–46. D, Plasmacytoma. Same case as in Figure 3–46C. There is dense dermal infiltration with pleomorphic round cells. Note the multinucleated cells in left center. (H & E; ×250.)

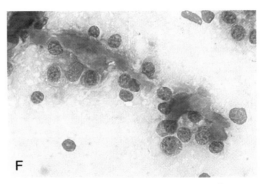

FIGURE 3–46. F, Plasmacytoma with amyloid. Same case as in Figure 3–46E. Note the abundant pink amorphous material associated with plasmacytoid cells. (Wright; ×250.) (Courtesy of Gail Walter et al., Michigan State University; presented at the 1992 ASVCP case review session.)

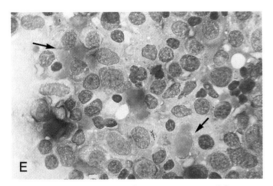

FIGURE 3–46. E, Plasmacytoma with amyloid. Hock mass imprint. Cat. The specimen is densely cellular with marked anisocytosis and anisokaryosis. Several cells have a plasmacytoid appearance while others appear histiocytic with abundant pale cytoplasm. Small amount of amyloid is present between cells (*arrows*). (Wright; ×250.) (Courtesy of Gail Walter et al., Michigan State University; presented at the 1992 ASVCP case review session.)

cases with a polymorphous-blastic type of morphology associated with recurrence and metastasis (Platz et al., 1999).

Cytologic differential diagnosis: **lymphoma, histiocytoma, amelanotic melanoma, neuroendocrine (Merkel cell) tumor.**

Epitheliotropic/Nonepitheliotropic Lymphoma

The disease may occur primarily in the skin or rarely as a manifestation of generalized lymphoma. It is more common in older dogs and cats. Prevalence of epitheliotropic lymphoma is 1% of skin tumors in dogs (Yager and Wilcock, 1994). Lesions are solitary to multiple in the form of nodules, plaques, ulcers, erythroderma, or exfoliative dermatitis in the form of excessive scaling (Fig. 3–47A & B). Pruritus may be common. Histologically, this group is divided into nonepitheliotropic and epitheliotropic types. B-lymphocytes are presumed involved in the infiltration of the dermis and subcutis with nonepitheliotropic lymphomas. Epitheliotropic lymphoma is characterized by

D). Amorphous eosinophilic material, representative of amyloid, is seen in less than 10% of plasmacytomas (Fig. 3–46E & F). Treatment involves wide surgical excision. Prognosis is generally good, but local recurrences may be common. One study found

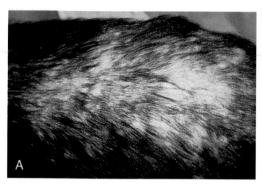

FIGURE 3–47.   A, Mycosis fungoides. Dog. Plaques and nodules are present over the back. (Courtesy of Janet Wojciechowski.)

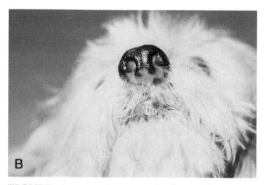

FIGURE 3–47.   B, Mycosis fungoides. Dog. Depigmentation and crusting are noted around the nose and mouth. (Courtesy of Janet Wojciechowski.)

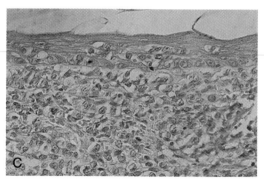

FIGURE 3–47.   C, Mycosis fungoides. Skin on chest. Dog. Neoplastic lymphocyte infiltrates involve the epidermis and dermis. Small focal collections of neoplastic cells, termed *Pautrier microabscesses,* are present within the epidermis. (H & E; ×125.)

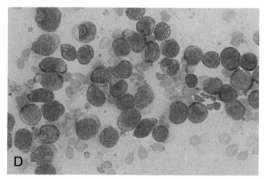

FIGURE 3–47.   D, Mycosis fungoides. Same case as in Figure 3–47C. Lymphocytes are variable, ranging in size from small to large, with round, indented, or convoluted nuclei. Cytoplasm is scant to moderate and lightly basophilic. (Wright-Giemsa; ×250.)

neoplastic lymphocyte infiltrates of the epidermis and adnexa (Fig. 3–47C). Sometimes focal collections of the neoplastic cells, termed *Pautrier microabscesses,* are formed within the epidermis. The cell of origin is usually a T-lymphocyte and this form of cutaneous T-cell lymphoma is sometimes termed *mycosis fungoides.* When these neoplastic T-lymphocytes are present in the epidermis and peripheral blood, it is then referred to as *Sézary syndrome* (Foster et al., 1997) based on a similar presentation in people. Cytologically, lymphocytes are variable ranging in size from small to large with round, indented, or convoluted nuclei (Fig. 3–47D & E). Nucleoli are usually indistinct but may be prominent. Cytoplasm is scant to moderate and lightly basophilic. Uniformity of the lymphoid population without significant inflammation or plasma cell infiltration is suggestive of cutaneous lymphoma. In general, treatment involving

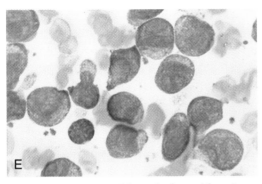

FIGURE 3–47. E, Mycosis fungoides. Same case as in Figure 3–47C. Nuclear folds are common. Nucleoli are usually indistinct but occasionally prominent. Note the small lymphocyte at bottom left for comparison of cell size. (Wright-Giemsa; ×500.)

chemotherapy, radiotherapy, and immunotherapy has been unsuccessful in achieving long-term remission. Surgical excision may be helpful for solitary lesions. Prognosis is poor as the disease rapidly progresses, necessitating euthanasia. Nodal involvement usually occurs late in both types, when present. Laboratory abnormalities such as monoclonal gammopathy, serum hyperviscosity, and hypercalcemia have been associated with cutaneous lymphoma.

Cytologic differential diagnosis: **chronic inflammatory dermatitis, histiocytoma.**

Canine Transmissible Venereal Tumor

This is a tumor of dogs, most often in free-roaming sexually active animals living in temperate climates, related to transplantation of intact cells. Immunocytochemistry supports a histiocytic origin (Mozos et al., 1996), although they appear not to be of canine origin, having an abnormal karyotype with 59 chromosomes compared with a normal karyotype of 78 in dogs. It appears on the skin of the external genitalia as well as the mucous membranes associated with sexual contact. Grossly, the tumor is pink to red, poorly circumscribed, multinodular, raised to pedunculated, soft, friable, ulcerated, and hemorrhagic, with frequent necrosis and superficial bacterial infection. The mass exfoliates easily by tissue impression, giving rise to a monomorphic population of large round cells with a round nucleus, coarse chromatin, and one to two prominent nucleoli (see Figs. 11–25 and 11–26). The cytoplasm is abundant and lightly basophilic, and frequently contains multiple punctate vacuoles. Mitotic figures may be seen. Associated with the tumor are small lymphoid cells and inflammatory cells, often with evidence of bacterial sepsis. Treatment involves chemotherapy, particularly with vincristine, radiotherapy, and surgical excision. Prognosis is good with chemotherapy. The tumors may regress on their own, presumably related to lymphocyte infiltration. Metastasis is rare, but recurrence is high with surgical intervention.

Cytologic differential diagnosis: **other round cell tumors, amelanotic melanoma.**

Naked Nuclei

Normal Thyroid

Subcutaneous masses located adjacent to the trachea may be confirmed as thyroid glands by fine-needle aspiration. Classically, they consist of small sheets of closely or loosely attached cells, some of which contain black granular intracytoplasmic material (Fig. 3–48). The cytoplasmic border may or may not be apparent with the appearance of floating nuclei. See Chapter 15 for further information.

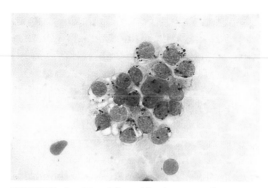

FIGURE 3–48. Thyroid tissue. Subcutaneous tissue aspirate. Dog. Subcutaneous masses located adjacent to the trachea may be confirmed as thyroid glands by fine-needle aspiration. Note the cohesive sheet of cells, many of which contain black granular intracytoplasmic material thought to be tyrosine.

RESPONSE TO TISSUE INJURY

Calcinosis Cutis and Calcinosis Circumscripta

Calcinosis cutis is an uncommon condition associated with glucocorticoid use or hyperadrenocorticism in dogs (Esplin and Carr, 1983). It involves dystrophic mineralization of collagen or elastin of the skin. Sites of predilection include the dorsal neck, inguinal area, and axillary region. Grossly, erythematous papules or firm gritty plaques develop and often ulcerate. Cytologically, dense granular material is present in the background and a mixed inflammatory response occurs, including macrophages, giant multinucleated cells, neutrophils, lymphocytes, and plasma cells. Prognosis is good as these benign lesions resolve untreated over several months.

A clinical subgroup of calcinosis cutis is calcinosis circumscripta, which is uncommon in dogs and rare in cats. This is a well-circumscribed solitary lesion within the deep dermis and subcutis formed by dystrophic mineralization, the etiology of which is unknown. It is mostly associated with young German shepherd dogs. The lesions often occur over joint areas or pres-

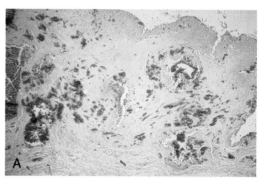

FIGURE 3–49. A, Calcinosis circumscripta. Skin mass. Dog. Multinodular dermal and subcutaneous mass is composed of central areas of mineralization, which stain intensely red. These areas are surrounded by macrophages, giant cells, dense fibrous connective tissue. (H & E; ×10.)

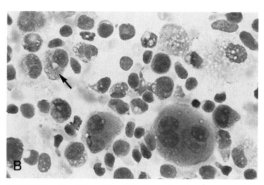

FIGURE 3–49. B, Calcinosis circumscripta. Tuber coxae mass aspirate. Dog. Same case as in Figure 3–49A. Fluid from elbows and hip areas contained similar fluid, which was aspirated, sedimented, and smeared onto a slide. Highly cellular sample contained macrophages, giant cells, and lymphocytes. Within the background and phagocytic cells (arrow) are numerous clear refractile structures consistent with calcium crystals. (Aqueous-based Wright; ×250.)

sure points, at sites of previous trauma, or under the tongue. Mass texture is firm and gritty. Histologically, the lesion is distinguished by large lakes of mineralized deposits surrounded by dense fibrous connective tissue and foreign body giant cells (Fig. 3–49A). Cytologically, it is similar to calcinosis cutis except fibroblasts may be more frequently observed. Mineral deposits often present as refractile yellow-green granules of irregular size and shape that are best observed with a lowered microscope condenser (Fig. 3–49B). Purple fine granular material present in the background likely represents necrotic tissue, which may be prominent. These are benign lesions that are treated by surgical excision (Bevier and Goldschmidt, 1981b).

Granulation Tissue

Firm subcutaneous swellings may arise from an exuberant fibroblastic response to tissue injury. Histologically, this mass is composed of horizontally arranged proliferating fibroblasts transected by vertically proliferating endothelium from small blood vessels (Fig.

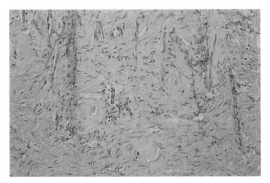

FIGURE 3–50. Granulation tissue. Dorsum mass. Dog. Dense fibrous connective tissue is layered horizontally with capillaries coursing through the tissue vertically. The reaction was secondary to noninfectious panniculitis. (H & E; ×50.)

3–50). Mitoses and macrophages are commonly found. The plump reactive fibroblasts seen on cytology have an ovoid vesicular nucleus and may resemble the fusiform cells seen in fibrosarcoma. Histopathology is recommended to distinguish the two conditions.

Hematoma

Grossly, these blood-filled masses can resemble neoplastic conditions such as hemangioma or hemangiosarcoma. Initially, when formed, the hematoma contains fluid identical in cell content to blood except that it lacks platelets (Hall and MacWilliams, 1988). Shortly afterward, macrophages engulfing erythrocytes (erythrophagocytosis) are common. Over time, the hemoglobin material breaks down, appearing as blue-green to black hemosiderin granules within the macrophage cytoplasm. On occasion, hematoidin crystals, which appear as rhomboid golden crystals, may form from iron-poor hemoglobin pigment. As the healing continues, plump fibroblasts may be seen which can mimic a neoplastic mesenchymal cell population.

Hygroma

This swelling within the subcutaneous tissues forms over bony prominences, commonly the elbow, of large-breed dogs secondary to repeated trauma or pressure. A cystlike structure forms from dense connective tissue that contains a serous to mucinous, clear, yellow or red fluid, depending on the degree of hemorrhage. Cytologically, the fluid appears clear to lightly basophilic and cells other than blood contamination include macrophages (Fig. 3–51) and reactive fibrocytes. Pathophysiology is similar to that seroma formation.

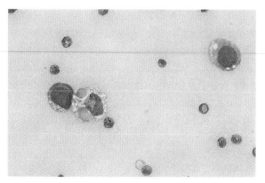

FIGURE 3–51. Hygroma. Aspirate of swelling over elbow. Dog. The fluid obtained was orange/hazy with WBC < 400/μl and protein 3.3 g/dl. The background is lightly granular related to increased protein content. Cells were mononuclear phagocytes and exhibited erythrophagia as shown. (Wright-Giemsa; ×250.)

Mucocele or Sialocele

Duct rupture related to trauma or infection leads to an accumulation of saliva within the subcutaneous tissues. The presence of a fluctuant mass containing clear to bloody fluid with stringlike features grossly suggests a salivary gland duct rupture. The cytologic specimen often stains uniformly purple from the high protein content. The background may contain scattered, pale basophilic, amorphous material, consistent with saliva. The fluid is often bloody with evidence of both acute and chronic hemor-

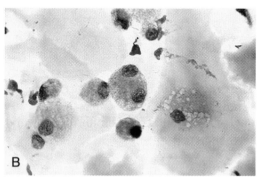

FIGURE 3–52. B, Sialocele. Cervical mass aspirate. Dog. The nucleated cells are predominately highly vacuolated mononuclear cells which are not easily identified as salivary gland epithelium or macrophages. Amorphous material in the background is consistent with mucus. (Aqueous-based Wright; ×250.)

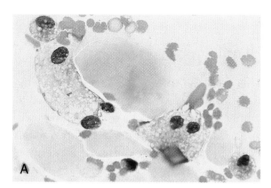

FIGURE 3–52. A, Sialocele. Cervical mass aspirate. Dog. Chronic hemorrhage is noted by the presence of a large yellow rhomboid crystal, termed *hematoidin*. The background contains pale-pink material and vacuolated mononuclear cells are abundant. (Wright; ×250.)

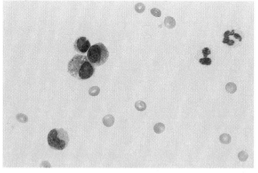

FIGURE 3–53. Seroma. Neck swelling aspirate. Dog. Fluid obtained was bloody with WBC 3,800/μl and protein 2.5 g/dl. Blood elements composed the majority of cell types found. Mononuclear phagocytes as shown accounted for 24% of the cell population. (Wright-Giemsa; ×250.)

rhage. Erythrophagocytosis is common and occasional yellow rhomboid crystals may be seen (Hall and MacWilliams, 1988). These are termed *hematoidin crystals* and are associated with chronic hemorrhage (Fig. 3–52A). The nucleated cells are predominately highly vacuolated macrophages that display active phagocytosis (Fig. 3–52B). Distinction between these cells and secretory glandular tissue may be difficult, especially when cells are individualized and nonphagocytic. Nondegenerate neutrophils are common, becoming degenerate when bacterial infection occurs.

Seroma

Injury may lead to a seroma, which is composed of clear to slightly blood-tinged fluid. The leaked plasma originates from immature capillaries created during granulation tissue formation. Cytologically, the fluid is poorly cellular and may require sedimentation prior to examination. Phagocytic macrophages will predominate among a mixture of inflammatory cells (Fig. 3–53).

References

Baker R, Lumsden JH: The skin. In Baker R, Lumsden JH (eds): *Color Atlas of Cytology of the Dog and Cat.* CV Mosby, St. Louis, 2000, pp. 39–70.

Barnes JC, Stanley O, Craig TM: Diffuse cutaneous leishmaniasis in a cat. J Am Vet Med Assoc 1993; 202:416–418.

Bevier DE, Goldschmidt MH: Skin tumors in the dog. Part I. Epithelial tumors and tumorlike lesions. Comp Cont Educ Pract Vet 1981a; 3: 389–400.

Bevier DE, Goldschmidt MH: Skin tumors in the dog. Part II. Tumors of the soft (mesenchymal) tissues. Comp Cont Educ Pract Vet 1981b; 3: 506–520.

Beyer TA, Pinckney RD, Cooley AC: Massive *Dracunculus insignis* infection in a dog. J Am Vet Med Assoc 1999; 214:366–368.

Carakostas MC, Miller RI, Woodward MG: Subcutaneous dermatophilosis in a cat. J Am Vet Med Assoc 1984; 185:675–676.

Day DG, Couto CG, Weisbrode SE, et al: Basal cell carcinoma in two cats. J Am Anim Hosp Assoc 1994; 30:265–269.

Desnoyers M, St-Germain L: What is your diagnosis? Vet Clin Pathol 1994; 23:89, 97.

Elliott GS, Whitney MS, Reed WM, et al: Antemortem diagnosis of paecilomycosis in a cat. J Am Vet Med Assoc 1984; 184:93–94.

Esplin DG, Carr SH: Skin tumors and other cutaneous masses. Mod Vet Pract 1983; 64:5–10.

Foil CS: Miscellaneous fungal infections. In Greene CE (ed): *Infectious Diseases of the Dog and Cat,* 2nd ed. WB Saunders, Philadelphia, 1998, pp. 420–430.

Foster AP, Evans E, Kerlin RL, et al: Cutaneous T-cell lymphoma with Sézary syndrome in a dog. Vet Clin Pathol 1997; 26:188–192.

Garma-Avina, A: The cytology of squamous cell carcinomas in domestic animals. J Vet Diagn Invest 1994; 6:238–246.

Gibson KL, Blass CE, Simpson M, et al: Malignant fibrous histiocytoma in a cat. J Am Vet Med Assoc 1989; 194:1443–1445.

Giovengo SL: Canine dracunculiasis. Comp Contin Educ Pract Vet 1993; 15: 726–729.

Goldschmidt M, Bevier DE: Skin tumors in the dog. Part III. Lymphohistiocytic and melanocytic tumors. Compend Contin Educ Pract Vet 1981; 3:588–597.

Goldschmidt MH, Shofer FS: *Skin Tumors of the Dog and Cat.* Pergamon Press, Oxford, UK, 1992, pp. 1–3, 50–65, 103–108, 271–283.

Greene CE, Gunn-Moore DA: Tuberculous mycobacterial infections. In Greene CE (ed): *Infectious Diseases of the Dog and Cat.* WB Saunders, Philadelphia, 1998, pp. 313–321.

Grieshaber TL, McKeever PJ, Conroy JD: Spontaneous cutaneous (eruptive) xanthomatosis in two cats. J Am Anim Hosp Assoc 1991; 27:509–512.

Grindem CB, Riley J, Sellon R, et al: Myxosarcoma in a dog. Vet Clin Pathol 1990; 19:119–121.

Gross TL, Ihrke PJ, Walder EJ: *Veterinary Dermatopathology. A Macroscopic and Microscopic Evalu-*

ation of Canine and Feline Skin Disease. CV Mosby, St. Louis, 1992, pp. 374–385.

Hall RL, MacWilliams PS: The cytologic examination of cutaneous and subcutaneous masses. Semin Vet Med Surg (Sm Anim) 1988; 94–108.

Hargis AM, Ihrke PJ, Spangler WL, et al: A retrospective clinicopathologic study of 212 dogs with cutaneous hemangiomas and hemangiosarcomas. Vet Pathol 1992; 29:316–328.

Hendrick MJ, Brooks JJ: Postvaccinal sarcomas in the cat: histology and immunohistochemistry. Vet Pathol 1994; 31:126–129.

Kravis LD, Vail DM, Kisseberth WC, et al: Frequency of argyrophilic nucleolar organizer regions in fine-needle aspirates and biopsy specimens from mast cell tumors in dogs. J Am Vet Med Assoc 1996; 209:1418–1420.

Lester SJ, Kenyon JE: Use of allopurinol to treat visceral leishmaniasis in a dog. J Am Vet Med Assoc 1996; 209:615–617.

McCarthy PE, Hedlund CS, Veazy RS, et al: Liposarcoma associated with a glass foreign body in a dog. J Am Vet Med Assoc 1996; 209:612–614.

Miller MA, Greene CE, Brix AE: Disseminated *Mycobacterium avium-intracellulare* complex infection in a miniature schnauzer. J Am Anim Hosp Assoc 1995; 31:213–216.

Miller MA, Nelson SL, Turk JR, et al: Cutaneous neoplasia in 340 cats. Vet Pathol 1991; 28:389–395.

Miller MA, Ramos JA, Kreeger JM: Cutaneous vascular neoplasia in 15 cats: clinical, morphologic, and immunohistochemical studies. Vet Pathol 1992; 29:329–336.

Moisan PG, Watson GL: Ceruminous gland tumors in dogs and cats: A review of 124 cases. J Am Anim Hosp Assoc 1996; 32:449–453.

Molander-McCrary H, Henry CJ, Potter K, et al: Cutaneous mast cell tumors in cats: 32 cases (1991–1994). J Am Anim Hosp Assoc 1998; 34: 281–284.

Moore PF: Utilization of cytoplasmic lysozyme immunoreactivity as a histiocytic marker in canine histiocytic disorders. Vet Pathol 1986; 23:757–762.

Moriello KA, Mason IS: *Handbook of Small Animal Dermatology.* Elsevier Science, Oxford, UK, 1995, p 315.

Mozos E, Mendez A, Gomez-Villamandos, et al: Immunohistochemical characterization of canine transmissible venereal tumor. Vet Pathol 1996; 33:257–263.

Pace LW, Kreeger JM, Miller MA, et al: Immunohistochemical staining of feline malignant fibrous histiocytomas. Vet Pathol 1994; 31:168–172.

Panciera DL, Stockham SL: *Dracunculosis insignis* infection in a dog. J Am Vet Med Assoc 1988; 192:76–78.

Peaston A: Clinical vignette: sporotrichosis. J Vet Intern Med 1993; 7:44–45.

Platz SJ, Breuer W, Pfleghaar S, et al: Prognostic value of histopathological grading in canine extramedullary plasmacytomas. Vet Pathol 1999; 36:23–27.

Rakich PM, Latimer KS, Mispagel ME, et al: Clinical and histologic characterization of cutaneous reactions to stings of the imported fire ant (*Solenopsis invicta*) in dogs. Vet Pathol 1993; 30: 555–559.

Roccabianca P, Caniatti M, Scanziani E, et al: Feline leprosy: Spontaneous remission in a cat. J Am Anim Hosp Assoc 1996; 32:189–193.

Ross JT, Scavelli TD, Matthiesen DT, et al: Adenocarcinoma of the apocrine glands of the anal sac in dogs: A review of 32 cases. J Am Anim Hosp Asset 1991; 27:349–355.

Tyler RD, Cowell, Meinkoth JH: Cutaneous and subcutaneous lesions: masses, cysts, ulcers, and fistulous tracts. In Cowell RL, Tyler RD, Meinkoth JH (eds): *Diagnostic Cytology and Hematology of the Dog and Cat.* 2nd ed. CV Mosby, St. Louis, 1999, pp. 20–51.

Waters CB, Morrison WB, DeNicola DB, et al: Giant cell variant of malignant fibrous histiocytoma in dogs: 10 cases (1986–1993). J Am Vet Med Assoc 1994; 205:1420–1424.

Werner AH, Werner BE: Feline sporotrichosis. Compend Contin Educ Pract Vet 1993; 15: 1189–1197.

Wilcock BP, Yager JA, Zink MC: The morphology and behavior of feline cutaneous mastocytomas. Vet Pathol 1986; 23:320–324.

Yager JA, Wilcock BP: *Color Atlas and Text of Surgical Pathology of the Dog and Cat. Dermatopathology and Skin Tumors.* CV Mosby, London, 1994, pp. 243–244, 245–248, 257–271, 273–286.

CHAPTER 4

Lymphoid System

Rose E. Raskin

The lymphoid organs commonly examined by cytology include the peripheral and internal lymph nodes, spleen, and occasionally the thymus. As a result of their similar cell populations, the following cytodiagnostic categories are used. It should be noted that more than one presentation might occur in a specimen at a time.

GENERAL CYTODIAGNOSTIC GROUPS FOR LYMPHOID ORGAN CYTOLOGY

- Normal tissue
- Reactive or hyperplastic tissue
- Inflammation
- Metastatic disease
- Primary neoplasia
- Extramedullary hematopoiesis

LYMPH NODES

Indications for Lymph Node Biopsy

- *Lymphadenomegaly,* or enlargement of one or multiple lymph nodes, may be detected by palpation or by radiography and ultrasonography.

- *Evaluation of metastatic disease* involves evaluation of the lymph node(s) draining the primary lesion (Table 4–1).

- *Classification of lymphoma* may be enhanced by the cytologic features stained with Romanowsky stains, or by cytochemical and immunocytochemical stains to distinguish B- and T-cell subtypes; the latter stains may be performed at specialized laboratories.

TABLE 4–1	Selected Peripheral Lymph Nodes in the Dog	
Lymph Node	**Location**	**Drainage Features**
Submandibular	Group of two to four nodes located ventral to the angle of the jaw	Includes most of the head, including the rostral oral cavity
Prescapular	Group of two or three nodes located in front of the supraspinatus muscle	Includes the caudal part of the head (pharynx, pinna), most of the thoracic limb, and part of the thoracic wall
Axillary	One or two nodes located caudal and medial to the shoulder joint	Includes most of the thoracic wall, deep structures of the thoracic limb and neck, and the thoracic and cranial abdominal mammary glands
Superficial inguinal	Two nodes located in the furrow between the abdominal wall and the medial thigh	Includes the caudal abdominal and inguinal mammary glands, ventral half of the abdominal wall, penis, prepuce, scrotal skin, tail, ventral pelvis, and medial part of the thigh and stifle
Popliteal	One node located behind the stifle	Includes areas distal to the stifle

Aspirate and Impression Biopsy Considerations

Submandibular lymph nodes are frequently enlarged and reactive because of their constant exposure to antigens, making them a poor choice for biopsy in generalized lymphadenopathy.

KEY POINT: Popliteal and prescapular lymph nodes are the preferred biopsy sites for generalized lymphadenopathy.

The size of the lymph node should also be considered. Very large nodes may yield misleading information as they frequently contain necrotic or hemorrhagic tissue. A slightly enlarged lymph node is preferred and a sample from more than one location is desirable. If a large lymph node must be aspirated, the needle should be aimed tangentially to avoid the direct center.

KEY POINT: The center of a very large lymph node should be avoided during aspiration.

In performing aspirate smears, a 22-gauge needle is used alone or together with a 6- or 12-ml syringe. The needle is inserted into the node in several directions. With the syringe attached to the needle or butterfly catheter, quick and multiple withdrawal motions of the plunger are made to create negative pressure. The pressure on the plunger is released *before* removing the needle to avoid splattering the material within the syringe. An air-filled syringe is reattached and the needle contents expelled onto the approximate center of a glass slide. The aspirate appears creamy white, watery to viscous, indicating many leukocytes are present. The material is *gently* squashed with a second slide, sliding them apart horizontally. Smears are dried rapidly with a hair dryer to avoid crenation effects.

KEY POINT: Aspirates smears must be spread gently since immature lymphoid cells are often quite fragile.

When preparing impression smears from an excisional biopsy, it is important to blot excessive tissue fluids before touch preparations are made to increase the cellular yield. The cut surface of the excised lymph node is blotted on a paper towel, and then touched gently to a glass slide. Cytologic and histopathologic samples must be mailed separately when submitted to a referral laboratory to avoid the formalin artifact.

KEY POINT: Keep cytologic preparations away from formalin fumes to avoid premature fixation resulting in poor staining and cytologic detail.

Normal Histology and Cytology

The canine or feline lymph node consists of a thin connective tissue capsule that surrounds cortical and medullary lymphoid tissue and extends inward as trabeculae. The outer cortex contains variably sized lymphatic nodules (Fig. 4–1A) composed primarily of B-lymphocytes surrounded by a thin rim of small T-lymphocytes. The diffuse lymphoid tissue between the nodules composed primarily of T-lymphocytes extends deep into the paracortex where macrophages and dendritic reticular cells act as antigen-presenting cells. The diffuse lymphoid tissue extends inward to form medullary cords (Fig. 4–1B), which contain B-lymphocytes, plasma cells, macrophages, and other leukocytes. Between the cords are endothelial-lined sinuses in contact with dendritic reticular cells and reticular fibers. Lymph enters the afferent vessels that penetrate the capsule, through the subcapsular and cortical sinuses of the cortex, into the medullary sinuses and exits through efferent vessels at the hilus. Blood flow enters the

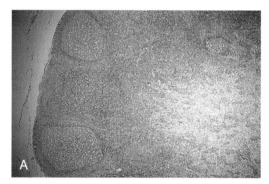

FIGURE 4–1.   A, Lymph node. Dog. Cortex contains variably sized lymphoid nodules and the medullary area contains cords of cells along endothelial-lined sinuses. (H & E; ×10.)

FIGURE 4–1.   B, Lymph node. Same case as in Figure 4–1A. Medullary cords appearing as dark bands are composed of lymphocytes, plasma cells, and macrophages and lie adjacent to pale-stained sinus spaces. (H & E; ×25.)

hilus through arterioles that branch into the cortex to perfuse the lymphatic nodules. In this region, vessels enlarge to form postcapillary or high endothelial venules of the paracortex (Fig. 4–1C). These venules are important sites for the travel of lymphocytes from blood into the lymph node parenchyma related to the selective binding of the lymphocyte with receptors on the endothelial cells. The venules drain into larger veins that exit via the hilus region.

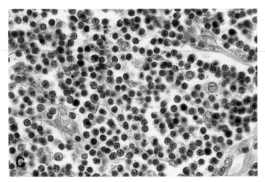

FIGURE 4–1. C, Lymph node. Same case as in Figure 4–1A. The deep cortex contains high endothelial venules shown in cross section (lower left) and longitudinal section (upper right). Lymphocytes selectively adhere to receptors on endothelium to leave the circulation and enter the lymph node. (H & E; ×250.)

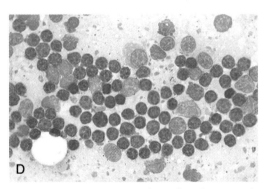

FIGURE 4–1. D, Lymph node. Tissue aspirate. Dog. This prescapular lymph node contains a majority of small lymphocytes. Low numbers of medium-sized lymphocytes are present as well as several lyzed cells that appear light-pink and lack cytoplasmic borders. (Wright-Giemsa; ×250.)

Cytologically, small, well-differentiated lymphocytes that measure 1 to 1.5 times the diameter of an erythrocyte in the dog and cat compose approximately 90% of the population (Fig. 4–1D). The chromatin of these cells is densely clumped with no visible nucleoli. Cytoplasm is scant. These cells

are the darkest staining of all the lymphocytes. Medium and large lymphocytes that measure two to three times erythrocyte diameter may be present in low numbers (<5% to 10%) (Fig. 4–1E & F). Their nuclei have a fine, diffuse and light chromatin pattern. Nucleoli may be prominent. The cytoplasm is more abundant and often basophilic. Mature plasma cells represent a small portion of the cells found. Their chromatin is densely clumped and often the

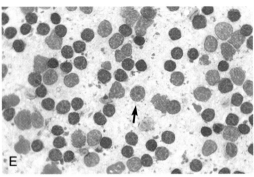

FIGURE 4–1. E, Normal lymph node. Tissue aspirate. Dog. This popliteal lymph node contains a majority of small lymphocytes. Note the medium-sized lymphocyte (*arrow*). (Wright-Giemsa; ×250.)

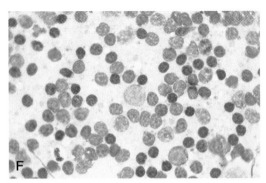

FIGURE 4–1. F, Normal lymph node. Tissue aspirate. Dog. Mixed cell population. Note the large lymphocyte in the center and occasional granulocytes. (Wright-Giemsa; ×250.)

nucleus is eccentrically placed within the abundant deeply basophilic cytoplasm. A pale area or halo is seen adjacent to the nucleus, which indicates the Golgi zone. Occasional macrophages (histiocytes) appear as large mononuclear cells with abundant light cytoplasm, often containing cellular debris. Nuclear chromatin is finely stippled and nucleoli may be found in activated macrophages. Mast cells and neutrophils also may be present in low numbers (Book-binder et al., 1992).

Reactive or Hyperplastic Lymph Node

Enlargement of a lymph node under this condition is due to any local or generalized antigenic response, which may include infection, inflammation, immune-mediated disease, or neoplasia from an area that drains into the lymph node. Histologically, lymphoid nodules form prominent germinal centers that develop following antigen stimulation (Fig. 4–2A). In addition to small lymphocytes, these centers contain dendritic reticular cells, macrophages, and larger lymphoid cells. In benign hyperplasia, a rim of small lymphocytes surrounds the germinal centers but with follicular or nodular lymphomas, only neoplastic cells are present within the nodule. The expanded follicles may press against the capsule but there is no destruction of the subcapsular sinus as occurs with lymphoma. Specialized paracortical blood vessels termed *high endothelial venules* in view of their cuboidal or columnar appearance increase in prominence and number (Valli and Parry, 1993). Plasma cells accumulate within follicles and infiltrate in large numbers into the medullary cords (Fig. 4–2B) and sinuses from which they are released into lymphatics.

Cytologically, small lymphocytes predominate, but there is an increase in medium and/or large cell types, to as much as 15% of the total cell population (Fig. 4–2C).

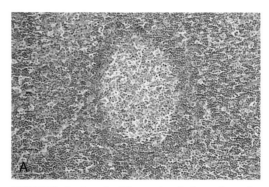

FIGURE 4–2. A, Hyperplastic lymph node. Dog. Prominent germinal center surrounded by a thin rim of small T-lymphocytes. (H & E; ×50.)

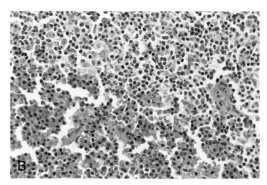

FIGURE 4–2. B, Reactive lymph node. Dog. Dense area at the bottom is composed of plasma cells within the medullary region that migrate from the follicles at top of picture. (H & E; ×125.)

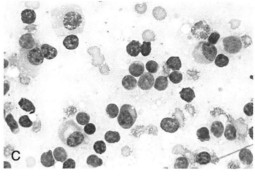

FIGURE 4–2. C, Reactive lymph node. Dog. Many small lymphocytes are present along with several well-differentiated plasma cells. Increased medium-sized lymphocytes are noted in the center. (Wright; ×250.)

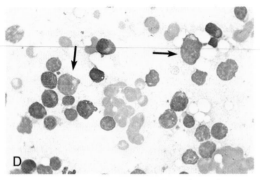

FIGURE 4–2. D, Reactive lymph node. Tissue aspirate. Dog. Plasma cells are moderately increased in number and two appear shifted toward immaturity (*arrows*). (Wright-Giemsa; ×250.)

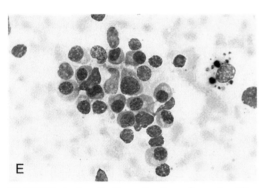

FIGURE 4–2. E, Reactive lymph node. Tissue imprint. Same case as in Figure 4–2B. Note the marked increased in plasma cell numbers composed of various degrees of differentiation. A hemosiderin-laden macrophage is present to the right of the field. (Aqueous-based Wright; ×250.)

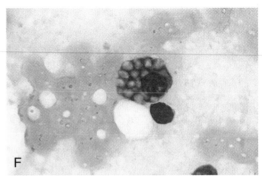

FIGURE 4–2. F, Mott cell. Same case as in Figure 4–2E. This plasma cell from a reactive lymph node is highly activated with an abundant basophilic cytoplasm that contains multiple large pale vacuoles. The vacuoles known as Russell bodies represent packets of immunoglobulin secretions. (Aqueous-based Wright; ×500.)

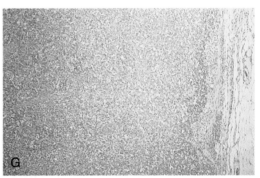

FIGURE 4–2. G, Hyperplastic lymph node. Cat. Peripheral node lymphadenopathy in this case is characterized by a paracortical expansion displacing normal lymphoid nodules and creating a homogenous appearance resembling lymphoma. At the right, a thin band of small dark lymphocytes from the nodule remains. (H & E; ×25.)

Plasma cells are mildly to markedly increased in number and may be shifted toward immaturity (Fig. 4–2D & E). Some highly activated plasma cells, termed *Mott cells,* are characterized by abundant cytoplasm filled with multiple large spherical pale vacuoles that represent immunoglobulin secretions known as *Russell bodies* (Fig. 4–2F). Macrophages, neutrophils, eosinophils, and mast cells also may mildly increase in response to antigen stimulation;

however, these cells occur in lower numbers than expected for lymphadenitis.

An idiopathic lymphadenopathy in young cats has been reported (Moore et al., 1986; Mooney et al., 1987). In this condition, peripheral lymph nodes show marked enlarge-

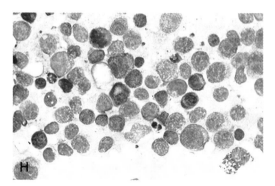

FIGURE 4–2. H, Reactive lymph node. Tissue imprint. Same case as in Figure 4–2G. This sample of prescapular lymph node contains a mixed population of small, medium, and large lymphocytes, plasma cells, and a mast cell (lower right). The majority of the lymphocytes are medium sized with moderately coarse chromatin and indistinct nucleoli. (Aqueous-based Wright; ×250.)

ment that histologically resembles lymphoma (Fig. 4–2G). Cells may be primarily medium and large lymphocytes with low numbers of small lymphocytes and plasma cells (Fig. 4–2H). High endothelial venules are prominent in the paracortex in this condition (Valli and Parry, 1993). These cases generally regress spontaneously in 1 to 17 weeks (Mooney et al., 1987). In one study, the majority of cats were feline leukemia virus (FeLV) positive and 1 of 14 cats progressed to lymphoma (Moore et al., 1986). Generalized lymphodenopathy is known to occur in cats infected with feline immunodeficiency virus (FIV), *Bartonella* sp. (Kordick et al., 1999) and with unidentified argyrophilic bacteria (Kirkpatrick et al., 1989) that morphologically resemble the organism causing bartonellosis (Valli and Parry, 1993).

Lymphadenitis

The predominant inflammatory cell population categorizes the type of inflammation in a lymph node.

Neutrophilic Lymphadenitis

Purulent or suppurative (Fig. 4–3A) lymphadenitis involves greater than 5% neutrophils and may be associated with bacterial (Fig. 4–3B & C), neoplastic, or immune-mediated conditions.

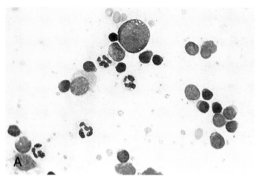

FIGURE 4–3. A, Neutrophilic lymphadenitis. Tissue aspirate. Cat. Four nondegenerate neutrophils are present along with small and medium lymphocytes. One large lymphocyte is also noted. (Wright; ×250.)

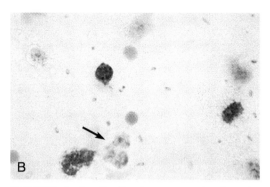

FIGURE 4–3. B, Septic suppurative lymphadenitis. Tissue aspirate. Cat. Bipolar coccobacillus bacteria confirmed as *Yersinia pestis* are present extracellularly adjacent to a degenerate neutrophil (*arrow*). (Wright-Giemsa.) (Photo courtesy of Kyra Royals et al., Colorado State University; presented at the 1996 ASVCP case review session.)

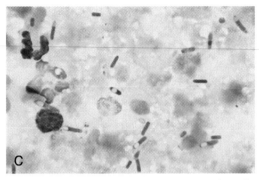

FIGURE 4–3.   C, Septic suppurative lymphadenitis. Tissue imprint. Dog. The history included a dog fight 2 months prior to the present lymphadenomegaly. Most of the lymphoid cells are necrotic and appear as amorphous basophilic material. Note two intact degenerate neutrophils and one small lymphocyte. Large bacilli with subterminal and terminal swellings are numerous in the background, which culture confirmed as *Clostridium* sp. (Wright-Giemsa; ×500.)

drome, and paraneoplastic syndrome for mast cell tumor (Fig. 4–4B) as well as certain lymphomas (Thorn and Aubert, 1999) and carcinomas (Fig. 4–4C).

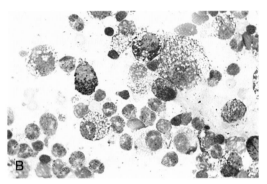

FIGURE 4–4.   B, Eosinophilic lymphadenitis. Tissue aspirate. Dog. Numerous eosinophils are present along with several mast cells displaying variable degrees of degranulation and pleomorphism in an animal with a mast cell tumor. (Aqueous-based Wright; ×250.)

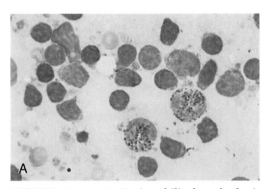

FIGURE 4–4.   A, Eosinophilic lymphadenitis. Tissue aspirate. Cat. Two eosinophils are shown within a population of small lymphocytes from an animal with a rodent ulcer of the mouth. (Wright-Giemsa; ×500.)

Eosinophilic Lymphadenitis

Greater than 3% eosinophils of the nucleated cell population are often related to flea bite hypersensitivity, feline eosinophilic skin disease (Fig. 4–4A), hypereosinophilic syn-

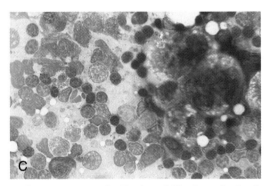

FIGURE 4–4.   C, Eosinophilic lymphadenitis. Tissue imprint. Dog. Small lymphocytes predominate along with increased numbers of medium lymphocytes and eosinophils. On the right is a cluster of pleomorphic epithelium from an animal with metastatic transitional cell carcinoma found within the sublumbar lymph node. (Wright-Giemsa; ×250.)

Histiocytic or Pyogranulomatous Lymphadenitis

Inflammation of the lymph nodes may involve increased numbers of macrophages, which is termed *histiocytic lymphadenitis* (Fig. 4–5A), or involve a mixture of neutrophils and macrophages, referred to *pyogranulomatous* lymphadenitis (Fig. 4–5B), even though a granuloma is best appreciated on histologic sections. Conditions associated with these inflammatory responses include systemic fungal infections, other fungal infections (Walton et al., 1994) (Fig.

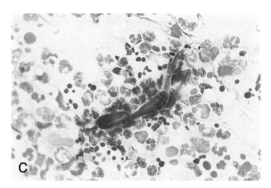

FIGURE 4–5. C, Pyogranulomatous lymphadenitis. Tissue aspirate. Dog. A mixed inflammatory cell infiltrate of degenerate neutrophils and macrophages is shown from an inguinal lymph node draining a mass on the digit. Note the septate fungal hyphae with bulbous appearance that was confirmed by culture as *Fusarium* sp. (Wright-Giemsa; ×250.)

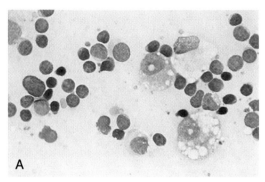

FIGURE 4–5. A, Histiocytic lymphadenitis. Cat. Several macrophages are present along with small and medium-sized lymphocytes. (Wright; ×250.)

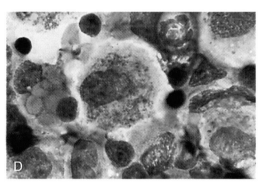

FIGURE 4–5. D, Salmon fluke poisoning disease. Peripheral lymph node aspirate. Dog. Numerous small basophilic granules are shown within a macrophage infected with *Neorickettsia helminthoeca.* (Romanowsky; ×500.) (Case material courtesy of Jocelyn Johnsrude.)

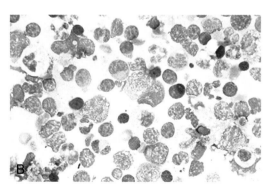

FIGURE 4–5. B, Pyogranulomatous lymphadenitis. Dog. Numerous macrophages and neutrophils appear among a mixed population of lymphocytes. (Wright-Giemsa; ×250.)

4–5C), mycobacteriosis (Grooters et al., 1995), leishmaniasis, salmon fluke poisoning disease (Fig. 4–5D & E), prototothecosis (Fig. 4–5F & G), pythiosis, vasculitis (Fig. 4–5H–J), and hemosiderosis (Fig. 4–5K & L). The systemic fungal diseases include blastomycosis (Fig. 4–5M), cryptococcosis (Lichtensteiger and Hilf, 1994) (Fig. 4–5N), histoplasmosis (Fig. 4–5O), and coccidioidomycosis.

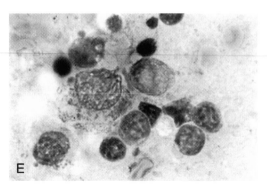

FIGURE 4–5. E, Salmon fluke poisoning disease. Same case as in Figure 4–5D. Lymph nodes display increased numbers of medium lymphocytes and plasma cell in addition to the inflammatory response. Note the rickettsial organism within the macrophage. (Romanowsky; ×500.) (Case material courtesy of Jocelyn Johnsrude.)

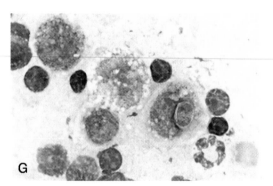

FIGURE 4–5. G, Protothecosis. Lymph node imprint. Dog. Note the single endospore engulfed by a macrophage. (Aqueous-based Wright; ×500.) (Photo courtesy of Peter Fernandes.)

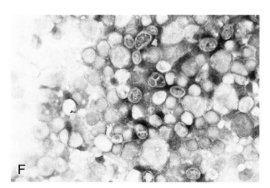

FIGURE 4–5. F, Protothecosis. Colonic lymph node imprint. Dog. Several round to oval structures are present that measure approximately 6 to 10 μm in length. These endospores have a basophilic granular cytoplasm and thin clear cell wall. Note the sporulated forms with multiple endospores. (Aqueous-based Wright; ×250.) (Case material courtesy of Karyn Bird et al., Texas A&M University; presented at the 1988 ASVCP case review session.)

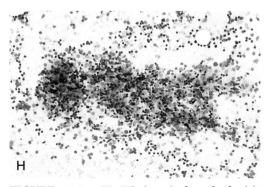

FIGURE 4–5. H, Histiocytic lymphadenitis with reticuloendothelial hyperplasia. Submandibular lymph node aspirate. Dog. Several aggregates of fibrohistiocytic elements are noted in this lymph node draining an inflamed skin mass. Histopathology supported the clinical diagnosis of an immune-mediated disease by finding lymphoplasmacytic and suppurative vasculitis in several subcutaneous tissues. (Wright-Giemsa; ×50.)

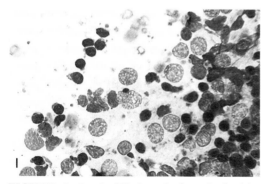

FIGURE 4–5. I, Histiocytic lymphadenitis. Same case as in Figure 4–5H. Higher magnification displays a cohesive mass of large mononuclear cells having abundant clear cytoplasm. Small lymphocytes are present in the background. (Wright-Giemsa; ×250.)

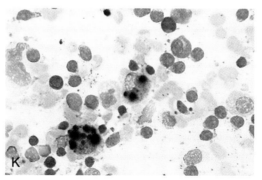

FIGURE 4–5. K, Histiocytic lymphadenitis with hemosiderosis. Lymph node aspirate. Dog. Numerous hemosiderin-laden macrophages are shown, characterized by large coarse black granules. The lymphoid cell population is mixed which is consistent with immune-stimulation. A malignant neoplasm was previously diagnosed in this area drained by this submandibular lymph node. (Aqueous-based Wright; ×250.)

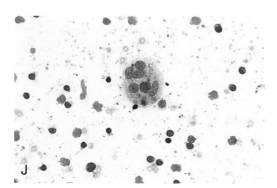

FIGURE 4–5. J, Histiocytic lymphadenitis. Same case as in Figure 4–5H. Multinucleated giant cells were present in low numbers in this generalized histiocytic proliferation within the lymph node. Mixed lymphoid cell population is noted in the background. (Wright-Giemsa; ×125.)

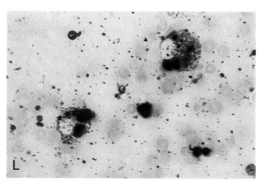

FIGURE 4–5. L, Hemosiderosis. Same case as in Figure 4–5K. Iron stain demonstrates a large amount of coarse blue-black granular material both intra- and extracellularly. (Prussian blue; ×250.)

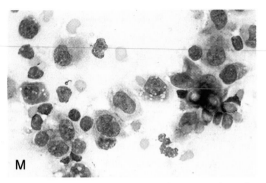

FIGURE 4–5. M, Pyogranulomatous lymphadenitis in blastomycosis. Tissue aspirate. Dog. Two round basophilic yeast structures are surrounded by a mixed inflammatory response, including macrophages, degenerate neutrophils, small and medium lymphocytes, and plasma cells. (Wright; ×250.)

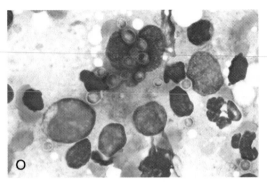

FIGURE 4–5. O, Pyogranulomatous lymphadenitis in histoplasmosis. Lymph node aspirate. Cat. Several intracellular small oval yeast forms are present within a macrophage. Extracellular yeast are also found, including a mixed population of lymphoid cells and degenerate neutrophils. (Aqueous-based Wright; ×500.)

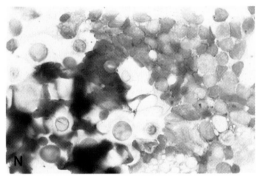

FIGURE 4–5. N, Histiocytic lymphadenitis in cryptococcosis. Lymph node aspirate. Cat. A subcutaneous mass behind the ear is present in this animal. A periauricular lymph node demonstrates numerous encapsulated yeast forms, consistent with *Cryptococcus* sp. Note the lymphocytes in the background with few inflammatory cells present. (Wright-Giemsa; ×250.)

Metastasis to the Lymph Node

Metastasis is suggested by the presence of a cell population not normally expected in a lymph node, which for epithelial cells is relatively easier to detect because of their large cell size and clustered appearance (Fig. 4–6A & B). These foreign cells often appear larger than surrounding lymphocytes and abnormal, displaying several cytologic features of malignancy (Fig. 4–6C). Histologically, metastasis to the lymph node may occur at the peripheral sinus or medullary sinuses related to lymphatic spread (Fig. 4–6D).

Mesenchymal-appearing neoplasms are most difficult to recognize because of their individualized cell presentation. The presence of anaplastic round to spindle-shaped cells in a lymph node aspirate can support a diagnosis of malignancy (Desnoyers and St-Germain, 1994). Tumors such as melanoma may be easily confused with hemosiderin-laden macrophages (Grindem, 1994) (Fig. 4–5K) related to the dark blue-black granules. Hemosiderin granules tend to be variable in size, large and coarse compared with melanin granules that are small and finely granular (Fig. 4–6E). Cytochemical staining may be necessary to distinguish the two, such as Fontana stain for melanin and Prussian blue for iron (Fig. 4–6F).

Metastatic hematopoietic neoplasms such as granulocytic leukemia cause mild to moderate lymphadenomegaly. The cell population appears mixed (Fig. 4–6G) and dysplastic cells or granulated precursors may be present (Fig. 4–6H). In some cases myeloblasts may be indistinguishable from lymphoid precursors (Fig. 4–6I) and cytochemical staining for granulocytic origin may be indicated (Fig. 4–6J). Well-granulated mast cells may appear in low numbers, up to 6

per slide in clinically healthy dogs (Bookbinder et al., 1992) but increased cell numbers and the appearance of poorly granulated mast cells suggest metastasis (Fig. 4–6K). Lymphoid malignancies originating from the bone marrow or solid tissue sites such as the spleen or gastrointestinal tract (Fig. 4–6L) may be easily recognized in lymph nodes when cells are granulated (Goldman and Grindem, 1997).

Inflammation may accompany metastasis

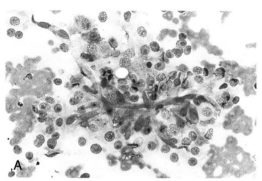

FIGURE 4–6. A, Metastatic renal carcinoma. Lymph node aspirate. Dog. An aggregate of capillaries are entwined around the malignant epithelial population. (Wright-Giemsa; ×125.)

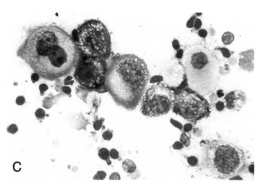

FIGURE 4–6. C, Metastatic squamous cell carcinoma. Same case as in Figure 4–6B. Higher magnification demonstrates the marked pleomorphism of the nuclei, coarse chromatin staining, and multiple, prominent, variably sized nucleoli. (Wright-Giemsa; ×250.)

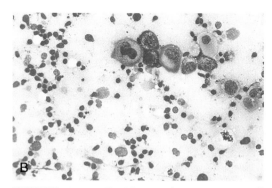

FIGURE 4–6. B, Metastatic squamous cell carcinoma. Lymph node aspirate. Dog. A sheet of neoplastic squamous epithelium is surrounded by numerous small lymphocytes. (Wright-Giemsa; ×125.)

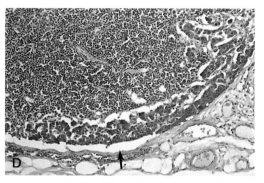

FIGURE 4–6. D, Metastatic carcinoma. Lymph node. Dog. Neoplastic population has infiltrated the cortex beginning at the subcapsular sinus region (arrow). (H & E; ×50.)

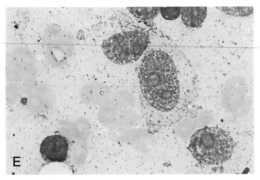

FIGURE 4–6. E, Metastatic melanoma. Lymph node aspirate. Dog. Fine black granules define the cell of origin. Prominent multiple nucleoli are also noted. Small lymphocytes are present in the background. (Aqueous-based Wright; ×500.)

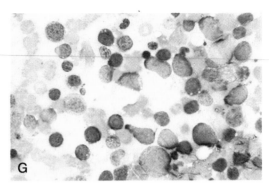

FIGURE 4–6. G, Granulocytic leukemia. Lymph node aspirate. Dog. A mixed cell population is present, with many large irregularly shaped cells. (Wright-Giemsa; ×250.)

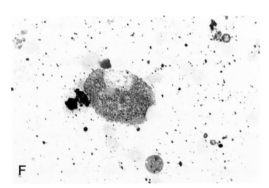

FIGURE 4–6. F, Metastastic melanoma. Lymph node aspirate. Dog. An iron stain helps to distinguish positive-staining background hemosiderin from a nonstaining cell containing melanin granules. Hemorrhage is often present in metastatic lesions. (Prussian blue; ×250.)

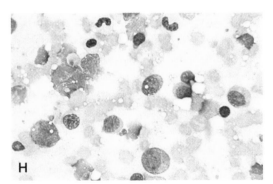

FIGURE 4–6. H, Granulocytic leukemia. Same case as in Figure 4–6G. Small granules are present in the granulocytic precursor in the cell at bottom of the field. Note the hyposegmented Pelger–Huet-type neutrophils at the top, indicating morphologic abnormalities in that cell line. (Wright-Giemsa; ×250.)

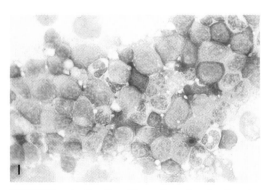

FIGURE 4–6. I, Granulocytic leukemia. Prescapular lymph node aspirate. Dog. Numerous large granulocytic precursors are present with irregularly shaped nuclei. (Wright-Giemsa; ×250.)

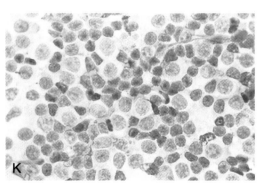

FIGURE 4–6. K, Metastatic mast cell tumor. Lymph node aspirate. Cat. Note the poorly granulated round cells among the small lymphocytes, suggesting a poorly differentiated mast cell tumor. (Aqueous-based Wright; ×250.)

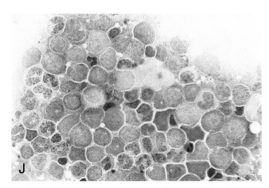

FIGURE 4–6. J, Granulocytic leukemia. Same case as in Figure 4–6I. Cytochemical staining indicates positive staining for this granulocytic marker stain. (Chloroacetate esterase; ×250.)

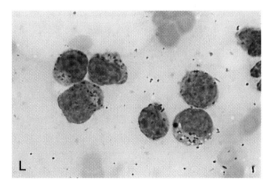

FIGURE 4–6. L, Metastatic large granular lymphoma. Intestinal lymph node aspirate. Cat. Nearly all cells present in this lymph node were medium sized with moderately basophilic cytoplasm containing prominent purple granules. (Wright-Giemsa; ×500.)

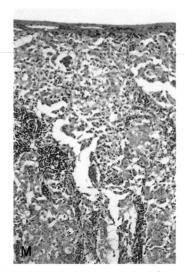

FIGURE 4–6. M, Metastatic islet cell tumor. Gastric lymph node. Dog. There is nearly complete effacement of the lymph node by an expansion of neoplastic cells. Note the remaining small dark-staining lymphocytes at left center. (H & E; ×50.) (Case material courtesy of Robin Allison et al., Colorado State University; presented at the 1998 ASVCP case review session.)

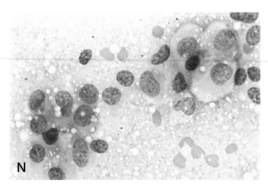

FIGURE 4–6. N, Metastatic islet cell tumor. Gastric lymph node imprint. Same case as in Figure 4–6M. Clusters of intact cells are occasionally found, with most cells present resembling those on the left side, having naked nuclei with indistinct cell borders, typical of endocrine tissue. (Wright-Giemsa; ×250.) (Case material courtesy of Robin Allison et al., Colorado State University; presented at the 1998 ASVCP case review session.)

to lymphoid tissue, with eosinophils most commonly present as a paraneoplastic syndrome in canine mast cell tumors (Fig. 4–4B) or some carcinomas (Fig. 4–4C). Neutrophils commonly occur with squamous cell carcinoma and may involve bacterial sepsis. The remaining lymphoid population often appears immune stimulated, with cell types present as described under Reactive or Hyperplastic Lymph Node. Early in the disease process, metastatic lesions will usually involve a small proportion of the entire cell population, usually less than 50%. In some cases, often late in the disease, the metastatic neoplasm may replace the lymph node parenchyma completely so as to interfere with the cytologic recognition of the tissue as lymph node (Fig. 4–6M & N).

Primary Neoplasia

These tumors originate from the lymph node and usually involve the lymphocyte population but rarely vascular tumors arising from the lymph node have been reported. HogenEsch and Hahn (1998) described eight hemangiomas and one lymphangioma, mostly in the popliteal lymph node of aged dogs from a research colony, which were found as incidental lesions at postmortem.

Lymphoma

Primary neoplasia most often involves the lymphocytes of the lymph node and is termed *lymphoma,* or formerly termed *lymphosarcoma.* It is generally recognized as lymphadenomegaly (Fig. 4–7A). The predominant cell in dogs and cats is usually an immature lymphocyte, since small well-differentiated lymphomas represent a minority of clinical cases. Medium- or large-sized lymphocytes often compose 60% to 90% of the total cells in lymphoma (Fig. 4–7B). An exception is the infrequent presentation of a T-cell-rich B-cell lymphoma in which reactive T lymphocytes represent the majority of the cell population. A report by Steele et al. (1997) demonstrated by using immuno-histochemistry that a parotid mass in a cat contained low numbers of large atypical B-cells among many small reactive T-lymphocytes.

A micrometer such as an erythrocyte is used to determine the size of the lymphocytes present (Fig. 4–7C). The nucleus of a small, medium, and large canine lymphocyte is 1 to 1.5, 2 to 2.5, and greater than

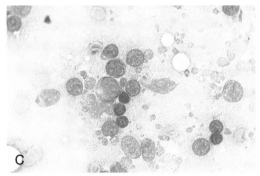

FIGURE 4–7. C, Lymphoma. Lymph node aspirate. Dog. A micrometer such as the erythrocyte at the top of the field is used to determine the size of the lymphocytes present. Note the three dark-staining small lymphocytes in the center along with two intact medium and one intact large lymphocyte. Basophilic cytoplasmic fragments termed *lymphograndular bodies* and pink remnants of lysed nuclei surround the intact cells. (Wright-Giemsa; ×250.)

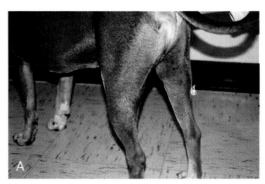

FIGURE 4–7. A, Lymphoma. Dog. Popliteal lymph node enlargement. (Courtesy of Leslie Fox, Gainesville, FL.)

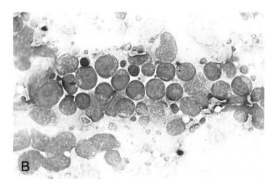

FIGURE 4–7. B, Lymphoma. Lymph node aspirate. Dog. B-cell, high grade. Centroblastic, monomorphic subtype. Medium and large lymphocytes compose 60% to 90% of the total cells. (Wright-Giemsa; ×250.)

three times a red blood cell (RBC) diameter, respectively.

Within the background of the preparation are lymphoglandular bodies (Fig. 4–7C), which result from the rupture of lymphocytes and appear as small platelet-sized basophilic cytoplasmic fragments. Although they may be seen in benign lymph node conditions, a higher frequency is expected in lymphoma because of the immaturity and fragility of these cells. The lyzed nuclei may appear as lacy amorphous eosinophilic material (Fig. 4–7C).

The population is often homogenous (Fig. 4–7D), although early in the disease there may be incomplete effacement of the lymph node. When cell populations are mixed with two cell sizes present such as small and large lymphocytes, the diagnosis of lymphoma may require additional procedures. Surgical removal and histologic examination of the lymph node is recommended in all equivocal cases to make a

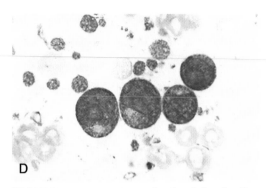

FIGURE 4–7. D, Lymphoglandular bodies. Lymph node aspirate. Dog. Prominent basophilic round structures of variable size indicate fragmentation of the cytoplasm. This appearance is often associated with lymphoma but may be found in other conditions having fragile cells. (Wright-Giemsa; ×500.)

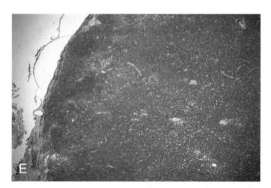

FIGURE 4–7. E, Lymphoma. Lymph node. Dog. A dense infiltration of neoplastic lymphocytes effaces the normal architecture, leaving no discernible cortex and medulla. (H & E; ×10.)

definitive diagnosis and classify the cell type of lymphoma for treatment and prognostic purposes. Clinical staging, particularly involving the blood, bone marrow, or miscellaneous sites (stage V), has prognostic importance for time to relapse following a complete remission and survival time (Teske et al., 1994).

Immunophenotyping the lymphoma into B-cell and T-cell types has been shown to assist in prognosis of canine lymphomas (Teske et al., 1994; Ruslander et al., 1997). In one study, B-cell types involved 76%, T-cell types involved 22%, and null cells involved 2% of the canine lymphoma cases (Ruslander et al., 1997). In this same report, dogs with T-cell lymphomas were at significantly higher risk of relapse (52 vs. 160 days) and early death (153 vs. 330 days) compared with B-cell lymphomas following therapy. Immunophenotyping of canine and feline lymphoid neoplasia may be performed by flow cytometry (Dean et al., 1995; Ruslander et al., 1997; Grindem et al., 1998), immunostaining of tissue sections (Teske et al., 1994; Fournel-Fleury et al., 1997a; Vail et al., 1998; Kiupel et al., 1999), or immunostaining of cytologic preparations obtained by free needle aspiration (Fisher et al., 1995; Caniatti et al., 1996). The study by Fisher et al. (1995) demonstrated an excellent correlation of immunophenotype between immunostained canine cytologic and histologic samples. Considering several studies (Table 4–2), B-cell lymphomas account for approximately 67% of the cases, while T-cell types involve 33%.

Another prognostic indicator involves use of cell proliferation markers in histologic and cytologic specimens to evaluate active cell turnover. The most commonly used are mitotic index, percent positive for Ki-67 antigen, percent positive for proliferation cell nuclear antigen (PCNA), and argyrophilic nucleolar organizing regions (AgNOR) quantitation (Vail et al., 1996; Vail et al., 1997; Fournel-Fleury et al., 1997b; Kiupel et al., 1998; Kiupel et al., 1999). Ki-67 recognizes an antigen expressed in all cell cycle phases except the resting stage (G0). PCNA increases during G1, becomes maximal at DNA synthesis (S), and decreases during

TABLE 4–2 Canine Lymphoma Cases Classified Using the Updated Kiel Classification Scheme

	Teske and van Heerde (1996) N = 67	Fournel-Fleury et al. (1997) N = 91	Raskin et al. (2000)† N = 61	Total Cases N = 219 (% of Total)
B-Cell Low-Grade				18 (8)
Lymphocytic/PLL	—	2	—	2
LP/immunocytoma	1	2	—	3
Plasmacytoma of LN	—	—	—	—
Mixed CB/centrocytic	2	1	—	3
Centrocytic	—	1	—	1
MMC	*	9	*	9 (4)
B-Cell High-Grade				129 (59)
Centroblastic (all types)	34	38	36	108 (49)
Immunoblastic	1	13	1	15 (7)
Lymphoblastic	—	—	3	3
Burkitt-like	—	1	—	1
Large cell anaplastic	—	—	2	2
T-Cell Low-Grade				26 (12)
Lymphocytic/PLL	—	6	1	7 (3)
Mycosis fungoides	—	7	1	8 (4)
T-zone lymphoma	—	—	3	3
Pleomorphic small	5	2	1	8 (4)
T-Cell High-Grade				46 (21)
Pleomorphic M/L	24	8	5	37 (17)
Immunoblastic	—	—	1	1
Lymphoblastic	—	1	7	8 (4)
Large cell anaplastic	—	—	—	—

PLL = prolymphocytic; LP = lymphoplasmacytic; LN = lymph node; CB = centroblastic; *MMC* = macronucleated medium-sized cells (not part of updated Kiel classification); M/L = medium and large cells; — = not noted; * = not recognized as a separate entity, similar appearing cells likely considered as Centroblastic category.
† Personal communication.

G2, mitosis (M), and G0. Mitotic index reflects only the M phase. The most comprehensive marker appears to be AgNOR, which indicates proteins associated with loops of DNA involved in ribosomal RNA transcription. The quantity of AgNOR not only reflects the percentage of cells cycling but also it increases when the cell cycle is faster. AgNOR counts correlated well with tumor grade (Kiupel et al., 1998). Studies on AgNOR frequency and area parameters demonstrated significant predictive potential for remission and survival time in treated and untreated cases of canine lymphoma (Vail et al., 1996; Kiupel et al., 1998; Kiupel et al., 1999).

Morphologic appearance of the neoplastic cells is used to further classify the lymphomas. Currently two classification schemes are used by cytopathologists to characterize lymphoma in veterinary medicine, which are derived from human classification schemes. These are the National Cancer Institute (NCI) Working Formulation (NCI, 1982; Carter et al., 1986) and the modified or updated Kiel Classification (Table 4–2) (Lennert and Feller, 1992; Callanan et al., 1996; Teske and van Heerde, 1996; Fournel-Fleury et al., 1997a), the latter scheme being most preferred. Teske and van Heerde (1996) found classification from needle aspiration biopsies closely correlated to that from histologic samples. Classification into low and high grades of malignancy using both schemes has been shown to have prognostic importance for canine lymphoma cases (Teske et al., 1994). Use of either scheme indicates that the morphologic types of lymphoma with a high grade of malignancy are most frequently encountered in dogs.

Of dogs displaying a high grade of malignancy, the most common morphologic type is the centroblastic form of B-cell origin, as it is called in the updated Kiel classification (Table 4–2), which represents approximately half of all lymphoma cases. Centroblasts are medium to large cells that originate from the follicular areas. A *monomorphic* subtype is composed of greater than 60% centroblasts (Fig. 4–7B). These cells have a round nucleus, fine chromatin pattern, and two to four small basophilic and prominent marginally placed nucleoli (Fig. 4–8A). The cytoplasm is scant and basophilic. Other follicular cell types such as centrocytes and immunoblasts may be present to a lesser extent.

A *polymorphic* subtype of the centroblastic category (Fig. 4–8B & C) contains an increased number of immunoblasts that ac-

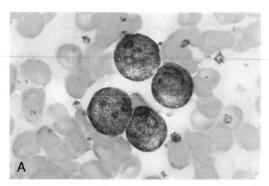

FIGURE 4–8. A, Lymphoma. Lymph node aspirate. Dog. B-cell, high grade. Centroblastic, monomorphic subtype. These medium to large cells have a round nucleus, fine chromatin pattern, two to four small prominent, generally marginally placed nucleoli. The cytoplasm is scant and deeply basophilic. Immunostaining was positive for CD21, CD79a, and IgG. (Wright-Giemsa; ×500.)

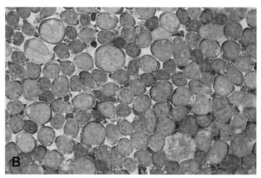

FIGURE 4–8. B, Lymphoma. Lymph node aspirate. Dog. B-cell, high grade. Centroblastic, polymorphic subtype. This population contains an increased number of immunoblasts. Note the mitotic figure at the bottom of the field. Mitotic activity was high in this case. Immunostaining was positive for CD79a and IgG. (Wright-Giemsa; ×250.)

count for greater than 10% and less than 90% of the cell population. Callanan et al. (1996) evaluated eight natural and experimental cases of FIV-associated lymphomas in cats, finding a high prevalence of B-cell types that under the updated Kiel classifica-

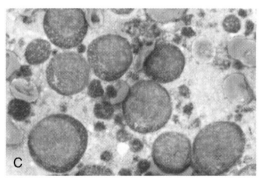

FIGURE 4–8.   C, Lymphoma. Lymph node aspirate. Dog. B-cell, high grade. Centroblastic, polymorphic subtype. A single prominent nucleolus can be seen in several cells. Numerous lymphoglandular bodies are present in the background. Immunostaining was positive for CD21, CD79a, and IgG. (Wright-Giemsa; ×500.)

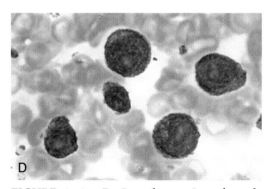

FIGURE 4–8.   D, Lymphoma. Lymph node aspirate. Dog. B-cell, high grade. Immunoblastic. Several immunoblasts are present, each containing one large centrally placed nucleolus. Immunostaining was positive for CD79a. (Wright-Giemsa; ×500.)

erythrocyte. There is one large centrally placed nucleolus (Fig. 4–8D).

A third subtype of the centroblastic category is termed *centrocytoid* because it is intermediate in size between the small centrocyte and the large centroblast (Fig. 4–8E). Generally the nucleus of this medium-sized cell contains two to five small basophilic centrally placed nucleoli. The cytoplasm is scant and moderately basophilic. In this subtype, centrocytoid cells should exceed 30% of the cell population. A unique-appearing cell type found in dogs and not recognized separately in human lymphoma cases resembles the centrocytoid cell except it contains only one large nucleolus instead of multiple nucleoli (Fig. 4–8E–G). This cell has been labeled macronucleated medium-sized cell (MMC) by Fournel-Fleury et al. (1997a), who suggest the cell arises from the marginal perifollicular zone. On

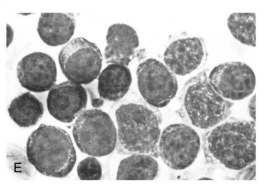

FIGURE 4–8.   E, Lymphoma. Lymph node aspirate. Dog. B-cell, high grade. Centroblastic, centrocytoid subtype. Many medium-sized cells are present that contain one or more nucleoli. A centrocyte is seen to the left of a medium-sized centrocytoid cell that has a single large centrally placed nucleolus. This centrocytoid cell sometimes has been referred to as a *macronucleated medium-sized cell* (MMC). Immunostaining was positive for CD21, CD79a, and IgG. (Wright-Giemsa; ×500.)

tion relate to the centroblastic, polymorphic subtype in five of the eight cases. Immunoblasts are large cells with abundant basophilic cytoplasm and a nucleus that measures at least three times the size of an

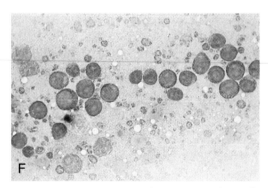

FIGURE 4–8. F, Lymphoma. Lymph node aspirate. Dog. B-cell, high grade. Centroblastic, centrocytoid subtype. In this subtype, medium-sized centrocytoid cells exceed 30% of the cell population. Immunostaining was positive for CD21 and CD79. (Wright-Giemsa; ×250.)

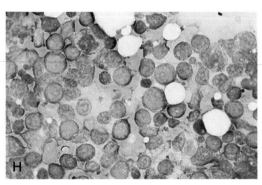

FIGURE 4–8. H, Lymphoma. Same case as in Figure 4–8D. The population is predominantly composed of large lymphoid cells that have a single large, centrally placed nucleolus. A mitotic figure is present at the top of the field. (Wright-Giemsa; ×250.)

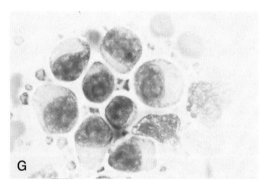

FIGURE 4–8. G, Lymphoma. Lymph node aspirate. Dog. Centroblastic, centrocytoid subtype. The nuclei measure 1.5 to 2 times RBC diameter, indicating these are medium-sized lymphocytes. The abundant cytoplasm in several cells produces a plasmacytoid appearance, which leads to the mistaken identification of these cells as immunoblasts since many have a single prominent, centrally placed nucleus present. (Wright-Giemsa; ×500.)

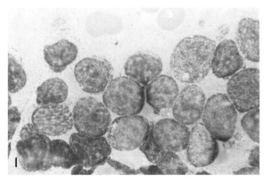

FIGURE 4–8. I, Lymphoma. Lymph node aspirate. Dog. B-cell, high grade. Lymphoblastic. Cells are small to medium-sized with round nuclei measuring 1.5 to 2.5 times RBC diameter. Nucleoli are generally indistinct. The cytoplasm is scant and moderately basophilic. Immunostaining was weakly positive for CD21 and IgG. (Wright-Giemsa; ×500.)

the basis of low mitotic activity and low expression of the Ki-67 (Fournel-Fleury et al., 1997b), MMC were considered to have a low grade of malignancy. However, cases with a predominant MMC appearance clini-cally present in stages IV or V at the time of initial diagnosis. Therefore it may be more appropriate to place them in the high grade of malignancy category based on their aggressive clinical behavior and larger cell size compared with other cases having a low grade of malignancy. It is further possible that despite the low Ki-67 expression, the cell may have a short cell cycle length when evaluated using AgNORs.

Other B-cell high-grade types that may be encountered include immunoblastic (Fig. 4–8D, H), lymphoblastic (Fig. 4–8I & J), and large-cell anaplastic (Fig. 4–8K & L). To define the cell of origin as B-cell, immunostaining of cytologic specimens may be positive with CD21, CD79a (Fig. 4–8M), and IgG (Fig. 4–8N).

Within the T-cell category, the pleomorphic medium- and large-cell category is most common and accounts for nearly 20%

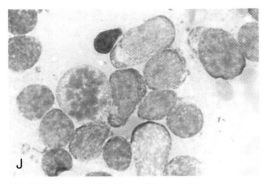

FIGURE 4–8. J, Lymphoma. Same case as in Figure 4–8I. Mitotic activity is high for this lymphoblastic category. Note the small darkstaining lymphocyte for size comparison. Most cells are medium sized with indistinct nucleoli and scant cytoplasm. (Wright-Giemsa; ×500.)

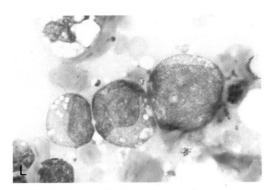

FIGURE 4–8. L, Lymphoma. Same case as in Figure 4–8K. Note the large histiocytic-appearing cells with cytoplasmic vacuolation. (Wright-Giemsa; ×500.)

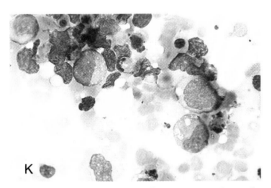

FIGURE 4–8. K, Lymphoma. Lymph node aspirate. Dog. B-cell, high grade. Large cell anaplastic. Among the necrotic debris several large intact cells are found that have histiocytic features. Immunostaining was positive only for IgG. (Wright-Giemsa; ×250.)

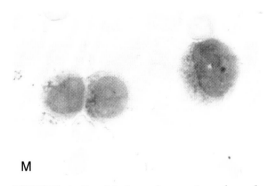

FIGURE 4–8. M, Lymphoma. Lymph node aspirate cytospin prep. Same case as in Figure 4–8D. B-cell. Immunostaining is positive as indicated by diffuse brown granular staining within the cytoplasm. (CD79a; ×500.)

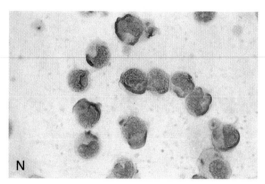

FIGURE 4–8. N, Lymphoma. Lymph node aspirate cytospin prep. Same case as in Figure 4–8C. B-cell. Immunostaining is positive as indicated by dark-brown granular staining within the cytoplasm. (IgG; ×250.)

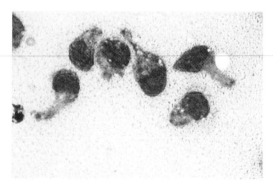

FIGURE 4–9. B, Lymphoma. Lymph node aspirate. Dog. T-cell, high grade. Pleomorphic medium/large cells. Animal also has cutaneous nodules, which appear similar cytologically, and on histopathology these lymphocytes infiltrate the epidermis. Cells display a hand-mirror shape with cytoplasmic pseudopods that extend in different directions. (Wright-Giemsa; ×500.)

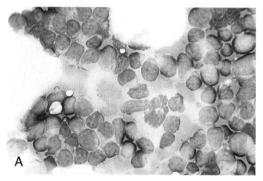

FIGURE 4–9. A, Lymphoma. Lymph node aspirate. Dog. T-cell, high grade. Pleomorphic medium/large cells. Medium-sized lymphocytes predominate displaying nuclear pleomorphism. Note the irregular nuclear shape often having multiple indentations or serrations on one side. Chromatin is finely granular and nucleoli are prominent in the large lymphocytes. The cytoplasm is moderately abundant and lightly basophilic. Immunostaining was positive for CD3. (Wright-Giemsa; ×250.)

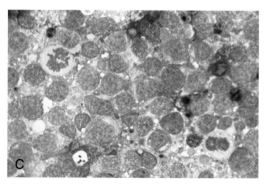

FIGURE 4–9. C, Lymphoma. Lymph node aspirate. Dog. T-cell, high grade. Lymphoblastic. The number of mitotic figures often exceeds three per five fields at 40× or 50× objectives. Cells have scant cytoplasm and nucleoli that are indistinct. (Wright-Giemsa; ×250.)

of all lymphoma cases (Table 4–2). This tumor is composed of medium, large, or mixed medium and large cells that display considerable nuclear pleomorphism (Fig.

4–9A & B). Often the nucleus is convex and smooth on one side while the opposite side is concave with many irregular indentations or serrations and may be described

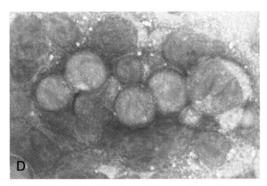

FIGURE 4–9.   D, Lymphoma. Lymph node aspirate. Dog. T-cell, high grade. Lymphoblastic. The predominant cell population is medium sized with multiple convolutions of the nucleus. Nucleoli are indistinct. Immunostaining was positive for CD3 and CD8. (Wright-Giemsa; ×500.)

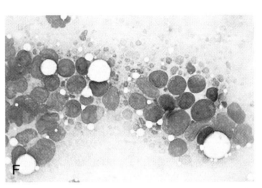

FIGURE 4–9.   F, Lymphoma. Lymph node aspirate. Dog. T-cell, high grade. Immunoblastic. There are several large cells present, with a single large, centrally placed nucleolus. Immunostaining was positive for CD3. (Wright-Giemsa; ×250.)

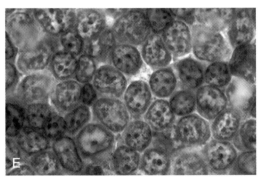

FIGURE 4–9.   E, Lymphoma. Lymph node aspirate. Dog. T-cell, high grade. Lymphoblastic. Use of a wet mount procedure easily demonstrates the round or irregularly round nuclear shape and the presence of small multiple nucleoli. (New methylene blue; ×500.)

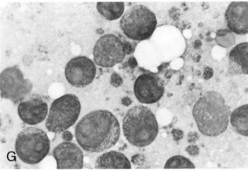

FIGURE 4–9.   G, Lymphoma. Same case as in Figure 4–9F. Higher magnification to demonstrate the irregularly round nuclear shape and prominent nucleolus. The cytoplasm is moderately abundant and basophilic. (Wright-Giemsa; ×500.)

as cerebriform. Nucleoli are large and of variable shape and number. The cytoplasm is moderately abundant and moderately basophilic. A few eosinophils may be present within these lesions in people. Other T-cell high-grade types that may be encountered include lymphoblastic (Fig. 4–9C–E) and immunoblastic (Fig. 4–9F & G).

The lymphoblastic type (Fig. 4–9C–E) is often associated with a mediastinal mass and a paraneoplastic syndrome of hypercalcemia (Carter et al., 1986). Both classification schemes recognize the lymphoblastic type with similar morphologic features, which involve cells that are usually small to medium-sized with nuclei measuring 1.5–2.5 times RBC diameter. The nucleus may be round or convoluted and the nucleoli

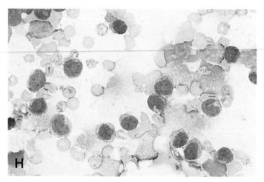

FIGURE 4–9. H, Lymphoma. Lymph node aspirate. Dog. T-cell, low grade. Pleomorphic small cell. A relatively monomorphic population of small cells with scant gray cytoplasm. Immunostaining was positive for CD3. (Wright-Giemsa; ×250.)

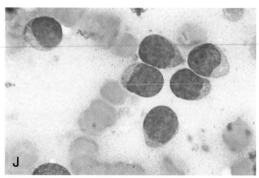

FIGURE 4–9. J, Lymphoma. Lymph node aspirate. Dog. T-cell, low grade. T-zone lymphoma. The tumor cells are small and monomorphic with small nucleoli. The nuclear surface is round to irregularly round without indentations. Immunostaining was positive for CD3. (Wright-Giemsa; ×500.)

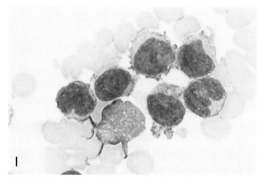

FIGURE 4–9. I, Lymphoma. Same case as in Figure 4–9H. The nucleus is characterized by a smooth surface on one side and serrations on the opposite side. (Wright-Giemsa; ×500.)

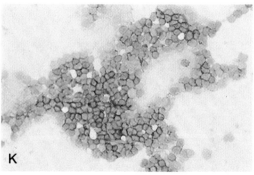

FIGURE 4–9. K, Lymphoma. Lymph node aspirate cytospin. Dog. T-cell, low grade. T-zone lymphoma. A strong positive reaction is indicated by the brown cytoplasmic stain. (CD3; ×125.)

are small and indistinct. The cytoplasm is often scant. Mitotic activity is high (Table 4–3). Another diagnostic tool is cytochemical staining that is distinctive with a focal or dot appearance with alpha naphthyl acetate esterase, alpha naphthyl butyrate esterase, and acid phosphatase (Carter et al., 1986; Raskin and Nipper, 1992). Prognosis for this morphologic type is poor owing to renal failure, which results from the hypercalcemia.

T-cell low-grade types are more frequent than B-cell low-grade types. They include mycosis fungoides or small cerebriform (see Fig. 3–47D & E), pleomorphic small (Fig. 4–9H & I), and T-zone lymphoma (Fig. 4–9J). To define the cell of origin as T-cell, immunostaining of cytologic specimens may be positive with CD3 (Fig. 4–9K), CD4, CD5, or CD8. Cytochemical staining with nonspecific esterases or acid phosphatase may also be used (Fig. 4–9L).

TABLE 4–3	Cytologic Protocol and Terms Used to Evaluate Lymphoma Cases

- Estimate the mitotic index by looking at five cellular fields under 40× or 50× objectives.
  Low: 0–1 mitotic figures per five fields
  Moderate: 2–3 mitotic figures per five fields
  High: >3 mitotic figures per five fields
- Determine the cell size in comparison to the size of an erythrocyte.
  Small: 1–1.5 × RBC
  Medium: 2–2.5 × RBC
  Large: >3 × RBC
- Determine the shape of the nucleus and its placement within the cytoplasm.
  Round: circular with no indentations
  Irregularly round: few indentations or convolutions
  Convoluted: several deep indentations
  Clefted: single deep indentation
  Central vs. eccentric placement
- Determine the number, size, visibility, and location of nucleoli within the neoplastic lymphocytes.
  Single vs. multiple
  Large vs. small
  Indistinct: not visible or barely perceivable
  Prominent: easily visible
  Central vs. marginal or peripheral placement
- Describe the cytoplasm by amount and color. Be sure to note presence of Golgi zone or granulation.
  Scant: small rim around nucleus
  Moderate size: amount intermediate between scant and abundant
  Abundant: nearly twice the size of the nucleus
  Pale: light basophilia or clear
  Moderate basophilia: color intermediate between pale and dark blue
  Deep basophilia: royal blue or darker
- Tumor grade is morphologically based on cell size and mitotic index.
  Low grade: Low mitotic index and small cell size
  High grade: Moderate or high mitotic index and medium or large cell size

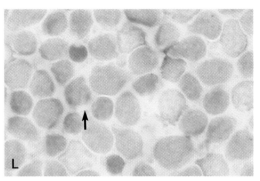

FIGURE 4–9. L, Lymphoma. Lymph node aspirate. Dog. T-cell, high grade. Lymphoblastic. Note the prominent focal staining of some lymphocytes such as the one identified with an arrow. Most of the other lymphocytes have trace focal staining. (Acid phosphatase; ×500.)

CYTOLOGIC ARTIFACTS

In attempting to aspirate the submandibular lymph node, it is quite common to sample salivary gland tissue (Fig. 4–10A & B). The submandibular lymph node is found directly ventral from the prominent part of the zygomatic arch, which is behind and below the eye, midway between the eye and ear. The mandibular salivary gland is located within the bifurcation of the external

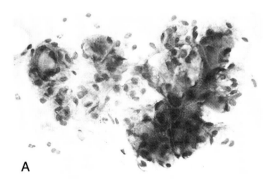

FIGURE 4–10. A, Salivary gland. Tissue aspirate. Dog. Attempted aspirate of the submandibular lymph node resulted in the collection of epithelial clusters. (Wright-Giemsa; ×125.)

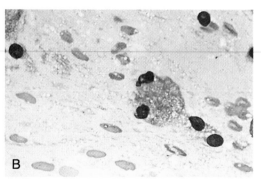

FIGURE 4–10. **B, Salivary gland. Tissue aspirate. Dog.** Individual salivary gland cell with abundant foamy basophilic cytoplasm. Free nuclei in the background are easily mistaken for small lymphocytes. Note the basophilic granular background consistent with mucin and the manner erythrocytes are caught in it resembling a string of cells. (Wright-Giemsa; ×250.)

FIGURE 4–10. **C, Diagram showing the location of the mandibular salivary gland and submandibular lymph node. Dog.** The asterisk (*) indicates the bony prominence of the zygomatic arch. The submandibular lymph node (L) is directly ventral or perpendicular to the arch. Note the more posterior and dorsal location of the mandibular salivary gland (S) located within the bifurcation of the external jugular vein (V).

jugular vein and is more posterior and dorsal to the lymph node. (Fig. 4–10C).

SPLEEN

Indications for Splenic Biopsy

■ *Splenomegaly* may be detected by palpation or by radiography and ultrasonography.

■ *Abnormal imaging features* suggest the presence of hyperplasia or infiltrative processes.

■ *Evaluation of hematopoiesis* may be indicated when bone marrow disease is present.

Aspirate Biopsy Considerations

Aspiration may be performed in cases of thrombocytopenia, but body movements should be minimized, either by manual restraint or sedation. The needle and syringe may be coated with sterile 4% disodium EDTA prior to aspiration to reduce the clotting potential of the specimen. A 1- to 1.5-inch, 22- or 23-gauge needle may be used alone or attached to a hand-held 12-ml syringe or aspiration gun. In some cases, it may be preferable to use a 2.5- to 3.5-inch spinal needle. The animal is placed in

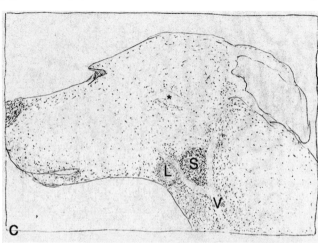

S salivary gland, mandibular
L lymph node, submandibular
V vein, external jugular
* zygomatic arch

right lateral or dorsal recumbency and the area over the site is prepared surgically. The site is carefully determined by palpation or ultrasonography.

KEY POINT: The nonaspiration method of biopsy is preferred with vascular sites such as the spleen to reduce blood contamination.

Normal Histology and Cytology

The spleen is enclosed by a thick, smooth muscle capsule that extends inward as trabeculae. The splenic parenchyma is divided into white pulp and red pulp. The white pulp consists of dense periarterial lymphatic sheaths and lymphatic nodules and the red pulp consists of erythrocytes contained within a reticular meshwork, within endothelial lined sinuses, or within blood vessels (Fig. 4–11A). The splenic artery enters the hilus of the spleen and branches into arteries that become the central arteries of the lymphatic sheaths. These vessels branch into pulp capillaries that are surrounded by concentric layers of macrophages within a reticular meshwork. The pericapillary macrophage sheaths, termed *ellipsoids,* are

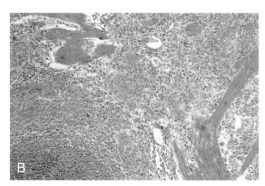

FIGURE 4–11. B, Normal spleen. Same case as in Figure 4–11A. An ellipsoid, located in the center, is a capillary that is surrounded by concentric layers of macrophages within a reticular meshwork. (H & E; ×50.)

abundant in the marginal zone surrounding periarterial lymphatic sheaths adjacent to the red pulp (Fig. 4–11B).

On cytology, aspirate preparations contain large amounts of blood contamination, as evidenced by many intact erythrocytes and platelet clumps. Lymphoid cells present are similar to those of the normal lymph node (see Fig. 4–1E). Small lymphocytes predominate with occasional medium and large lymphocytes present. A few macrophages and plasma cells may be seen along with rare neutrophils and mast cells. Macrophages may contain small amounts of granular debris, compatible with hemosiderin. Occasional groups of macrophages may be admixed with a reticular stroma representing the ellipsoids (Fig. 4–11C).

Reactive or Hyperplastic Spleen

Hyperplasia may result from antigenic reaction to infectious agents or the presence of blood parasites. Small lymphocytes still predominate but there is an increase in medium- and large-sized lymphocytes. Macrophages and plasma cells are commonly observed (Fig. 4–12A). Frequent large collections of reticular stroma with increased

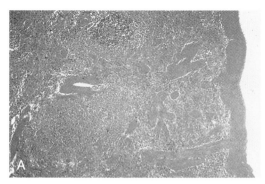

FIGURE 4–11. A, Normal spleen. Cat. A thick smooth muscle capsule that extends inward as trabeculae encloses the spleen. Note the dense periarterial lymphatic sheath at top center of the field. (H & E; ×25.)

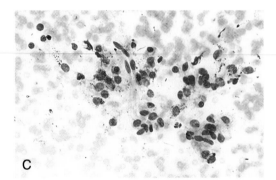

FIGURE 4–11. C, Normal spleen. Tissue aspirate. Dog. A collection of macrophages is shown mixed with a reticular stroma that represents an ellipsoid. (Wright-Giemsa; ×125.)

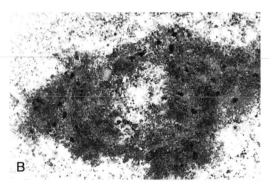

FIGURE 4–12. B, Hyperplastic spleen. Tissue aspirate. Dog. This animal was being treated with chemotherapy for lymphoma. A very large aggregate of reticular stroma is shown dotted by an increased number of mast cells that appear as dark-purple cells evenly dispersed throughout. (Wright-Giemsa; ×50.)

numbers of mast cells may be observed at low magnification (Fig. 4–12B). Hemosiderosis is often present with large amounts of coarse dark granules (Fig. 4–12C). Capillaries may be more commonly observed with increased endothelial elements in the spleen (Fig. 4–12D).

Splenitis

In addition to the inflammatory response associated with splenic hyperplasia, inflam-

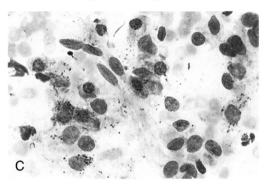

FIGURE 4–12. C, Hyperplastic spleen. Tissue aspirate. Dog. Hemosiderosis is recognized by the presence of hemosiderin-laden macrophages containing large amounts of coarse dark granules. (Wright-Giemsa; ×250.)

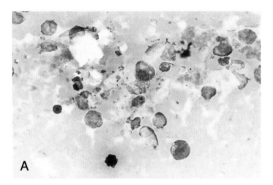

FIGURE 4–12. A, Reactive spleen. Tissue aspirate. Dog. An increase in medium-sized lymphocytes is present. In addition, several plasma cells are noted along with a macrophage. (Wright-Giemsa; ×250.)

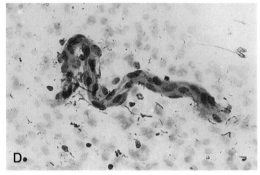

FIGURE 4–12. D, Hyperplastic spleen. Same case as in Figure 4–12C. An endothelial-lined capillary is noted as a result of endothelial hyperplasia. (Wright-Giemsa; ×125.)

matory cells will increase in number with other noninfectious or infectious causes of disease. Noninfectious causes such as malignancy or immune reaction can incite neutrophilic or eosinophilic infiltration (Thorn and Aubert, 1999) (Fig. 4–13A). The diagnosis of splenitis must be made cautiously if circulating neutrophilia or eosinophilia is present. Macrophagic or histiocytic inflam-

mation often occurs with the presence of systemic fungal infections such as histoplasmosis or protozoal infections such as cytauxzoonosis and leishmaniasis (Fig. 4–13B).

Primary and Metastatic Neoplasia

Differentiation between primary and metastatic neoplasia may not always be possible, especially if multiple organs are involved. Lymphoma will appear morphologically similar to that of the lymph node (see Figs. 4–7 to 4–9). Granular lymphocytic leukemia is thought to originate from the spleen (Vernau and Moore, 1999). The patient often presents with marked granular lymphocytosis in circulation that is present also within the spleen (Fig. 4–14A) (Lau et al, 1999). The bone marrow is usually not infiltrated by the neoplastic population. Clinical signs are variable and progression of the neoplastic disease may be slow. Granules may be very small and difficult to see with use of aqueous-based Wright stains (Fig.

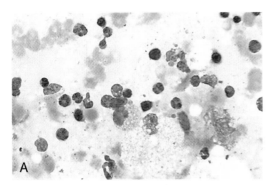

FIGURE 4–13. A, Splenitis. Tissue aspirate. Dog. Neutrophils, eosinophils, and activated macrophages compose the severe inflammatory response in this animal with a necrotizing splenitis. (Wright-Giemsa; ×250.)

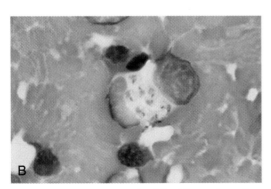

FIGURE 4–13. B, Splenitis. Tissue imprint. Dog. Macrophage with engulfed protozoal organisms confirmed as *Leishmania* sp. Note the organism contains a small round nucleus and a short rod-shaped kinetoplast. Various stages of erythroid precursors support a diagnosis of extramedullary hematopoiesis. (Wright-Giemsa; ×500.) (Photo courtesy of Cheryl Swenson and Gary Kociba, The Ohio State University; presented at the 1987 ASVCP case review session.)

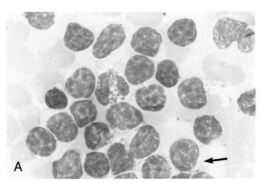

FIGURE 4–14. A, Granular lymphocyte lymphoma. Splenic aspirate. Dog. One small lymphocyte and an eosinophil surrounded by a monomorphic population of medium lymphocytes with clumped chromatin and moderately abundant clear cytoplasm. Some of the cells visibly contain several fine azurophilic granules that is best demonstrated by the cell indicated (*arrow*). The spleen was considered to be the primary organ of involvement and stained with CD3, a T-cell marker. (Wright-Giemsa; ×500.)

4–14B & C). Non-neoplastic conditions may produce a reactive granular lymphocytosis, which should be ruled out first.

In the study by Day et al. (1995), hematoma occurred in six cases and nonspecific changes such as extramedullary hemato-

poiesis, congestion, and hemosiderosis occurred in 16 of 87 canine biopsies. Hemangiosarcoma was the most commonly diagnosed splenic neoplasm (Day et al., 1995) involving 17 of 87 canine splenic biopsies. Hemangiosarcoma cells are similar

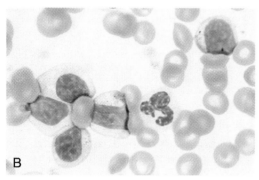

FIGURE 4–14. B, Granular lymphocyte leukemia. Blood smear. Same case as in Figure 4–14A. The history involved 2 months of persistent lymphocytosis of counts exceeding 20,000/µl. Rickettsial infections were ruled out by titer tests. Note the typical abundant clear cytoplasm with small red granules arranged in a focal paranuclear manner. The bone marrow was not infiltrated by this cell population. (Wright-Giemsa; ×500.)

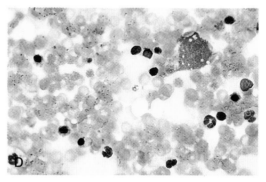

FIGURE 4–14. D, Hemangiosarcoma. Splenic aspirate. Dog. Scattered large mesenchymal appearing cells may be found scanning on low magnification such as the one shown. (Wright-Giemsa; ×250.)

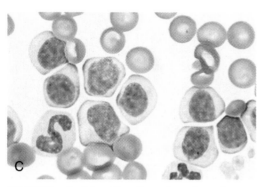

FIGURE 4–14. C, Granular lymphocyte leukemia. Same case and specimen as in Figure 4–14B. Use of this stain did not demonstrate the cytoplasmic granules. Alcohol-based Romanowsky stains are recommended. (Aqueous-based Wright; ×500.)

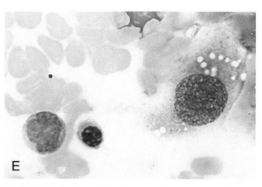

FIGURE 4–14. E, Hemangiosarcoma. Same case as in Figure 4–14D. Medium lymphocyte, rubricyte, and large malignant cell. Note the round nucleus with coarse chromatin, multiple large nucleoli, and vacuolated cytoplasm with indistinct cell borders. Extramedullary hematopoiesis and lymphoid reactivity are commonly found in this condition. (Wright-Giemsa; ×500.)

to those in other sites. Scattered large mesenchymal-appearing cells may be found scanning on low magnification (Fig. 4–14D). Extramedullary hematopoiesis (Fig. 4–14E), chronic hemorrhage, and lymphoid reactivity may accompany the tumor. Neoplastic cells are large with abundant cytoplasm having wispy indistinct borders and frequently multiple punctate vacuoles (Fig. 4–14F). The nucleus is round with coarse chromatin and multiple prominent nucleoli.

Other mesenchymal-appearing tumors in the canine spleen involve primarily fibrosarcoma, undifferentiated sarcoma (Fig. 4–14G), leiomyosarcoma, osteosarcoma, liposarcoma, myxosarcoma, and malignant fibrous histiocytoma (Spangler et al., 1994; Hendrick et al., 1992).

In cats, the most important cause of splenomegaly is mastocytoma, accounting for 15% of the total pathologic conditions submitted for diagnosis (Spangler and Culbertson, 1992). Diffuse enlargement of the spleen is detected on palpation or diagnostic imaging (Fig. 4–14H). Often a nearly pure population of highly granulated mast cells is present, several of which may display erythrophagocytosis (Fig. 4–14I). Other dis-

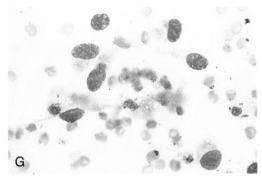

FIGURE 4–14. G, Poorly differentiated sarcoma. Splenic aspirate. Dog. Mesenchymal-appearing cells with wispy cell borders, round to oval nuclei, coarse chromatin, anisokaryosis, and prominent nucleoli are present. (Wright-Giemsa; ×250.)

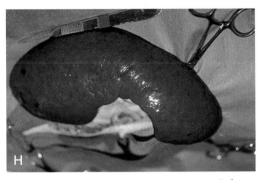

FIGURE 4–14. H, Mastocytoma. Spleen. Cat. Diffuse enlargement of the spleen is commonly found for this neoplasm.

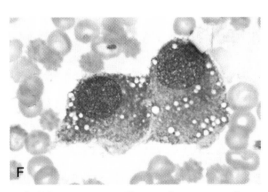

FIGURE 4–14. F, Hemangiosarcoma. Same case as in Figure 4–14D. Multiple punctate vacuoles are commonly found in the stellate cells of this neoplasm. (Wright-Giemsa; ×500.)

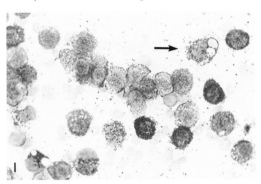

FIGURE 4–14. I, Mastocytoma. Spleen. Cat. A monomorphic population of moderately to highly granulated mast cells is present. Note the cell (*arrow*) demonstrating erythrophagocytosis, a feature common for splenic mastocytoma. (Wright-Giemsa; ×250.)

crete cell tumors found in the spleen include myeloid leukemia, extramedullary myeloma or plasmacytoma (Fig. 4–14J), and malignant histiocytosis (Fig. 4–14K & L).

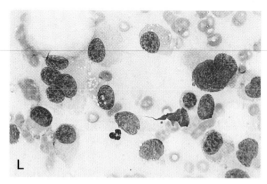

FIGURE 4–14. L, Malignant histiocytosis. Same case as in Figure 4–14K. Higher magnification demonstrates a lobulated cell (right) and a multinucleated cell (left). (Wright-Giemsa; ×250.)

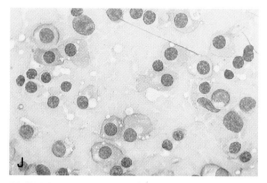

FIGURE 4–14. J, Plasmacytoma. Splenic imprint. Dog. Plasma cells composed the majority of cells present. Note the abundant eosinophilic cytoplasm typical for a "flame cell." Serum protein electrophoresis indicated a monoclonal gammopathy, which immunoelectrophoresis confirmed as an abnormal amount of IgA. (Romanowsky; ×250.) (Case material courtesy of Christine Swardson and Joanne Messick, The Ohio State University; presented at the 1989 ASVCP case review session.)

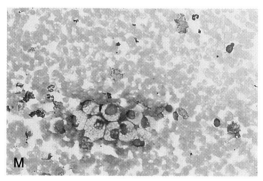

FIGURE 4–14. M, Metastatic prostatic carcinoma. Splenic asp. Dog. Cluster of individualized epithelial cells with marked anisokaryosis. (Wright-Giemsa; ×125.)

Occasionally, highly disseminated epithelial malignancies will be found in the spleen. An example of secretory epithelium with anaplastic features is shown in Figure 4–14M & N.

Extramedullary Hematopoiesis

Extramedullary hematopoiesis was the most common cytologic abnormality in one study, accounting for 24% of the patients (O'Keefe and Couto, 1987). While precursors from all three cell lines may be ob-

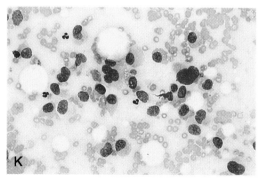

FIGURE 4–14. K, Malignant histiocytosis. Splenic aspirate. Dog. A cellular specimen shows a monomorphic population of individually arranged cells. The cells are round to oval with a moderate amount of basophilic cytoplasm, several of which contain few punctate vacuoles. (Wright-Giemsa; ×125.)

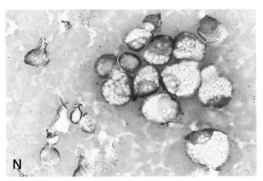

FIGURE 4–14. N, Metastatic prostatic carcinoma. Same case as in Figure 4–14M. Higher magnification demonstrates the secretory nature of the tumor cells from the presence of abundant vacuolated cytoplasm. A carcinoma with similar appearing cells was found in the prostate and thought to be the tumor's origin. (Wright-Giemsa; ×250.)

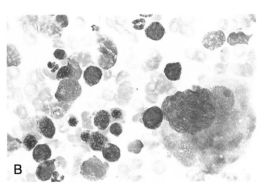

FIGURE 4–15. B, Extramedullary hematopoiesis. Same case as in Figure 4–15A. Higher magnification demonstrates low numbers of medium-sized lymphocytes with many rubricytes in addition to the mature megakaryocyte. (Wright-Giemsa; ×250.)

served, erythroid cells are the most common, with metarubricytes, rubricytes, and prorubricytes present (Fig. 4–15A–C). Care must be taken as erythroid precursors and lymphoid precursors appear very similar. Mature megakaryocytes are easily observed during scanning because of their large size. Conditions associated with extramedullary

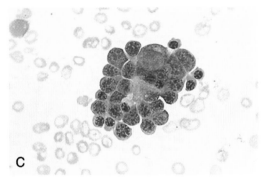

FIGURE 4–15. C, Extramedullary hematopoiesis. Same case as in Figure 4–15A. A nurse cell or a macrophage surrounded by various stages of erythroid development may be found in areas of increased erythropoiesis. (Wright-Giemsa; ×250.)

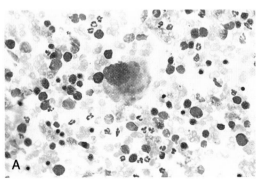

FIGURE 4–15. A, Extramedullary hematopoiesis. Splenic aspirate. Dog. A megakaryocyte and numerous erythroid precursors are detected in this sample from an animal that received chemotherapy 2 weeks earlier for lymphoma. (Wright-Giemsa; ×125.)

hematopoiesis include chronic hemolytic anemia, myeloproliferative disorders, and lymphoproliferative disorders.

Appearing similar to extramedullary hematopoiesis is myelolipoma, an uncommon tumor in both dogs and cats, occurring in the liver or spleen. The presence of hematopoietic precursors with large amounts of lipid vacuoles in the background is strongly suggestive of this benign neoplasm (Fig.

4–15D–F). It is often found unassociated with hematologic abnormalities. Ultrasound examination may demonstrate a small focal hyperechoic mass in the spleen.

Cytologic Artifacts

Samples collected with the assistance of ultrasound often produce magenta debris in the background. This granular material represents ultrasound gel particles (Fig.

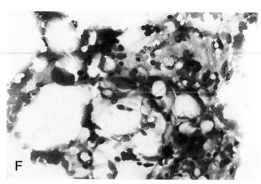

FIGURE 4–15. F, Myelolipoma. Same case as in Figure 4–15D. A megakaryocyte and collections of reticuloendothelial stroma are present within the small discrete nodule on the splenic tail. (Wright-Giemsa; ×125.)

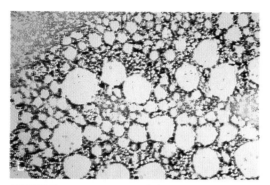

FIGURE 4–15. D, Myelolipoma. Splenic aspirate. Cat. Low magnification demonstrates the massive amounts of variably sized clear vacuoles, consistent with lipid. (Wright-Giemsa; ×25.)

4–16A) and can mimic necrotic tissue when mixed with blood. The material also may cause lysis or cellular swelling and therefore may create unsuitable preparations for cytologic examination.

Care should be taken when an incisional biopsy is taken of the spleen and impression smears are made. When the capsular

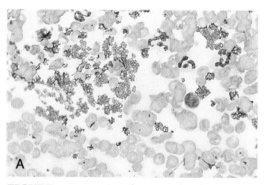

FIGURE 4–16. A, Ultrasound gel. Transabdominal needle aspirate. Dog. An attempt to sample the spleen produced a cytologic artifact. Note the pink to magenta coarse granular material in the background. (Wright; ×250.) (Case material courtesy of Kurt Henkel et al., Michigan State University; presented at the 1996 ASVCP case review session.)

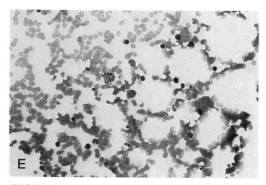

FIGURE 4–15. E, Myelolipoma. Same case as in Figure 4–15D. Dark-staining erythroid precursors are associated with the lipid material. (Wright-Giemsa; ×125.)

surface is mistakenly imprinted instead of the parenchyma, uniform sheets of loosely attached mesothelium are seen (Fig. 4–16B & C).

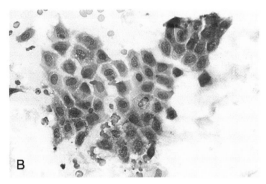

FIGURE 4–16. B, Mesothelium. Splenic imprint. Dog. Splenomegaly from suspected hypersplenism necessitated removal of the spleen. The outside surface was inadvertently imprinted on the slide. Note a large sheet of interlocking cells. (Aqueous-based Wright; ×125.)

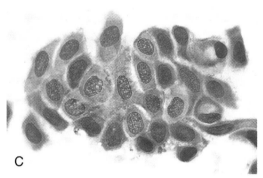

FIGURE 4–16. C, Mesothelium. Same case as in Figure 4–16B. Higher magnification demonstrates a uniform population of adherent cells with abundant basophilic cytoplasm. Clear spaces between cells represent cytoplasmic junctions. This benign sheet of cells is typical for mesothelial lining. The capsule on this spleen was prominently thickened grossly and histologically. (Aqueous-based Wright; ×250.)

THYMUS

Indications for Thymic Biopsy

■ *Enlargement* may be detected by radiography and ultrasonography, often producing signs of dyspnea, pleural effusions, and dysphagia (swallowing difficulties).

■ *Abnormal imaging features* suggest the presence of hyperplasia or infiltrative processes.

Normal Histology and Cytology

Before puberty, the thymus has a prominent parenchyma divided into cortical and medullary regions (Fig. 4–17A). The outermost cortex is composed of small, densely packed lymphocytes without formation of lymphoid nodules. The central medulla is continuous between lobules that are formed by the inward extension of the thin connective tissue capsule. The medulla contains fewer and larger vesicular lymphocytes. The thymus is supported by a reticular network of stellate epithelium that forms loose cuffs

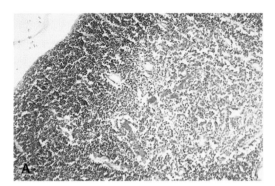

FIGURE 4–17. A, Normal thymus. Young dog. The dense cortical area is composed of packed lymphocytes (left), while the medulla is more pale staining (right). Note the dark-staining structures in the medulla called *Hassall's corpuscles.* (H & E; ×50.)

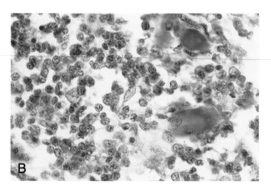

FIGURE 4–17. B, Normal thymus. Same case as in Figure 4–17A. The medulla contains eosinophilic Hassall's corpuscles that represent perivascular cuffs of flattened reticular stroma that becomes keratinized or calcified. The medullary lymphocytes are larger with vesicular nucleus. (H & E; ×250.)

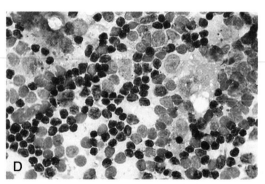

FIGURE 4–17. D, Normal thymus. Same case as in Figure 4–17C. Higher magnification to demonstrate the large stellate reticular epithelium with vesicular nuclei. (Wright-Giemsa; ×250.)

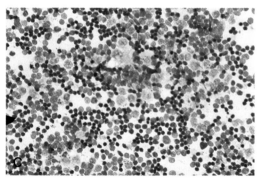

FIGURE 4–17. C, Normal thymus. Tissue aspirate. Young dog. Many small dark-staining lymphocytes are the predominant population, with fewer medium lymphocytes. Note the two large epithelial cells in the top center of the field. (Wright-Giemsa; ×125.)

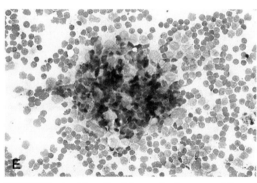

FIGURE 4–17. E, Normal thymus. Tissue aspirate. Young dog. Thymic epithelium may be found in tight balls, possibly representing perivascular cuffs. (Wright-Giemsa; ×125.)

around small vessels, termed *Hassall's corpuscles.* These concentric whorls of flattened reticular cells may become keratinized or calcified (Fig. 4–17A & B). The reticular epithelium also gives rise to a ductal system within the medulla that may become cystic and lined by ciliated epithelium. After puberty, the thymic parenchyma begins to atrophy, becoming replaced by adipose tissue.

Cytologically, the cell population of the cortex is similar to that of the lymph node with the predominance of small dense staining lymphocytes (Fig. 4–17C & D). Occasional mast cells are present. Large stellate cells with round vesicular nuclei representing the thymic epithelium may be found scattered between the lymphocytes or in tight balls (Fig. 4–17E & F), the latter

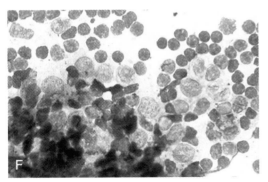

FIGURE 4–17. F, Normal thymus. Same case as in Figure 4–17E. Higher magnification to demonstrate the small lymphocytes and thymic epithelium. (Wright-Giemsa; ×250.)

arrangement become Hassall's corpuscles. These dense collections of epithelium resemble epithelioid macrophages having abundant pale-blue cytoplasm with cellular attachment to each other.

Primary Neoplasia

The two different cell populations, lymphocytes and reticular epithelium, become the origin for the two types of neoplasia that develops within the thymus. Neoplasia of the lymphoid cells of the thymus is termed *thymic lymphoma,* having the appearance of lymphoma in other lymphoid organs like the lymph node (see Fig. 4–7 to 4–9). The cell type involved most often is the lymphoblastic type and these tumors have been associated with hypercalcemia.

Neoplasia of the thymic epithelial cells is termed *thymoma* and usually takes one of three forms in dogs and cats; epithelial thymoma, mixed lymphoepithelial thymoma, and lymphocyte-predominant thymoma. The relative numbers of these two cell types histologically determine the specific diagnosis. In the epithelial thymoma, the reticular epithelium predominates, with low numbers

of mostly small lymphocytes remaining. The epithelial cells appear as large cohesive, pale, mononuclear cells that resemble epithelioid macrophages. In the mixed cell thymoma, variably sized clusters of neoplastic epithelium appear with many small lymphocytes and fewer medium or large lymphocytes (Fig. 4–18A & B). Large numbers of well-

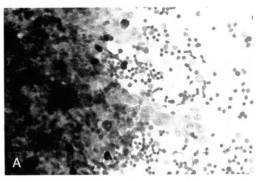

FIGURE 4–18. A, Thymoma. Tissue aspirate. Dog. Mixture of small lymphocytes and clusters of thymic epithelium suggest the lymphoepithelial histologic type. Note the scattered mast cells throughout the stroma at the left side seen as dark cells. (Wright-Giemsa; ×125.)

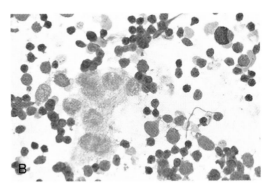

FIGURE 4–18. B, Thymoma. Same case as in Figure 4–18A. This animal presented with no clinical signs except radiographic evidence of an anterior mediastinal mass during screening for elective surgery. Note the small cluster of reticular epithelium that resembles spindle cells. A well-differentiated mast cell is shown in the upper right corner. (Wright-Giemsa; ×250.)

differentiated mast cells are commonly found within thymomas and may give the false impression of a mast cell tumor or metastatic mast cells into a lymph node. Eosinophilic material may be associated with cells in a thymoma (Andreasen et al., 1991), which closely resembles the colloid found in a thyroid tumor and may present a diagnostic dilemma. Immunohistochemistry when performed often indicates positive stain reactions for CD3 and cytokeratin markers.

Clinically, increased survival has been demonstrated for dogs greater than 8 years of age, dogs with the histologic subtype lymphocyte-rich, and dogs without concurrent megaesophagus (Atwater et al., 1994). Myasthenia gravis and pure red cell aplasia are paraneoplastic syndromes associated with thymoma in addition to hypercalcemia. Elevated serum antibodies against acetylcholine receptor has been demonstrated in a dog with megaesophagus (Lainesse et al., 1996). Because of the close association between megaesophagus and myasthenia gravis, it is recommended that all dogs with megaesophagus and thymoma be tested for myasthenia gravis. Chylous effusion has also been associated with thy-

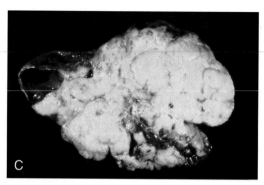

FIGURE 4–18. C, Thymoma. German shepherd dog. This large cranial mediastinal mass measured 12 × 10 × 8 cm. It was partially encapsulated, slightly firm, and tan with occasional mucus-containing cysts. (Photo courtesy of Lois Roth, Angell Memorial Hospital; presented at the 1997 ASVCP case review session.)

moma related to the infiltration of the tumor into the lymphatics. Cats with thymoma were reported to have exfoliative skin lesions (Scott et al., 1995; Day, 1997). These masses are often large (Fig. 4–18C) but because of their localized and often encapsulated appearance, surgical excision is recommended. Metastasis to the lung and liver is uncommon and has been reported in three of eight malignant cases in one study (Bellah et al., 1983).

References

Andreasen CB, Mahaffey EA, Latimer KS: What is your diagnosis? Vet Clin Pathol 1991; 20:15–16.

Atwater SW, Powers BE, Park RD, et al: Thymoma in dogs: 23 cases (1980–1991). J Am Vet Med Assoc 1994; 205:1007–1013.

Bellah JR, Stiff ME, Russell RG: Thymoma in the dog: Two case reports and review of 20 additional cases. J Am Vet Med Assoc 1983; 183: 306–311.

Bookbinder PF, Butt MT, Harvey HJ: Determination of the number of mast cells in lymph node, bone marrow, and buffy coat cytologic specimens from dogs. J Am Vet Med Assoc 1992; 11:1648–1650.

Callanan JJ, Jones BA, Irvine J, et al: Histologic classification and immunophenotype of lymphosarcomas in cats with naturally and experimentally acquired feline immunodeficiency virus infections. Vet Pathol 1996; 33:264–272.

Caniatti M, Roccabianca P, Scanziani E, et al: Canine lymphoma: Immunocytochemical analysis of fine-needle aspiration biopsy. Vet Pathol 1996; 33:204–212.

Carter RF, Valli VEO, Lumsden JH: The cytology, histology, and prevalence of cell types in canine lymphoma classified according to the National Cancer Institute Working Formulation. Can J Vet Res 1986; 50:154–164.

Day MJ: Review of thymic pathology in 30 cats and 36 dogs. J Sm Anim Pract 1997; 38: 393–403.

Day MJ, Lucke VM, Pearson H: A review of pathological diagnoses made from 87 canine splenic biopsies. J Sm Anim Pract 1995; 36:426–433.

Dean GA, Groshek PM, Jain NC, et al: Immunophenotypic analysis of feline haemolymphatic neoplasia using flow cytometry. Comp Haematol Int 1995; 5:84–92.

Desnoyers M, St-Germain L: What is your diagnosis? Vet Clin Pathol 1994; 23:89,97.

Fisher DJ, Naydan D, Werner LL, et al: Immunophenotyping lymphomas in dogs: A comparison of results from fine needle aspirate and needle biopsy samples. Vet Clin Pathol 1995; 24: 118–123.

Fournel-Fleury C, Magnol JP, Bricaire P, et al: Cytohistological and immunological classification of canine malignant lymphomas: Comparison with human non-Hodgkin's lymphomas. J Comp Pathol 1997a; 117:35–59.

Fournel-Fleury C, Magnol JP, Chabanne L, et al: Growth fractions in canine non-Hodgkin's lymphomas as determined *in situ* by the expression of the Ki-67 antigen. J Comp Path 1997b; 117: 61–72.

Goldman EE, Grindem CB: What is your diagnosis? Seven-year-old dog with progressive lethargy and inappetence. Vet Clin Pathol 1997; 26:187, 195–197.

Grindem CB: What is your diagnosis? Vet Clin Pathol 1994; 23:72, 77.

Grindem CB, Page RL, Ammerman BE, et al: Immunophenotypic comparison of blood and lymph node from dogs with lymphoma. Vet Clin Pathol 1998; 27:16–20.

Grooters AM, Couto CG, Andrews JM, et al: Systemic *Mycobacterium smegmatis* infection in a dog. J Am Vet Med Assoc 1995; 206:200–202.

Hendrick MJ, Brooks JJ, Bruce EH: Six cases of malignant fibrous histiocytoma of the canine spleen. Vet Pathol 1992; 29:351–354.

HogenEsch H, Hahn FF: Primary vascular neoplasms of lymph nodes in the dog. Vet Pathol 1998; 35:74–76.

Kirkpatrick CE, Moore FM, Patnaik AK, et al: Argyrophilic, intracellular bacteria in some cats with idiopathic peripheral lymphodenopathy. J Comp Pathol 1989; 101:341–349.

Kiupel M, Bostock D, Bergmann V: The prognostic significance of AgNOR counts and PCNA-positive cell counts in canine malignant lymphomas. J Comp Pathol 1998; 119:407–418.

Kiupel M, Teske E, Bostock D: Prognostic factors for treated canine malignant lymphoma. Vet Pathol 1999; 36:292–300.

Kordick DL, Brown TT, Shin K, et al: Clinical and pathologic evaluation of chronic *Bartonella henselae* or *Bartonella clarridgeiae* infection in cats. J Clin Microbiol 1999; 37:1536–1547.

Lainesse MFC, Taylor SM, Myers SL, et al: Focal myasthenia gravis as a paraneoplastic syndrome of canine thymoma: Improvement following thymectomy. J Am Anim Hosp Assoc 1996; 32: 111–117.

Lau KWM, Kruth SA, Thorn CE, et al. Large granular lymphocytic leukemia in a mixed breed dog. Can Vet J 1999; 40:725–728.

Lennert K, Feller AC: *Histopathology of Non-Hodgkin's Lymphoma (Based on the Updated Kiel Classification)*, 2nd ed. Springer-Verlag, New York, 1992, pp 13–18, 22–39, 115–126.

Lichtensteiger CA, Hilf LE: Atypical cryptococcal lymphadenitis in a dog. Vet Pathol 1994; 31: 493–496.

Mooney SC, Patnaik AK, Hayes AA, et al: Generalized lymphadenopathy resembling lymphoma in cats: Six cases (1972–1976). J Am Vet Med Assoc 1987; 190:897–899.

Moore FM, Emerson WE, Cotter SM, et al: Distinctive peripheral lymph node hyperplasia of young cats. Vet Pathol 1986; 23:386–391.

National Cancer Institute: The non-Hodgkin's lymphoma pathologic classification project: NCI sponsored study of classifications of non-Hodgkin's lymphomas: Summary and description of a working formulation for clinical usage. Cancer 1982; 49:2112–2135.

O'Keefe DA, Couto CG: Fine-needle aspiration of the spleen as an aid in the diagnosis of splenomegaly. J Vet Int Med 1987; 1:102–109.

Raskin RE, Nipper MN: Cytochemical staining characteristics of lymph nodes from normal and lymphoma-affected dogs. Vet Clin Pathol 1992; 21:62–67.

Ruslander DA, Gebhard DH, Tompkins MB, et al: In Vivo 1997; 11:169–172.

Scott DW, Yager JA, Johnston KM: Exfoliative dermatitis in association with thymoma in three cats. Feline Pract 1995; 23:8–13.

Spangler WL, Culbertson MR: Prevalence and type of splenic diseases in cats: 455 cases (1985–1991). J Am Vet Med Assoc 1992; 201:773–776.

Spangler WL, Culbertson MR, Kass PH: Primary mesenchymal (nonangiomatous/nonlymphomatous) neoplasms occurring in the canine spleen: Anatomic classification, immunohistochemistry, and mitotic activity correlated with patient survival. Vet Pathol 1994; 31:37–47.

Steele KE, Saunders GK, Coleman GD: T-cell-rich B-cell lymphoma in a cat. Vet Pathol 1997; 34:47–49.

Teske E, van Heerde P: Diagnostic value and reproducibility of fine-needle aspiration cytology in canine malignant lymphoma. Vet Quart 1996; 18:112–115.

Teske E, van Heerde P, Rutteman GR, et al: Prognostic factors for treatment of malignant lymphoma in dogs. J Am Vet Med Assoc 1994; 205:1722–1728.

Thorn CE, Aubert I. Abdominal mass aspirate from a cat with eosinophilia and basophilia. Vet Clin Pathol 1999; 28:139–141.

Vail DM, Kisseberth WC, Obradovich JE, et al: Assessment of potential doubling time (Tpot), argyrophilic nucleolar organizing regions (AgNOR) and proliferating cell nuclear antigen (PCNA) as predictors of therapy response in canine non-Hodgkin's lymphoma. Exp Hematol 1996; 24:807–815.

Vail DM, Kravis LD, Kisseberth WC, et al: Application of rapid CD3 immunophenotype analysis and argyrophilic nucleolar organizer region (AgNOR) frequency to fine needle aspirate specimens from dogs with lymphoma. Vet Clin Pathol 1997; 26:66–69.

Vail DM, Moore AS, Ogilvie GK, et al: Feline lymphoma (145 cases): Proliferation indices, cluster of differentiation 3 immunoreactivity, and their association with prognosis in 90 cats. J Vet Intern Med 1998; 12:349–354.

Valli VEO, Parry BW: The Hematopoietic System. In: Jubb KVF, Kennedy PC, Palmer N (eds): Pathology of Domestic Animals. 4th ed. Vol. 3, Academic Press, San Diego, CA, 1993, pp 209–257.

Vernau W, Moore PF: Canine chronic lymphocytic leukemia is predominantly a T cell disease (Abstract). Vet Pathol 1999; 36:482.

Walton R, Thrall MA, Wheeler S: What is your diagnosis? Vet Clin Pathol 1994; 23:117, 128.

CHAPTER 5

Respiratory Tract

Mary Jo Burkhard

Amy Valenciano

Anne Barger

Cytologic evaluation of the respiratory tract in correlation with history, clinical data, and imaging results provides invaluable diagnostic information that directly impacts patient management. Cytologic features seen in the respiratory tract following injury, disease, and primary or metastatic neoplasia are dependent largely on the normal underlying structure and function of the cellular elements. Thorough examination of a quality sample is critical for obtaining meaningful cytology results. This chapter describes appropriate sampling techniques and cytologic interpretation of samples from the respiratory tract, including the nasal cavity, larynx, airways, and lung parenchyma.

THE NASAL CAVITY

Normal Anatomy and Histologic Features

Beginning at the nares, the nasal cavity is composed of mucous membrane-lined passages through bony and cartilaginous sinuses divided by the nasal septum and terminating caudally as the osseous ethmoid plate. The vestibule encompasses the nares and narrow anterior portion of the nasal cavity, while the posterior portion, or nasal cavity proper, consists of extensive, delicate, mucous membrane-lined turbinates. The nasolacrimal duct opens through the ventral lateral wall of the vestibule, allowing serous secretion to flow from the conjunctival sac to the rostral nasal cavity. Communicating with the nasal cavity are several paired, air-filled, mucosa-lined paranasal sinuses.

The vestibule is contiguous with the external skin and is lined by keratinized squamous epithelium that transitions into nonkeratinized squamous epithelium followed by ciliated pseudostratified columnar epithelium of the nasal cavity proper, nasal septum, and paranasal sinuses. Serous, mucous, and mixed tubuloalveolar glands are present in the rostral nasal cavity, while olfactory glands, albeit in low numbers in carnivores, are found in the caudal nasal cavity. Nasal-associated lymphoid tissue

(NALT) and lymphoid follicles are found in the submucosa of the caudal nasal cavity and are especially numerous in the nasopharynx.

Collection Techniques and Sample Preparation

When history and clinical signs suggest intranasal disease, the first step toward diagnosis is further characterization of the lesion or disease process by thorough inspection of the external and internal nasal cavity, pharynx, hard and soft palates, and oral cavity including the gingiva and upper dental arcade for oronasal fistulation and periodontal disease. Additionally, palpation for enlarged regional lymph nodes and subsequent aspiration and/or biopsy may provide a valuable indirect means of achieving a diagnosis if disseminated or metastatic disease is present. Adequate visual inspection of the nasal cavity endoscopically and localization via radiographs will enable the appropriate collection techniques to be employed. If an endoscope is unavailable, an otoscope may be used to examine the rostral nasal cavity and with aid of a dental mirror and light, the nasopharynx can also be visualized. Radiography and rhinoscopy should be performed prior to sampling as hemorrhage may hinder radiographic interpretation and obscure visualization during endoscopy.

A complete blood count (CBC) and coagulation profile should be performed prior to sampling as the majority of collection techniques result in hemorrhage owing to the rich venous plexuses underlying the nasal mucosa. Proper patient restraint is tantamount to successful procurement of tissue samples. General anesthesia allows appropriate restraint and placement of an endotracheal tube that, with the cuff properly inflated, together with packing the oropharynx with gauze and tilting the patient's nose downward protect against aspiration during sample collection.

Nasal Swabs

The presence of an acute or chronic nasal discharge indicates upper respiratory tract disease but is nonspecific and may be present with inflammatory, infectious, or neoplastic disorders. Nasal discharge may be unilateral or bilateral and range from serous, suppurative, mucoid to serosanguineous depending on the underlying cause(s). Superficial and deep nasal swabs, although easy to obtain and relatively nontraumatic, often do not provide much information beyond identifying superficial inflammation, secondary bacterial infection, hemorrhage, necrosis, and mucus, often while the underlying disease process remains obscure. As a general rule, invasive techniques allowing collection of tissue deep to the nasal mucosa increase diagnostic potential. However, occasionally the simplest technique can be rewarding, such as the cytologic examination of a nasal swab for the diagnosis of cryptococcosis infection in cats. Therefore, examination of nasal exudate should be performed initially in any nasal disease.

Nasal Flush

Nasal flushing methods have been reviewed elsewhere (Smallwood and Zenoble, 1993). A definitive diagnosis may be made in 50% of the cases unless a more invasive and aggressive flush procedure is used to obtain material for cytologic evaluation. A 6 to 10 French polypropylene or soft red rubber urinary catheter is inserted into the external nares to flush sterile, nonbacteriostatic, physiologic saline or lactated Ringer's solution through the nasal cavity (Fig. 5–1A). A traumatic nasal flush can be accomplished

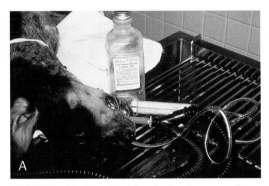

FIGURE 5–1. A, Nasal flush procedure.
Shown is the placement of a flexible tube within the nasal cavity of an anesthetized dog and use of sodium chloride irrigation fluid. (Courtesy of Robert King, Gainesville, FL.)

The fluid and particulate matter retrieved should be placed into an EDTA-anticoagulant tube. If the fluid is turbid, direct smears can be prepared for cytologic evaluation by placing a drop of the fluid on a clean glass slide and placing a second slide on top. After the fluid has spread between the slides, the two slides are pulled apart in a horizontal fashion, with a slight amount of vertical pressure applied if small tissue fragments are present. If the fluid is relatively clear, the sample can be concentrated by centrifugation and smears prepared from the sediment material resuspended in a small volume of remaining supernatant. Further concentration of the sample may be achieved via cytocentrifugation if the equipment is available. If large tissue chunks are retrieved, touch or squash preparations may be prepared for cytologic evaluation. A small aliquot of fluid can be placed in a tube without any additives for culture and sensitivity, or the fluid may be applied to a culture transport swab.

by beveling or nicking the tubing or catheter, creating a rough surface to aid in dislodging tissue. As with any instrument placed into the nasal cavity, penetration through the cribriform plate into the cranial vault can be avoided by measuring the distance from the external nares to the medial canthus of the eye and cutting the tubing or catheter to the appropriate length, or marking the instrument with tape.

Small aliquots (5 to 10 ml) of fluid are introduced into the nasal cavity via a 20- to 35-ml syringe with alternating positive and negative pressure. As the fluid enters the cavity, the tubing or catheter is aggressively moved back and forth against the nasal turbinates in an attempt to free tissue fragments that can be collected on gauze sponges held below the external nares or reaspirated into the collection syringe. An alternative method involves directing a Foley catheter into the oral cavity and retroflexing it around the soft palate into the nasopharynx, inflating the bulb, and lavaging the saline such that the fluid passes through the nasal cavity and out the external nares for collection (Fig. 5–1B).

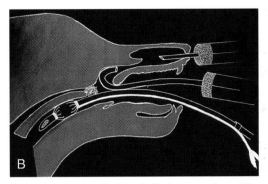

FIGURE 5–1. B, Nasal flush procedure. Diagram of an alternate technique demonstrating placement of a flexible tube retroflexed below and around the soft palate with collection of fluid from the external nares. (From Meyer DJ: The Management of Cytology Specimens. Compend Contin Educ Pract Vet 9:10–16, 1987. Reprinted with permission.)

Fine-Needle Aspiration

Fine-needle aspiration biopsy is most rewarding when mass lesions are present. If a visible external nasal mass is present, direct aspiration may be performed. To sample masses within the nasal cavity, the location is best identified by imaging techniques prior to aspiration. For fine-needle aspiration, a 1- to 1½-inch, 22- to 23-gauge needle is attached to a 3- to 12-ml syringe. The needle is introduced into the mass while strong negative pressure is applied and released several times. The needle should be redirected and the procedure repeated; negative pressure is released prior to withdrawing the needle from the mass. Frequently, only minimal material is collected into the needle hub, which can be expelled onto slides for cytologic evaluation.

Imprint and Brush Cytology

Alligator biopsy forceps are used to obtain a pinch biopsy for impression cytology and histopathology, while an endoscopic brush is used to collect tissue to roll on a glass slide for cytology. Both sampling techniques are typically performed with endoscopic guidance. Imprint cytology can also be performed on core biopsy samples obtained using a Tru-Cut Disposable Biopsy Needle (Travenol Laboratories, Inc., Deerfield, IL). Similarly, the polypropylene portion of an indwelling catheter with the needle removed, or a polypropylene urinary catheter with the end cut at a 45-degree angle, can also be used to obtain tissue specimens. The catheter is pushed into the mass and rotated while applying negative pressure. Tissue can then be rolled on a glass slide or used to make touch imprints for cytologic evaluation before placing in 10% neutral buffered formalin.

If the above procedures yield nondiagnostic results, or are unable to be per-formed secondary to the nature of the lesion or small patient size, exploratory rhinotomy may be necessary to obtain an excisional biopsy in which impression smears for cytology can be prepared, reserving the remainder of the tissue for histopathologic examination. In one study of 54 dogs with nasal tumors, brush and imprint cytology determined correctly an epithelial origin in 88% and 90%, respectively (Clercx et al., 1996). However, in the same study relative to mesenchymal tumors, sensitivity was significantly less, with the histologic type determined in only 20% of brush cytology and 50% of imprint cytology.

Normal Nasal Cytology

Nasal swabs and flushes of healthy animals contain few cells, small amounts of mucus, and low numbers of a mixed population of extracellular bacteria (normal flora) found colonizing the surface of epithelial cells. Ciliated respiratory epithelial cells typically predominate, with lesser numbers of squamous epithelial cells originating from the anterior nasal cavity. Occasionally, basal epithelial cells are present that are round to cuboidal with scant deeply basophilic cytoplasm and round centrally placed nuclei. Respiratory epithelial cells can be seen singly or in small clusters, are columnar, and contain a round, basally located nucleus. Cilia, if present, are located opposite the nucleus and can be an indistinct to a prominent eosinophilic brush border (Fig. 5–2). Goblet cells, similar to columnar respiratory cells, contain a basally located nucleus and are columnar, but lack cilia. These cells are plump with a moderate amount of cytoplasm that appears mostly lightly basophilic and foamy but may on occasion contain numerous prominent, round, purple-staining cytoplasmic mucin granules, similar to the goblet cells of the trachea, bronchi, and

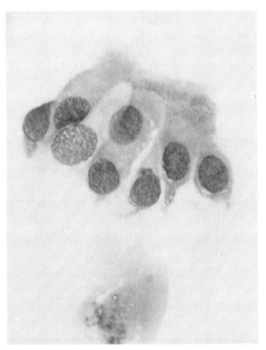

FIGURE 5–2. Normal nasal epithelium. Tissue aspirate. Ciliated columnar epithelium having basally located nuclei is found normally in the upper respiratory tract. (Wright-Giemsa; ×250.)

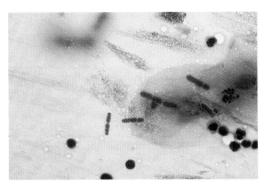

FIGURE 5–3. Oropharyngeal contamination. TTW. Presence of squamous epithelial cells with closely associated *Simonsiella* bacteria suggests contamination by normal microflora or an oronasal fistula. (Wright-Giemsa; ×125.)

large bronchioles. Mucus on cytologic specimens appears as a light basophilic to eosinophilic, amorphous extracellular material that often entraps cells. The degree of hemorrhage observed is contingent upon the collection procedure. Erythrocytes with platelet clumps and white blood cells in numbers and cell type proportions consistent with blood (approximately one white cell per 500 to 1000 red cells) indicate iatrogenic contamination of the sample or peracute hemorrhage. The nasal cavity of the dog and cat harbor large numbers of a mixed population of both aerobic and anaerobic bacteria that are considered normal microflora, including, *Streptococcus* sp., *Staphylococcus* sp., *Escherichia coli*, *Pseudomonas* sp., *Proteus* sp., and *Bordetella bronchiseptica*.

Oropharyngeal Contamination

Oropharyngeal contamination can be seen most frequently in samples collected by flushing techniques and is identified by the presence of a mixed population of bacteria found extracellularly and colonizing the surface of epithelial cells. The presence of *Simonsiella* sp., a characteristic large, rod-shaped bacterium that aligns in rows upon cell division resembling stacked coins, is a hallmark of oropharyngeal contamination (Fig. 5–3).

Hyperplasia/Dysplasia

Chronic inflammation secondary to various infectious and noninfectious etiologies (e.g., trauma, chronic irritation, or neoplasia) is common in the nasal cavity and can have a profound effect upon the integrity and function of normal cellular constituents. Several adaptive mechanisms are employed by cells to survive amid the pathologic stimulus provided by inflammation. Increased numbers of cells, or hyperplasia, is one such mechanism often accompanied by

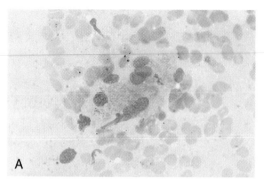

FIGURE 5–4. A, Serous mucous glands of frontal sinus. Tissue imprint. Dog. Clusters of hyperplastic glandular epithelium have an abundant, pale-blue to gray, foamy cytoplasm. (Wright-Giemsa; ×250.) (Courtesy of Rose Raskin, Gainesville, FL.)

dysplasia (Fig. 5–4A). Dysplasia is characterized by loss of architectural organization and is readily identified histologically but less often cytologically. Samples from an inflamed nasal cavity are thus likely to contain numerous clusters and sheets of epithelial cells showing an increased nuclear-to-cytoplasmic ratio, mild to moderate anisocytosis, and increased cytoplasmic basophilia (Fig. 5–4B). Mitotic figures, while

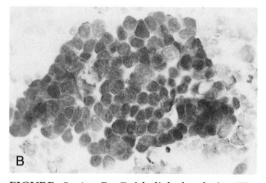

FIGURE 5–4. B, Epithelial dysplasia. Tissue aspirate. This cluster of cells is characterized by increased cytoplasmic basophilia and moderate anisocytosis and anisokaryosis. (Wright-Giemsa; ×125.)

normal in appearance, may be increased as well. Hyperplasia and dysplasia are reversible but may represent early neoplastic changes and can be difficult to cytologically differentiate from well-differentiated carcinoma.

Metaplasia

Another adaptive response to chronic irritation or chronic inflammation is metaplasia, which is a change in cellular differentiation where the susceptible specialized normal cell type is transformed to one that is better able to endure the environmental stress while losing specialized function. In the case of the respiratory system, the columnar respiratory epithelium undergoes squamous metaplasia, resulting in a loss of the ability to produce and secrete protective mucus. Cytologically, metaplasia is detected by the presence of squamous epithelial cells seen individually and in sheets as the primary cell type or admixed with more normal respiratory epithelial cells (French, 1987). Keratinized squamous cells have angular borders and contain abundant hyalinized, basophilic cytoplasm with small, occasionally pyknotic or karyorrhectic nuclei. One must rule out surface epithelial cell contamination as a source of keratinized squamous cells. As with hyperplasia, neoplastic transformation of the squamous cells may occur.

Noninfectious Inflammatory Disease

Foreign Bodies

Nasal foreign bodies occur most commonly in dogs and are usually of plant origin such as plant awns, foxtails, and twigs. Foreign bodies may be directly inhaled into the nasal cavity, or they may enter the cavity traumatically (e.g., buckshot) through the nares or nasal planum, or via the oral cavity by penetrating the palate. Cytologically, specimens are characterized by marked inflammatory reactions ranging from suppurative to pyogranulomatous often with significant hemorrhage and foreign material such as plant material or fibers. Secondary bacterial infection is common.

Allergic Rhinitis

Hypersensitivity reaction may occur in the nasal cavity alone or concurrent with involvement of the lower airways. The inflammation is characterized predominantly by eosinophils, with fewer neutrophils, and occasional mast cells and plasma cells (Fig. 5–5). Increased numbers of goblet cells and abundant mucus may also be seen along with rafts of respiratory epithelial cells secondary to epithelial hyperplasia. Differentials for eosinophilic inflammation include parasitic and fungal infection. Mast cell tumors should also be considered; however, allergic rhinitis often has low numbers of mast cells as part of the inflammatory response, while mast cells are the predominant cell present in mast cell tumors with fewer eosinophils. A few cases of lymphoplasmacytic rhinitis have been reported causing chronic nasal disease in dogs and is

suspected to be immune mediated rather than allergic in origin (Burgener, 1987).

Nasal Polyps

Nasal polyps occur most commonly in cats and are defined as hyperplasia of the mucous membranes or exuberant proliferation of fibrous connective tissue. Polyps originate within the nasopharyngeal region from the eustachian tube, middle ear, or nasopharynx. Nasal polyps are speculated to develop from chronic irritation, although etiology remains unclear. Inflammatory polyps are similar, however these contain a chronic inflammatory infiltrate (Fig. 5–6A). Polyps appear grossly as small, smooth, well-circumscribed, pedunculated masses arising from the mucosal surface of the nasal cavity. Clinical signs are usually apparent when the polyp enlarges enough to occlude the nasopharynx. Cytologically, a mixture of mature lymphocytes and plasma cells are observed commonly admixed with rafts of epithelial cells occasionally with small numbers of neutrophils and macrophages. Evidence of squamous metaplasia and/or dysplasia is frequently seen, which can make the distinction from epithelial neoplasia difficult.

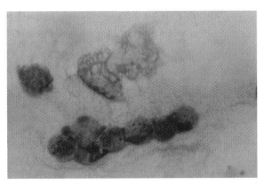

FIGURE 5–5. Allergic rhinitis. Nasal flush. Dog. Several eosinophils are enveloped in basophilic mucus that affects the stain quality of the cells. (Wright-Giemsa; ×250.)

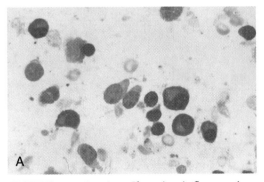

FIGURE 5–6. A, Chronic inflammation. Tissue aspirate. This mononuclear cell population is composed of small and medium-sized lymphocytes and well-differentiated plasma cells. (Wright-Giemsa; ×250.)

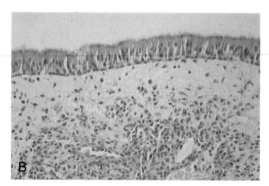

FIGURE 5–6. B, Chronic rhinitis. Nasal mucosa. Cat. Tissue section demonstrating intact respiratory epithelium with mild to moderate infiltration of mononuclear cells into the lamina propria. (H & E; ×100.) (Courtesy of Rose Raskin, Gainesville, FL.)

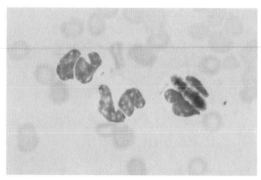

FIGURE 5–7. Septic suppurative rhinitis. Nasal swab. Cat. Three karyolytic neutrophils are present; one of which has phagocytized *Simonsiella* sp. bacteria. An active bacterial infection was present in this animal with chronic sneezing and nasal discharge. (Wright-Giemsa; ×500.) (Courtesy of Rose Raskin, Gainesville, FL.)

Chronic Sinusitis

Recurrent clinical signs of sneezing and nasal congestion may be related to infectious agents, parasites, allergies, foreign bodies, or neoplasia. A cause may not be demonstrated on cytology or histology in some of these cases. Cytologically, respiratory epithelium appears reactive as evidenced by hyperplasia, dysplasia, or metaplasia. Inflammatory infiltrates often consist of mixed mononuclear cells, including small to medium-sized lymphocytes, plasma cells, and macrophages (Fig. 5–6B).

Infectious Causes

Bacteria

With the exception of *Bordetella bronchiseptica* and *Pasteurella multocida,* which may cause acute rhinitis in the dog, primary bacterial rhinitis is rare. Secondary bacterial infection may accompany multiple etiologies, including neoplastic, viral, fungal or parasitic infections, trauma, foreign bodies, dental disease, and oronasal fistulation (Fig.

5–7). Infection with *Mycoplasma* sp. and *Chlamydia* sp. in cats may cause mild upper respiratory signs concurrently with conjunctivitis.

Primary bacterial infection of the nasal cavity is determined by finding large numbers of a fairly monomorphic bacterial population on cytology accompanied by a marked suppurative inflammatory response with numerous phagocytosed bacteria (Fig. 5–8). Culture of the nasal exudate reveals heavy growth of one type of organism. In contrast, normal flora is characterized by low numbers of a heterogeneous population of bacteria found colonizing squamous epithelial cells, lack of an inflammatory response, and mixed bacterial growth on culture. Identification of the bacteria as bacilli or cocci may aid initial institution of antimicrobial therapy, as cocci are typically Gram positive and bacilli are typically Gram negative. Culture and sensitivity are necessary for proper identification of microorganisms. Again, it is emphasized that great care be taken to rule out all possible under-

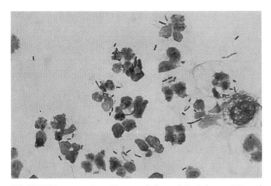

FIGURE 5–8. Bacterial rhinitis. Nasal flush. Large numbers of degenerate neutrophils and a monomorphic population of intracellular and extracellular bacteria, consistent with septic suppurative inflammation. (Wright-Giemsa; ×250.)

lying causes before primary bacterial rhinitis is diagnosed, because it is uncommon.

Viral

Viral infections involving the upper airways usually manifest as acute inflammation that is transient unless there is resultant secondary bacterial infection. In the cat, feline rhinotracheitis virus (feline herpesvirus I) and feline calicivirus are the most common viral agents causing moderate to severe upper respiratory tract signs. Infection with reovirus is associated with mild symptoms. Chronic rhinitis is a common sequela of acute viral infection that has resulted in turbinate damage and subsequent epithelial and glandular hyperplasia. Diagnosis of viral rhinitis is based on patient signalment, history (lack of appropriate vaccination, contact with other animals), clinical signs (mucopurulent nasal discharge, presence of oral ulcers, conjunctivitis, and fever), and direct fluorescent antibody testing of cells obtained from conjunctival scrapings, virus isolation, and serology. Severe and recurrent

rhinitis is common in cats infected with feline leukemia virus (FeLV) and feline immunodeficiency virus (FIV). Canine distemper, adenovirus types 1 and 2, and parainfluenza are the most common causes of canine viral rhinitis, with rare disease resulting from infection with herpes virus and reovirus. Cytologic findings in viral rhinitis include variable amounts and types of inflammatory cells depending on duration and the presence of secondary bacterial infection. Viral inclusions are very rarely observed within the epithelial cells.

Fungal

The diagnosis of fungal rhinitis can be complicated for the same reasons as for bacterial rhinitis, as fungi are common secondary and opportunistic invaders. In addition, *Aspergillus* sp. and *Penicillium* sp. can be cultured from the nasal cavity of some healthy dogs as well as from dogs with neoplasia of the nasal cavity. *Aspergillus* sp. and *Penicillium* sp. are the most common fungal agents in mycotic rhinitis in the dog, whereas *Cryptococcus* sp. occurs most frequently in cats. Upper respiratory tract involvement with *Histoplasma capsulatum* or *Blastomyces dermatitidis* has also been reported but is rare (Table 5–1).

Nasal, lower respiratory tract, and disseminated infection in dogs and cats can occur with aspergillosis and penicilliosis. Aspergillosis often appears as a secondary or opportunistic infection and German shepherd dogs appear over-represented in cases of systemic aspergillosis, but there are reported cases with no clear predisposition. Both fungi are morphologically similar, necessitating culture for differentiation. Because these two fungi are frequent contaminants of the respiratory tract, positive culture should be supported by cytologic or histologic identification of the organism

TABLE 5–1 Mycotic and Protozoal Organisms Commonly Seen in the Respiratory Tract of Dogs and Cats

Organism	Common Locations	Forms Seen	Size	Typical Cellular Location	Typical Inflammation	Cytologic Features
Fungal						
Aspergillus sp.	Nasal cavity Lung	Hyphae	5–7 μm	Extracellular	Granulomatous Pyogranulomatous	Septate, branching hyphae
Blastomyces dermatitidis	Airways Lung	Yeast	5–20 μm	Extracellular	Granulomatous Pyogranulomatous	Broad-based budding
Coccidioides immitis	Lung	Spherules Endospores	10–100 μm 2–5 μm	Extracellular	Granulomatous Pyogranulomatous	Spherules often seen
Cryptococcus neoformans	Nasal cavity Lung	Yeast Unencapsulated forms	8–40 μm 4–8 μm	Extracellular Intracellular (rare)	Variable	Mucoid capsule Narrow-based budding
Histoplasma capsulatum	Nasal cavity Airways Lung	Yeast	1–4 μm	Intracellular Extracellular	Granulomatous Pyogranulomatous	Thin clear capsule
Penicillum sp.	Nasal cavity	Hyphae	5–7 μm	Extracellular	Granulomatous Pyogranulomatous	Cytologically similar to Aspergillus
Pneumocystis carinii	Lung	Cysts Trophozoites	5–10 μm 1–2 μm	Intracellular Extracellular	Granulomatous Pyogranulomatous	Free trophozoites difficult to identify
Sporothrix schenkii	Airways Lung	Yeast	2–7 μm	Intracellular Extracellular	Granulomatous Pyogranulomatous	Cigar-shaped organisms
Rhinosporidium seeberi	Nasal cavity	Endospores Sporangia	5–15 μm 30–300 μm	Extracellular	Mixed	Sporangia rare
Protozoa						
Neospora caninum	Lung	Tachyzoites	1–7 μm	Intracellular Extracellular	Mixed Suppurative	Cytologically similar to Toxoplasma
Toxoplasma gondii	Airways Lung	Tachyzoites	1–4 μm	Intracellular Extracellular	Mixed Suppurative	Banana-shaped forms, single or clustered

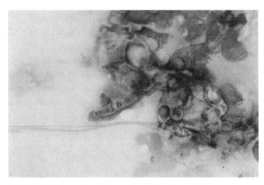

FIGURE 5–9. Fungal rhinitis. Tissue aspirate. Mat of branching fungal hyphae stain intensely basophilic with prominent septations and globose terminal ends. (Wright-Giemsa; ×250.)

with an associated inflammatory reaction in establishing a diagnosis. Cytologically, fungal hyphae are branching, septate, 5 to 7 μm in width, with straight parallel walls and globose terminal ends. Hyphae are found in low numbers or in dense mats often admixed with mucus, inflammatory cells, cellular debris, and necrosis. Hyphae can either stain intensely basophilic with a thin, clear, outer cell wall or appear as negatively staining images against a cellular background (Fig. 5–9). In the latter case, periodic acid-Schiff or silver stains (e.g., GMS) may be used. Occasionally, round to ovoid blue-green fungal spores may be observed and the diagnosis of fungal rhinitis needs to be correlated with clinical signs, associated inflammatory response, and the environmental surroundings of the patient. Infection with *Aspergillus* sp. can be associated with purulent, granulomatous, or pyogranulomatous inflammation. While cytologic characteristics are suggestive of aspergiliosis, culture is necessary for a definitive diagnosis. Similar to bacterial rhinitis, the presence of fungal elements does not rule out underlying neoplasia or other disorders.

Cryptococcus sp. is a common fungal agent causing chronic upper respiratory tract disease primarily in cats but also in dogs. Inhalation is the suspected route of infection. Ocular, cutaneous, and neurologic disease may be present concurrently with rhinitis. Immunity is speculated to play a role in development of infections as well as in spread of the disease, and corticosteroid therapy during infection causes worsening of the symptoms as well as disease progression (Greene, 1998; Medleau et al., 1990). However, underlying diseases, in particular those that are immunosuppressive (e.g., FeLV, FIV), have not been proven to be predisposing factors to infection (Medleau et al., 1990; Flatland et al., 1996). Organisms are readily identified in swabs of nasal exudates or imprints and aspirates from nasal masses (Fig. 5–10A). Positive identification of the organism via cytology is diagnostic, however, serologic testing and fungal culture may also be useful. New methylene blue (Fig. 5–10B) and India ink can be used to demonstrate the negative-staining capsule; however, care must be taken not to mistake air bubbles and fat droplets for organisms. *Cryptococcus* sp. yeast forms are

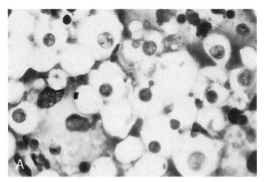

FIGURE 5–10. A, Cryptococcal rhinitis. Nasal swab. Numerous yeast forms with distinctive nonstaining, variably thick, mucoid capsules surrounding granular internal structures. Occasionally, narrow-based budding may be seen. (Wright-Giemsa; ×250.)

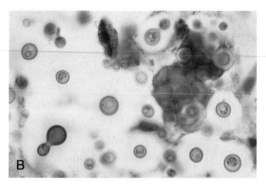

FIGURE 5–10. B, Cryptococcal rhinitis. Nasal discharge. Cat. Prominent budding and internal structure along with the capsule are highlighted by a water-soluble stain. (New methylene blue; ×250.) (Courtesy of Rose Raskin, Gainesville, FL.)

round to oval structures that stain intensely basophilic and, including the capsule, range in diameter from 8 to 40 μm. The organism has a thick, nonstaining mucoid capsule and a granular internal structure that stains red to purple. The capsule material can give the sample a mucinous texture. Occasionally, narrow-based budding may be seen. Unencapsulated or rough forms are 4 to 8 μm and are difficult to distinguish from *H. capsulatum*. Fungal culture and serology are useful in this situation. Cytologic specimens can contain variable degrees of pyogranulomatous inflammation, sometimes with engulfed organisms identified within the macrophages. Occasionally, scant inflammatory cells are observed amid full fields of organisms.

Rhinosporidium seeberi is a fungal organism that is occasionally associated with nasal infection in dogs, appearing grossly as singular or multiple polyps in which numerous small, white, miliary sporangia can be observed on the surface. Pathogenesis of infection is incompletely known but contact with water and trauma to the nasal mucous membranes are predisposing factors. Cytologically, preparations consist of few to large numbers of blue- to magenta-staining spores that range in diameter from 5 to 15 μm and have a slightly refractile capsule and contain numerous, round eosinophilic structures (spherules). In some cases, the spores stain deeply eosinophilic, preventing visualization of the internal structures. Sporangia are not commonly observed in stained smears, however, can be observed in unstained direct preparations (Caniatti et al., 1998). Sporangia are variably sized but often are very large (range 30 to 300 μm), well-defined, globoid structures that undergo sporulation to contain numerous small, round endospores (Fig. 5–11A). The wall of the sporangia is slightly refractile and does not stain, whereas the endospores are lightly basophilic with Romanowsky stains (Fig. 5–11B & C). The endospores within the sporangia are brown when observed microscopically prior to staining. Rhinosporidiosis incites mixed inflammation consisting of neutrophils, plasma cells

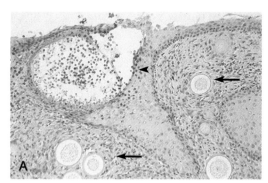

FIGURE 5–11. A, Rhinosporidia sporangia. Nasal mass. Dog. Large mature sporangium with numerous endospores expels its contents to the surface (*arrowhead*). Smaller variably sized sporangia are present within the lamina propria (*arrows*). (H & E; ×50.) (Glass slide material courtesy of John Bentinck-Smith et al., Mississippi State University; presented at the 1984 ASVCP case review session.)

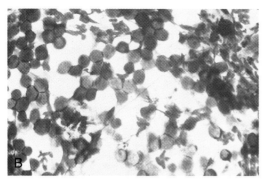

FIGURE 5–11. B, Rhinosporidia endospores. Nasal flush. Dog. Large numbers of round, eosinophilic staining endospores of *Rhinosporidium seeberi*. Sporangia are rarely seen cytologically. (Wright-Giemsa; ×250.)

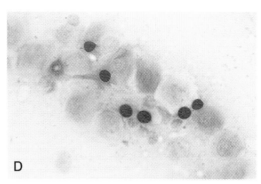

FIGURE 5–11. D, Rhinosporidia endospores. Same case as in Figure 5–11C. Seven magenta stained endospores are prominent. (Periodic acid-Schiff; ×250.)

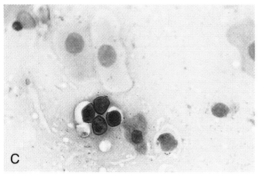

FIGURE 5–11. C, Rhinosporidia endospores. Tissue imprint. Same case as in Figure 5–11A. The capsule outline of four endospores is visible along with associated squamous epithelium. (Wright; ×250.)

and lymphocytes with macrophages, mast cells, and eosinophils less commonly observed. Rosettes of inflammatory cells, particularly neutrophils, around the spores have been observed and considered a useful feature in finding the spores during cytologic examination (Gori and Scasso, 1994). PAS staining enhances finding the spores in cytologic or histologic specimens (Fig. 5–11D).

Parasitic

Parasitic rhinitis is uncommon in dogs and cats and can be asymptomatic or associated with clinical signs (King et al., 1990). Infection with *Capillaria aerophila* is diagnosed by finding the adult nematodes or characteristic ova in nasal secretions. The ova are large (60 × 35 μm), ovoid, with two asymmetrical terminal plugs, and are associated with mixed inflammation often containing eosinophils. The nasal cavity and frontal sinuses of dogs may be inhabited by several forms of the arthropod parasite, *Linguatula serrata*, which is most readily diagnosed by direct visualization via rhinoscopy as the ova are often not readily observed in nasal exudates. The ova are 90 × 70 μm, larvae up to 500 μm, and nymphs 4 to 6 mm. Infection with this parasite most commonly elicits mild signs such as sneezing and nasal discharge, but occasionally results in severe clinical signs. The nasal mite *Pneumonyssus caninum* also is best diagnosed by direct visualization of off-white, 1- to 2-mm adult mites inhabiting the nasal cavity and paranasal sinuses of dogs. Infection results in a mild, transient rhinitis.

TABLE 5–2	Neoplasia of the Nasal Cavity	
Tissue of Origin	**Benign Neoplasia**	**Malignant Neoplasia**
Epithelial	Adenoma	Adenocarcinoma*
	Papilloma	Squamous cell carcinoma*
		Undifferentiated carcinoma
Mesenchymal	Fibroma	Fibrosarcoma*
	Chondroma	Chondrosarcoma*
	Osteoma	Osteosarcoma*
	Leiomyoma	Leiomyosarcoma
		Undifferentiated sarcoma
		Fibrous histiocytoma
		Hemangiosarcoma
		Liposarcoma
		Melanoma
Round (discrete) cell		Lymphoma*
		Transmissible venereal tumor*
		Mass cell tumor*
		Plasmacytoma

* Indicates most common tumor types.

Neoplasia of the Nasal Cavity and Paranasal Sinuses

While neoplasia of the nasal cavity and paranasal sinuses is uncommon in dogs and cats, a diagnosis of upper respiratory tract neoplasia usually carries a poor prognosis, as the majority of nasal tumors are malignant. In both dogs and cats, carcinomas predominate. Dogs are more commonly affected by tumors of the upper respiratory tract than cats, and neoplasia is more commonly diagnosed in older animals (lymphoma and transmissible venereal tumor are notable exceptions). Although no sex predilection has been observed in dogs, male cats are more often affected than females. Tumors can arise from any of the numerous tissue types found in the nasal cavity and paranasal sinuses (Table 5–2). Identification of the site of origin can be difficult, as most malignant tumors are locally invasive and destructive, having ex-

tended into surrounding tissues at the time of diagnosis. The majority of tumors involve the caudal two thirds of the nasal cavity near or adjacent to the cribriform plate, with fewer tumors localized to the paranasal sinuses. Malignant neoplasia often involves the nasal turbinates and septum and can extend through the maxilla into the oral cavity. Extension into the orbit and cranial vault via erosion through the cribriform plate can occur but is uncommon. Metastasis to regional lymph nodes occurs late in the disease process and is most often associated with epithelial tumors. Cytologic evaluation of the regional lymph nodes can provide significant diagnostic information if neoplasia of the nasal cavity is suspected.

The cytologic and even histopathologic diagnosis of malignant neoplasia should be based only on highly diagnostic samples. Emphasis is placed on evaluation of samples obtained from deep tissues as secondary necrosis, inflammation, and hemorrhage are often prominent features of tumors involving the upper airways and can confound the cytologic diagnosis.

Epithelial Neoplasia

Malignant epithelial tumors occur more frequently than their benign counterparts. The most common epithelial tumors of the nasal cavity include adenocarcinomas, squamous cell carcinomas, and anaplastic or undifferentiated carcinomas. Adenocarcinomas and squamous cell carcinomas predominate in dogs and cats, respectively. Cytologic samples from carcinomas tend to be moderately cellular. Neoplastic epithelial cells are present in small aggregates to larger sheets (Fig. 5–12). Adenocarcinomas can be identified by the presence of ring or rosette acinar arrangements that are best visualized at low magnification (e.g., 10×) (Fig. 5–13). Malignant epithelial cells are round to polygonal and typically display numerous criteria of malignancy such as macrocytosis, moderate to marked anisocytosis, anisokaryosis, and an increased nuclear-to-cytoplasmic ratio. The deeply basophilic cytoplasm may contain numerous discrete clear cyto-

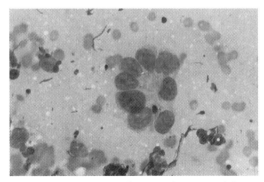

FIGURE 5–13. Adenocarcinoma. Tissue imprint. Glandular origin may be identified by the presence of acinar arrangements. (Wright-Giemsa; ×250.)

plasmic vacuoles or one large clear vacuole (signet ring form) suggestive of secretory product. Nucleolar criteria of malignancy should also be assessed, evaluating for the number of nucleoli per nucleus and any size or shape variations. Anaplastic cells may individualize and appear similar to lymphoid cells but large cell size and periodic sheet formation are helpful in distinguishing the two types of neoplasms (Fig. 5–14A & B). Extracellular secretory material such as mucus may also be identified as eosinophilic amorphous to fibrillar material.

Squamous cell carcinomas (SCC) are distinguished by the presence of cells with angular borders containing abundant, homogenous, glassy cytoplasm, and centrally placed nuclei. The neoplastic cells display a wide range in maturation, ranging from immature small, cuboidal nucleated epithelial cells with deeply basophilic cytoplasm to more mature cells, identified as anucleate, fully keratinized cells with abundant pale basophilic cytoplasm and sharply angulated borders. Evidence of asynchronous development is a useful feature, as fully keratinized cells can be observed with retained large nuclei. Prominent anisokaryosis and variable chromatin patterns ranging from

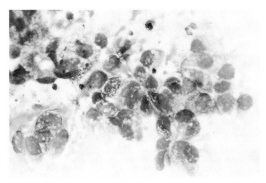

FIGURE 5–12. Nasal carcinoma. Nasal flush. Demonstration of cohesive sheets of pleomorphic cells with highly vacuolated cytoplasm. (Wright-Giemsa; ×125.)

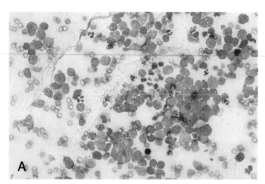

FIGURE 5-14. A, Anaplastic nasal carcinoma. Mass imprint. Dog. Many individualized cells with minimal cohesiveness are present in this highly invasive nasal cavity tumor giving it a "round cell" appearance. (Wright-Giemsa; ×125.) (Courtesy of Rose Raskin, Gainesville, FL.)

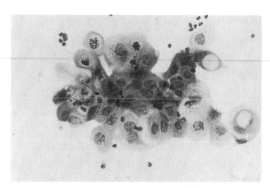

FIGURE 5-15. Squamous cell carcinoma. Nasal flush. Asynchronous keratinization, moderate pleomorphism, and perinuclear vacuolation are typical features of squamous cell carcinoma. The associated suppurative inflammation is commonly seen with this type of tumor. (Wright-Giemsa; ×125.)

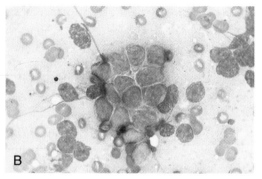

FIGURE 5-14. B, Anaplastic nasal carcinoma. Same case as in Figure 5-14A. Areas of the slide demonstrate a cohesive sheet-like epithelial appearance. (Wright-Giemsa; ×250.) (Courtesy of Rose Raskin, Gainesville, FL.)

smooth (immature) to clumped (mature) may be seen. A few neoplastic squamous cells may also show a perinuclear clearing (perinuclear "halo") or even a few, small, clear, punctate perinuclear vacuoles (Fig. 5-15). Abundant keratinaceous debris represented as amorphous basophilic extracellular material is often scattered about the slides. A common characteristic of SCC is

the presence of a moderate to marked accompanying neutrophilic inflammatory response.

Careful documentation of the above characteristics and criteria of malignancy is critical to a diagnosis of neoplasia of the nasal cavity. If numerous criteria of malignancy are not readily apparent, caution should be used in the diagnosis of neoplasia, as cytologic differentiation of a well-differentiated carcinoma from benign epithelial neoplasia, epithelial hyperplasia, or squamous metaplasia may be impossible, particularly in the presence of inflammation.

Mesenchymal Neoplasia

Mesenchymal neoplasia of the nasal cavity is uncommon. The most common mesenchymal tumors involving the nasal cavity are osteosarcoma, fibrosarcoma, and chondrosarcoma. Cytologic samples are typically of low cellularity consisting of individualized and occasionally small, loose aggregates of oval, plump, or spindle-shaped cells (Fig. 5–16A & B). Cytoplasmic borders are typically ill defined and neoplastic cells may contain few to moderate numbers of fine eosinophilic to purple cytoplasmic granules. Matrix may be observed as streaming, brightly eosinophilic fibrillar material often intimately associated with the neoplastic

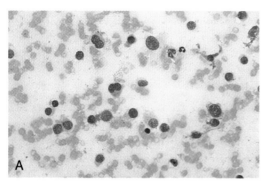

FIGURE 5–16. A, Nasal chondrosarcoma. Tissue imprint. Dog. There was a 3-month history of serous nasal discharge and gurgling sounds from nares. Present are pleomorphic individualized cells that display high nuclear-to-cytoplasmic ratios. Several binucleate forms are noted. (Wright-Giemsa; ×125.) (Courtesy of Rose Raskin, Gainesville, FL.)

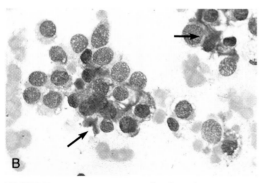

FIGURE 5–16. B, Nasal chondrosarcoma. Same case as in Figure 5–16A. Matrix is observed as streaming magenta, fibrillar material intimately associated with the aggregated neoplastic population (arrows). (Wright-Giemsa; ×250.)

cells. This material is easily confused with mucus.

Often, cytology of mesenchymal cell tumors of the nose, as in other areas of the body, yield equivocal results as the slides are markedly hemodiluted with only a few pleomorphic spindle-shaped cells for evaluation. Also, if significant inflammation is present, reactive fibroblasts are difficult to distinguish from fibrosarcoma. In this case, cytologic evaluation coupled with physical exam and historical and radiographic information raises the index of suspicion for mesenchymal neoplasia, warranting biopsy with histopathologic examination for definitive diagnosis. Additionally, histopathology is often necessary for classification of mesenchymal neoplasia, as the various types do not have many distinguishing cytologic features. Other types of mesenchymal tumors involving the upper airways (see Table 5–2) are uncommon but have cytologic features resembling soft tissue sarcomas in more common sites.

Round (Discrete) Cell Neoplasia

Round (discrete) cell tumors such as lymphoma, mast cell tumors, and transmissible venereal tumors can occur in the nasal cavity. These tumors yield highly cellular preparations composed of individualized neoplastic discrete round cells with distinct cytoplasmic borders. The morphology resembles those seen in other sites.

Lymphoma is the most common discrete cell tumor reported in the nasal cavity of dogs and cats. Lymphoma of the nasal cavity tends to be characterized by a monomorphic population of medium-sized or large immature lymphoblasts with scant deeply basophilic cytoplasm, large round nuclei, finely granular chromatin, and single to multiple nucleoli (Fig. 5–17). Anaplastic nasal carcinomas (see Fig. 5–14A) can indi-

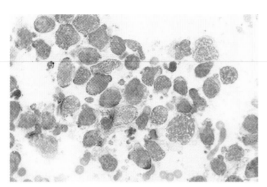

FIGURE 5–17. Nasal lymphoma. Mass imprint. Cat. Monomorphic population of large round cells with scant cytoplasm, irregularly round nuclei, and single prominent single nucleolus. History included 1-year duration of nasal congestion. (Wright-Giemsa; ×250.) (Courtesy of Rose Raskin, Gainesville, FL.)

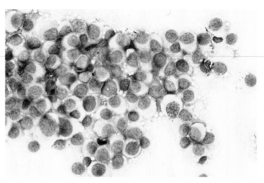

FIGURE 5–18. Transmissible venereal tumor. Nasal mass imprint. Dog. Highly cellular, moderately pleomorphic population of discrete cells with abundant pale cytoplasm, ropy chromatin, and distinct nucleoli. (Wright-Giemsa; ×125.)

vidualize and resemble lymphoma but the presence of very large cells and occasional sheet formation will assist in making the proper diagnosis. Care to distinguish lymphoma from lymphoid hyperplasia, or an inflammatory polyp, is also important (see Fig. 5–6A). In lymphoid hyperplasia, a heterogeneous population of lymphocytes and plasma cells are present, with a predominance of small mature lymphocytes and fewer medium-sized or large lymphoid cells. In some cases, lymphoma is characterized by a predominance of medium-sized lymphocytes with an increased amount of cytoplasm and smooth chromatin lacking nucleoli. Even more problematic are cases where the neoplastic population consists of small, well-differentiated lymphocytes. In such questionable cases, biopsy is imperative for definitive diagnosis of lymphoma.

Canine transmissible venereal tumor (TVT) is a contagious neoplasm involving the external genitalia of both sexes with a low occurrence of metastasis. Spread to the nasal cavity is thought to occur secondary to implantation from a primary genital tumor, however, there are a few cases in which nasal TVTs have been observed as primary tumors without evidence of genital involvement (Peréz et al., 1994; Ginel et al., 1995). Cytologic preparations reveal large numbers of a monomorphic population of large round cells with abundant light to moderately basophilic cytoplasm containing numerous distinct small vacuoles. Nuclei are round with coarse to ropy chromatin with one or two large, prominent nucleoli. Mitoses are frequently observed (Fig. 5–18).

LARYNX

Normal Histologic and Cytologic Features

The larynx is a musculocartilaginous portion of the upper respiratory tract that encompasses the vocal folds, arytenoid cartilage, and glottis. The larynx is composed of an elastic cartilage lined by a stratified squamous epithelium with collections of lymphoid tissue scattered throughout the lamina propria.

Sample Collection

Respiratory stridor, dyspnea, and changes in or loss of vocal tone suggest laryngeal disease. Cytologic evaluation of the larynx is most useful for the characterization of mass lesions, infiltrative processes, or inflammatory disease and depends on obtaining adequate, representative samples. Laryngeal masses, while uncommon, may be detected and stabilized for sampling by palpation. Radiographs may also detect and localize mass lesions, but may be difficult to interpret because of breed variations and superimposition of soft tissues. Ultrasonographic evaluation affords superior visualization of laryngeal masses and guidance for fine-needle aspiration. Ultrasound-guided aspiration through the ventral laryngeal cartilage has not been associated with significant complications even in cats (Rudorf and Brown, 1998).

Laryngoscopy allows direct visualization and sampling of laryngeal masses but requires anesthesia. Lidocaine spray may be necessary in the examination and sampling process, especially in cats, because of laryngospasm. Masses observed during laryngoscopy can be sampled by fine-needle aspiration or brush cytology, or alligator biopsy forceps may be used to obtain pinch biopsies for cytologic touch imprints. Intraluminal sampling may be associated with significant hemorrhage and edema, particularly in cats, which can obstruct the larynx.

Normal Laryngeal Cytology

Samples from the normal larynx are sparsely cellular, typically with only scattered squamous epithelial cells observed. Occasional aspirates or brush techniques may demonstrate small aggregates of well-differentiated lymphocytes in addition to the epithelial cells.

Inflammation

The most common causes of laryngitis in dogs and cats are infectious (e.g., infectious tracheobronchitis, rhinotracheitis) or due to local irritation from inhalation, intubation, or chronic coughing. The laryngeal mucosa and vocal folds are reddened, thickened, and frequently edematous without evidence of mass lesions. Suppurative inflammation is commonly present although observation of etiologic agents is rare. Hemorrhage is identified by the presence of erythrophagocytic macrophages, while a basophilic, granular, proteinaceous fluid background characterizes edema. In chronic inflammation, fibrosis or ossification of the larynx often occurs, resulting in sparsely cellular aspirates containing rare spindle-shaped cells.

Granulomatous Laryngitis

Granulomatous laryngitis is a distinct, but uncommon syndrome seen in dogs, which may mimic the appearance of neoplasia both grossly and cytologically (Oakes and McCarthy, 1994). Mass lesions can be large and may obstruct the laryngeal lumen. The cytologic appearance is similar to that of other granulomatous lesions and is characterized by the presence of large numbers of epithelioid macrophages. In chronic lesions, fibroplasia is prominent and aspiration reveals increased numbers of plump, moderately pleomorphic, and spindle-shaped cells easily confused with mesenchymal neoplasia. Etiologic agents are not observed and the underlying cause of granulomatous laryngitis is unknown.

Reactive Lymphoid Hyperplasia

Reactive lymphoid hyperplasia may occur secondary to infectious, inflammatory, or neoplastic disorders of the larynx. Reactive hyperplasia is differentiated from lymphoma by the heterogeneity of the lymphocyte population, orderly progression from lymphoblasts to small lymphocytes, and the presence of plasma cells and/or other inflammatory cells such as neutrophils, macrophages, and eosinophils.

NEOPLASIA

Tumors of the larynx are uncommon in small animals, however, primary laryngeal tumors have been identified in both dogs and cats. These tumors can arise from the epithelial or musculocartilaginous components of the larynx, or from the lymphoid nodules. Lymphoma is the most commonly reported laryngeal tumor in the cat, followed by squamous cell carcinoma. In dogs, carcinomas and squamous cell carcinomas predominate.

Lymphoma

Lymphoma of the larynx has the same diversity of appearance as lymphoma in other sites. Typically, a uniform population of lymphoblasts is observed (Fig. 5–19). Lymphoma composed of small, well-differentiated, or intermediate-sized lymphocytes may occur but is difficult to diagnose cytologically, necessitating histologic examination of the architecture for invasion.

Squamous Cell Carcinoma

Because the larynx is lined by squamous epithelial cells, it is necessary to ensure that a deep sample is obtained as swabs, scrapings, or shallow aspiration will result in exfoliation of the surface squamous lining. Aspirates from squamous cell carcinomas (SCCs) tend to be of moderate cellularity. Individual cell morphology ranges from basal to fully keratinized squamous epithelial cells (Figs. 5–20A & B). Basal cells are immature cuboidal to round epithelial cells with deeply basophilic cytoplasm, large central nuclei, coarse chromatin, and prominent nucleoli. Mature squamous cells are large with angular borders and contain abundant homogenous cytoplasm and pyknotic or karyorrhectic nuclei. The presence of mature squamous cells alone in a laryngeal sample should not be interpreted as SCC. Multiple stages of epithelial cell development, cellular pleomorphism, and the

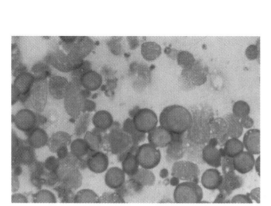

FIGURE 5–19. Lymphoma. Tissue aspirate. Large lymphoblasts with scant deeply basophilic cytoplasm, smooth chromatin, and prominent nucleoli. (Wright-Giemsa; ×250.)

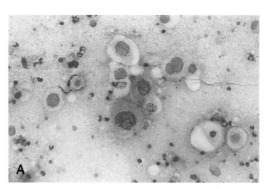

FIGURE 5–20. A, Squamous cell carcinoma. Tissue aspirate. Pleomorphic squamous epithelium in several stages are evident in association with suppurative inflammation. (Wright-Giemsa; ×50.)

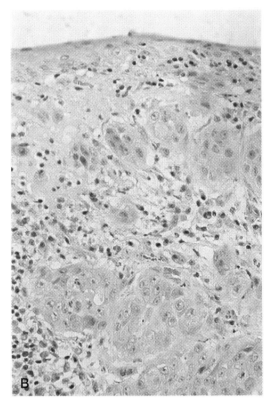

FIGURE 5–20. B, Squamous cell carcinoma. Laryngeal mass. Cat. Clinical signs included brief duration of dyspnea. Tissue section demonstrates islands of neoplastic squamous cells that extend into the deeper tissues. Lymphocytes, plasma cells, and neutrophils are also present indicating chronic active inflammation. (H & E; ×100.) (Courtesy of Rose Raskin, Gainesville, FL.)

presence of asynchronous cytoplasmic and nuclear maturation are necessary for a cytologic diagnosis of SCC. Suppurative inflammation is commonly associated with SCCs and can confound the diagnosis as inflammation can induce squamous dysplasia.

Carcinoma

Carcinoma of the larynx is more prevalent in dogs than in cats. Aspirates are moderately cellular and contain small clusters to sheets of cohesive epithelial cells containing round, centrally located nuclei with coarsely clumped chromatin and basophilic cytoplasm. Well-differentiated carcinomas are characterized by a relatively uniform population of epithelial cells with only mild to moderate anisocytosis and anisokaryosis and single or indistinct nucleoli. Poorly differentiated carcinomas show moderate to marked pleomorphism between clumps of cells as well as within cells of the same cluster. Laryngeal adenocarcinomas are extremely rare, thus acinar formation or ductular structures are not an expected cytologic feature of laryngeal carcinomas.

Mesenchymal Neoplasia

Tumors arising from the musculocartilaginous component are infrequent but include rhabdomyosarcoma, rhabdomyoma, leiomyoma, leiomyosarcoma, fibrosarcoma (Figs. 5–21A & B), chondrosarcoma, and osteosarcoma. These tumors often resemble their counterparts arising in more common sites. In addition, perilaryngeal thyroid carcinomas can invade the larynx. Malignant mela-

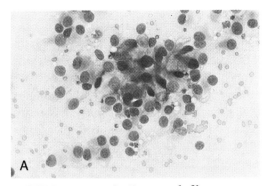

FIGURE 5–21. A, Laryngeal fibrosarcoma. Mass imprint. Cat. Aggregate of mesenchymal-appearing cells in an animal with month-long duration dysphonia and recent dyspnea. (Aqueous-based Wright; ×125.) (Courtesy of Rose Raskin, Gainesville, FL.)

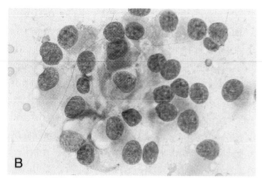

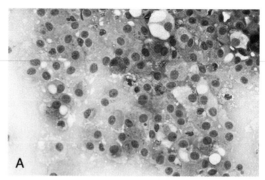

FIGURE 5–21. B, Laryngeal fibrosarcoma. Same case as in Figure 5–21A. An eosinophilic intercellular matrix is associated with the neoplastic cells. Nuclei are oval to round with granular chromatin and small nucleoli. Cytoplasmic borders are wispy and indistinct. Immunohistochemistry was negative for muscle markers. (Aqueous-based Wright; ×250.) (Courtesy of Rose Raskin, Gainesville, FL.)

FIGURE 5–22. A, Laryngeal rhabdomyoma. Mass imprint. Dog. Highly cellular sample with a monomorphic population of large epithelioid-appearing cells having abundant eosinophilic cytoplasm. Large distinct clear vacuoles are present within the cytoplasm of several cells. (Aqueous-based Wright; ×125.) (Courtesy of Rose Raskin, Gainesville, FL.)

noma and granular cell tumors may also arise from the laryngeal region in dogs. Earlier reports of a laryngeal oncocytoma in dogs (Pass et al., 1980; Calderwood-Mays, 1984) have been later reviewed (Meuten et al., 1985) and found to be of muscle origin. Laryngeal rhabdomyomas (Figs. 5–22A & B) have plump, large cells with abundant granular or foamy to vacuolated cytoplasm. Nuclei are large, round to oval, and centrally located with finely clumped chromatin and typically contain a single indistinct nucleolus. Anisocytosis and anisokaryosis are common. The tumor frequently contains large areas of hemorrhage, which may result in hemodiluted specimens with few neoplastic cells. Rhabdomyomas are similar cytologically to oncocytomas in other sites. Ultrastructurally, oncocytomas and rhabdomyomas or rhabdomyosarcomas contain numerous mitochondria and may be distinguished by finding myofibrils and Z-bands as evidence of muscle origin (Tang et al., 1994; Madewell et al., 1988). Definitive di-

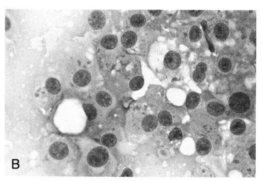

FIGURE 5–22. B, Laryngeal rhabdomyoma. Same case as in Figure 5–22A. Nuclei are generally round with coarse chromatin and small prominent single or multiple nucleoli. The cytoplasm may contain large vacuoles that displace the nucleus or large pink granules. Vacuoles were negative for lipid or glycogen. The neoplastic cells were positive for sarcomeric actin, confirming its muscle origin. (Aqueous-based Wright; ×250.) (Courtesy of Rose Raskin, Gainesville, FL.)

agnosis of muscle origin tumors is best accomplished with immunohistochemical staining for desmin, myoglobin, or actin (Meuten et al., 1985; Madewell et al., 1988).

LARYNGEAL CYSTS

Laryngeal cysts are an uncommon finding in the larynx. Fluid aspirated from the cyst may range from clear to milky and typically has low cellularity.

TRACHEA, BRONCHI, AND LUNGS

Normal Anatomy and Histology of the Airway

The anatomic components of the remaining air passages include the trachea, bronchi, bronchioles, and alveoli. The trachea extends from the base of the larynx to the carina and is composed of incomplete cartilaginous rings supported by connective tissue and smooth muscle lined by ciliated, pseudostratified epithelium. The transition to pseudostratified epithelium begins as the larynx merges with the trachea and extends to the bronchi. Goblet cells are commonly found within the tracheal epithelium. Bronchi are similar in structure to the trachea, however, bronchial cartilaginous rings are complete rather than C-shaped. Smaller airways, or bronchioles, have no cartilaginous support, are composed of smooth muscle, and are lined by ciliated and nonciliated cuboidal epithelium. Terminal bronchioles branch into respiratory bronchioles that further divide into alveolar ducts, alveolar sacs, and alveoli. Alveoli are lined by flattened epithelium (type I pneumocytes) with lesser numbers of more rounded epithelial cells (type II pneumocytes). There is a support network of connective tissue underlying the epithelium consisting of fine reticular, collagenous, and elastic fibers with occasional fibroblasts. Intermingling between the alveoli are numerous capillaries. The lung has a resident population of mac-rophages, which exist primarily in the alveoli. Airways contain foci of bronchus-associated lymphoid tissue (BALT) as well as serous and mucous secreting submucosal glands located in the submucosa and lamina propria. These may be sampled during evaluation of the respiratory tract if the overlying epithelium is damaged.

Collection Techniques

Transtracheal wash and bronchoalveolar lavage are two fairly easy and inexpensive tests with a high diagnostic yield. The samples can be used for cytologic examination of airway disease as well as for culture and sensitivity. In animals with respiratory disease, it is important to obtain a cytologic sample in a manner that will give a large number of well-preserved cells. Indications for sampling the airways are clinical and/or radiographic evidence of respiratory disease. Tracheal washes are helpful for examining the larger airways, whereas bronchoalveolar lavage focuses on the smaller airways and alveoli. Samples of lung parenchyma may be obtained by direct aspiration, especially if the lesion is focal. These diagnostic procedures allow determination of inflammatory processes in the lungs without the risk of lung biopsy. Complications are minimal. There are multiple techniques for collection from the tracheobronchial tract; the two most common will be reviewed for each.

Transtracheal Wash

The purpose of a transtracheal wash (TTW) is to collect fluid and/or cells from the trachea in a sterile fashion. Airway sampling can be achieved by direct penetration through the tracheal wall or via an endotracheal tube. The former technique is usually reserved for larger dogs and the latter is performed in smaller dogs and cats.

Direct aspiration of the tracheal lumen can be performed directly through the cricothyroid ligament or by entering between tracheal rings. The animal should be placed in sternal recumbency for either technique. Sedation is optional depending on the demeanor of the patient. General anesthesia should not be used, as it is essential to maintain the cough reflex to retrieve an adequate sample. Sterility should be maintained, therefore the area of the cricothyroid ligament should be clipped and surgically prepared, and sterile gloves should be worn during the procedure. The cricothyroid ligament is palpable as an indentation between the thyroid and cricoid cartilage of the larynx. Lidocaine should be injected in the skin and underlying subcutaneous tissue of this area. A 16- to 19-gauge jugular catheter is used for the wash depending on the size of the animal. Generally, for dogs greater than 50 lbs, a 16-gauge catheter is recommended, while an 18- or 19-gauge catheter is used in dogs 20 to 50 lbs and a 19-gauge catheter for cats and dogs less than 20 lbs. The needle of the catheter should be inserted, bevel down, through the area of skin where the lidocaine was injected. The needle is passed through the ligament at a downward angle to avoid laceration of the larynx and to decrease risk of oropharyngeal contamination. The catheter is passed over the needle, approximately to the level of the carina (fourth intercostal space). At this time, the needle is removed leaving the catheter in place. Approximately 0.1 to 0.2 ml/kg of warm, sterile, nonbacteriostatic saline is used for the wash. Half of the volume is injected rapidly to induce coughing; the syringe is disconnected and replaced with an empty syringe for aspiration (Fig. 5–23). Aspiration is repeated until no more fluid is obtained. The procedure is then repeated with the remainder of the saline.

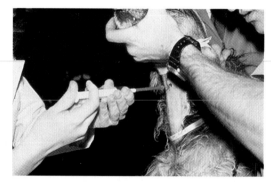

FIGURE 5–23. Transtracheal wash procedure. Injection of saline fluid following proper placement of catheter through the cricoid ligament in a dog. (Courtesy of Robert King, Gainesville, FL.)

This method has the advantage that general anesthesia is not required and the chance of oropharyngeal contamination is low, although still possible if the catheter goes cranially and through the vocal folds of the larynx. Complications with this technique are uncommon but include subcutaneous emphysema, tracheal laceration, hemorrhage, hemoptysis, pneumomediastinum, and/or pneumothorax (Rakich and Latimer, 1989).

An alternative method that is frequently utilized is to perform the TTW by way of an endotracheal tube. General anesthesia is required for this procedure, as an endotracheal tube must be placed. Care must be taken not to contaminate the tip of the endotracheal tube in the oropharynx. After intubation, the cuff is inflated and the animal is placed in lateral recumbency. A jugular catheter or sterile polypropylene urinary catheter is then inserted into the endotracheal tube and extended to the carina. A red rubber feeding tube should not be used because these easily collapse during aspiration of viscous material such as mucus (Smallwood and Zenoble, 1993). Once the catheter is placed, saline is instilled and collected as described above.

Bronchoalveolar Lavage

Bronchoalveolar lavage (BAL) is used to sample the smaller airways and alveoli and is therefore more effective than TTW at sampling the lower respiratory tract. As for tracheal washes, there are multiple techniques for BAL, each with variable advantages. All techniques yield highly diagnostic samples. The two techniques that will be described are bronchoscopy and BAL via an endotracheal tube.

Bronchoscopy is an excellent method for obtaining a BAL, but specific equipment is necessary to utilize this method and the animal must be of adequate size to allow placement of the bronchoscope beyond the mainstream bronchus. The animal must be maintained under general anesthesia. After placement of the endotracheal tube the fiberoptic bronchoscope is passed through the endotracheal tube to allow visualization of the trachea and main stem bronchi (Fig. 5–24). If radiographs have been taken prior to bronchoscopy, a specific lobe(s) of the lung may be selected based upon localization or severity of the lesion. Warmed, sterile saline is injected through the biopsy channel in a volume equaling 5 ml/kg and can be aspirated in the same syringe by applying gentle suction (Hawkins et al.,

1995). Saline can be injected as one large bolus or in 2 to 3 aliquots (Rakich and Latimer, 1989). Multiple lung lobes should be lavaged to increase opportunity to identify etiologic agents or cells with criteria of malignancy. It is advisable to keep animals on supplemental oxygen after the procedure, if not during, to decrease the risk of hypoxia. Advantages of this technique include the ability to visualize the airway, choose the lobe to be lavaged, and biopsy masses, if observed (McCauley et al., 1998).

If a bronchoscope is unavailable or the patient is too small for the scope to pass through the endotracheal tube or beyond the main stem bronchus, a BAL may be performed via an endotracheal tube (Moise and Blue, 1983; Hawkins et al., 1994). The procedure has been well described in cats but may also be performed in dogs. Again, general anesthesia is required. After intubation, the animal should be placed in lateral recumbency, with the most severely affected side down. Following inflation of the endotracheal tube cuff, a syringe adapter is attached to the end of the tube. Three separate aliquots of fluid (warm, sterile saline) should be used, totaling 5 ml/kg. The first aliquot should be injected rapidly and followed immediately by application of suction using the same syringe until no more fluid is obtained. This procedure is repeated for the second and third aliquots. The rear of the animal may be elevated to assist with fluid retrieval.

BAL results in localized edema, alveolar distention, mild to moderate congestion, and alveolar collapse. The prevailing complications of BAL techniques are transient hypoxia, primarily associated with decreased compliance and ventilation/perfusion mismatch (Hawkins et al., 1995). The patient should be supplemented with oxygen for 5 to 20 minutes after the BAL and monitored with a pulse oximeter if available.

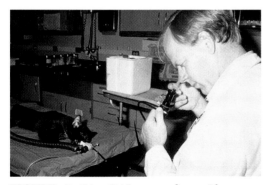

FIGURE 5–24. BAL procedure. Placement of the fiberoptic scope through the endotracheal tube followed by injection of a saline fluid. (Courtesy of Robert King, Gainesville, FL.)

The sample should be immediately placed on ice until it can be examined. Cell counts can be performed on a standard hemocytometer. The accuracy of these counts may be questionable because of increased mucus and lack of standardization of techniques, however, cell counts are crucial following a BAL to establish adequacy of the sample (Hawkins et al., 1990). If fewer than 250 cells/ml are observed, the procedure should be repeated.

The sample should be examined grossly and if large mucus plugs are observed, squash preparations should be made, as cells and organisms are frequently embedded within the mucus. The cellular component of the fluid should be concentrated. Cytocentrifugation is the preferred technique, if available. Alternatively the sample may be centrifuged 10 minutes at 150 $\times$ g, approximately 1000 RPM; the supernatant removed, reserving 50 to 100 μl to resuspend the cell pellet. A direct smear of the concentrated fluid can be made from this sample.

Transthoracic Fine-Needle Aspiration

Transthoracic fine-needle aspiration (FNA) is an excellent diagnostic method for obtaining material from the lung parenchyma for cytologic evaluation. This technique is most useful when diffuse parenchymal disease or discrete mass or masses are identified via radiography or ultrasonography, with discrete lesions yielding higher quality specimens over those with diffuse interstitial involvement. While a specific diagnosis may not be established in all cases, FNA is useful to categorize the lesion as inflammatory or neoplastic (Wood et al., 1998).

While aspiration of the lung parenchyma has the potential for complications, especially in moribund patients or those in severe respiratory distress, these complications are less than with thoracotomy or transtho-

racic biopsy and are typically minimal if a mass lesion is located closely adjacent to the thoracic wall (Teske et al., 1991). Coagulation screening should be performed prior to transthoracic FNA, including a platelet count, prothrombin time (PT), and activated partial thromboplastin time (APTT). Patients with abnormal hemostasis have significantly increased risk of severe hemorrhage following FNA of the lung.

The patient may be placed in sternal recumbency or allowed to stand, however, proper restraint is critical. If the patient is distressed or struggling, sedation may be necessary to minimize risks. Local anesthetic may be injected into the anterior edge of the intercostal space as the intercostal vessels and nerves are located just posterior to each rib. Visualizing the mass or site to be aspirated by ultrasound is ideal as ultrasound guidance allows direct placement of the needle into the lesion, enhancing the likelihood that a diagnostic sample is obtained. If ultrasound is not available, careful localization of the lesion using at least two radiographic views is essential. The right caudal lung lobe is typically sampled with diffuse disease; the standard sampling site is the seventh to ninth intercostal space, one third of the distance from the spinal column to the costochondral junction. The most common mistake is to enter the chest too far caudally and aspirate the liver.

If the lesion to be sampled is close to the body wall, a 22- to 25-gauge, 2-inch needle attached to a 3-ml syringe can be used. If the lesion is deeper, a 22-gauge spinal needle may be required to reach the site. In either case, the needle is introduced through the skin and intercostal muscles at a 90-degree angle to the chest wall in one controlled thrust. Once the chest cavity has been entered, negative pressure is applied to the syringe by pulling back on the plunger slightly. The needle tip is advanced to the appropriate depth as estimated by examination of radiographs or by ultrasonography. The needle should be advanced, withdrawn slightly, and readvanced through the lesion while maintaining negative pressure. Advancing at slightly different angles will enhance the likelihood of obtaining a representative and diagnostic sample, however, it also increases the potential for complications. After sampling the lesion, the syringe is withdrawn, releasing the negative pressure in the syringe just before the needle leaves the chest cavity. Aspiration should be performed quickly, but in a controlled manner. Because the risk of complications increases with the length of time the needle is in the chest cavity, it is usually safer to perform multiple aspirations than to aspirate continuously from a single needle placement.

Typically, only a small amount of material is aspirated into the needle, with little or no material seen in the hub of the needle. The syringe is detached from the needle, filled with air, then reattached to the needle. The air is used to expel the aspirated material within the needle of hub onto slides for preparation and staining. If fluid is aspirated, it should be transferred into an EDTA-anticoagulant tube for fluid analysis, including protein concentration and cell counts as well as cytologic evaluation. If blood or hemorrhagic fluid is aspirated, the procedure should be halted and reattempted at another site. Aspiration of air alone may occur in cases of significant small airway disease. In this instance, aspiration should be repeated with caution, as there is an increased risk of pneumothorax.

The patient should be checked frequently for the first few hours following aspiration to assess respiratory and cardiac function. A chest radiograph should be examined 1 hour after lung aspiration, or at any time following aspiration if the patient's respiration worsens, to evaluate for the presence of pneumothorax, particularly tension pneumothorax.

Normal Cytology of the Trachea and Bronchial Tree

The trachea and bronchi are lined by pseudostratified, ciliated epithelial cells, which are customarily observed in fluid from tracheal but not bronchoalveolar samples (Table 5–3). These cells are elongated with a round, prominent nucleus, and basophilic cytoplasm with cilia at the apical surface (Fig. 5–25). Cuboidal epithelium lines the bronchioles, therefore these cells may be seen in both TTW and BAL samples. Bronchiolar epithelium appear individually or in sheets, and are round to cuboidal with moderate amounts of basophilic cytoplasm and a round, centrally placed nucleus.

Macrophages are the primary cell type observed in both TTW and BAL (Table 5–4). These cells often appear "activated" and contain numerous small, discrete vacuoles in the cytoplasm filled with phagocytized debris (Fig. 5–26). Other leukocytes may be seen less frequently. Neutrophils typically represent less than 5% of the nucleated cell population (Rebar et al., 1980; Hawkins et al., 1990; Vail et al., 1995) although more than 20% has been reported (Lécuyer et al., 1995; Padrid et al., 1991). Other cell types observed in lesser numbers include lymphocytes (5% to 14%), eosinophils in dogs (<5%), and mast cells (<2%) (Rebar et al., 1980; Padrid et al., 1991; Lécuyer et al., 1995; Vail et al., 1995). Rare goblet cells may be observed and are not considered an abnormal finding unless numbers are markedly increased. Goblet cells are approximately the size of macrophages but contain abundant cytoplasm filled with distinctive deeply basophilic, uniform granules (Fig. 5–27). Immunophenotypic studies of canine lymphocytes found in BAL fluid determined the lymphocyte subpopulations were 52% pan T-positive, 22% CD4-positive, and 18% CD8-positive (Vail et al., 1995).

TABLE 5–3	Comparison of Normal and Inflammatory Airway Cytology

Normal cytology of the airway

Ciliated columnar epithelial cells

Cuboidal epithelial cells

Macrophages, often activated

Mucus

Rare goblet cells

Common changes with inflammation

Deeply basophilic, hyperplastic epithelial cells, frequently in sheets

Goblet cell hyperplasia

Inflammatory cells (e.g., neutrophils, macrophages)

Increased mucus and Curschmann's spirals

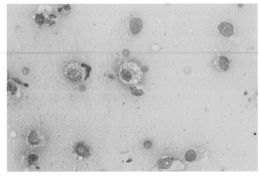

FIGURE 5–26. Macrophages. TTW. The phagocytic cells have abundant cytoplasm with numerous small discrete vacuoles. Mononuclear cells compose the majority of cells in the tracheal and bronchiolar washes. (Wright-Giemsa; ×125.)

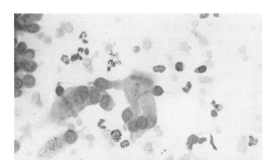

FIGURE 5–25. Normal epithelium. TTW. Several elongate columnar epithelial cells with eosinophilic cilia at the apical surface. (Wright-Giemsa; ×125.)

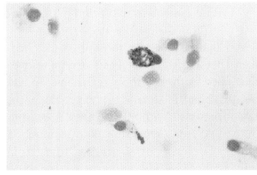

FIGURE 5–27. Goblet cells. BAL. These granulated cells may be observed along with respiratory epithelial cells. Note the distinct large purple intracytoplasmic globules in two central cells. (Wright-Giemsa; ×125.)

TABLE 5–4	Expected Total Cell Count and Percent Range for Cell Types Seen in Bronchoalveolar Lavage Samples from Clinically Healthy Dogs and Cats*					
	Total Cells/μl	Macrophage	Lymphocyte	Eosinophil	Neutrophil	Mast Cell
Dog	<500	70%–80%	6%–14%	<5%	<5%	1%–2%
Cat	<400	70%–80%	<5%	up to 25%	<6%	<2%

* Actual values may differ between techniques. These counts were compiled from the mean values of several references to be used as a general guide.

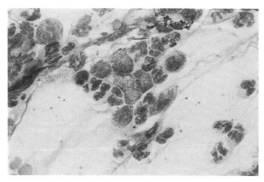

FIGURE 5–28. Eosinophils. TTW. Cells are trapped in mucus and subsequently do not stain well, allowing granules to stain brown, characteristic of tracheal and bronchiolar washes. (Wright-Giemsa; ×250.)

Eosinophil numbers vary markedly between the dog and the cat. Whereas less than 5% is typical of samples from dogs, a range of 5% to 28% eosinophils may be seen in BAL samples from healthy cats (Padrid et al., 1991; Hawkins et al., 1994; Lécuyer et al., 1995; Dye et al., 1996). The percentage of eosinophils in the airways of apparently healthy cats is extremely variable and thus should be interpreted carefully and in correlation with clinical signs and other diagnostic results. Eosinophils are often overlooked in samples because they can appear differently from the typical eosinophil observed in blood. It is not uncommon for the nucleus to be nonsegmented. Eosinophils frequently become entrapped in aggregates of mucus and are unable to stain completely, resulting in dark-red- to brown-staining granules rather than the expected bright-pink-orange granules (Rakich and Latimer, 1989) (Fig. 5–28). In samples that have dried slowly, usually the samples with thick clumps of mucus, the granules also darken.

Normal Histologic and Cytologic Features of the Lung

The lung parenchyma is composed of alveoli, which are lined by type I and type II alveolar epithelial cells or pneumocytes. Type I pneumocytes are flattened epithelial cells that typically cover greater than 90% of the alveolar surface. Type II pneumocytes are cuboidal cells responsible for synthesizing pulmonary surfactant. Alveolar macrophages are commonly seen and when activated become large, highly vacuolated, and highly phagocytic. Aggregates of lymphoid tissue reside in the bronchial submucosa and may be sampled during evaluation of the lung.

Samples from healthy pulmonary tissue are sparsely cellular, and contain primarily respiratory epithelial cells. Respiratory epithelial cells are lightly basophilic, columnar to cuboidal cells containing oval nuclei with granular chromatin situated toward the basilar aspect of the cell (Fig. 5–29). Cilia are

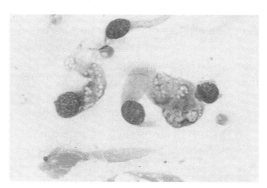

FIGURE 5–29. Upper airway epithelium. Ciliated columnar epithelium and goblet cells shown here are representative of those found in the trachea, bronchi, or large bronchioles. Epithelium becomes cuboidal in the small bronchioles. Two mucus-secreting cells with gray-blue foamy cytoplasm are shown. (Wright-Giemsa; ×250.)

commonly seen on the apical surface. Goblet cells may contain pink to purple granules. Small number of alveolar macrophages, erythrocytes, and white blood cells may also be seen. Mucus is often present in respiratory samples as ribbons of eosinophilic material but is typically sparse in aspirates from normal lung tissue. Obtaining a sample that is cytologically "normal" does not preclude the possibility of pulmonary disease but instead suggests that the lesion was not sampled. Reaspiration should be considered.

Oropharyngeal Contamination

Oropharyngeal contamination is a complication associated with several procedures for sampling the airways. Cytologically this is observed as the presence of mature, keratinized, squamous epithelial cells, often coated with a mixed population of bacteria, including colonies of *Simonsiella* sp., which are considered normal flora of the oropharyngeal cavity or esophagus (see Fig. 5–3). Neutrophils are a common inhabitant of the oral cavity, particularly associated with dental disease. Airway samples with evidence of oropharyngeal contamination cannot be properly evaluated, as it is impossible to determine the source of the inflammation. The procedure should be repeated, with further effort to decrease the potential for oropharyngeal contamination.

One case demonstrated the presence of *Simonsiella* sp. in the transtracheal aspirate of a dog with a congenital bronchoesophageal fistula (Burton et al., 1992). Initially the presence of normal microflora suggested oropharyngeal contamination of the sample or aspiration of pharyngeal material. Although rare, this should be considered when the TTW fluid contains mature squamous epithelium and oral cavity bacteria.

Inflammation of the Tracheobronchial Tract and Lungs

Inflammatory cell populations change dramatically depending on the inciting cause of the inflammation. Neutrophils and eosinophils are observed in more acute processes, whereas increasing numbers of macrophages and lymphocytes, in addition to the neutrophils or eosinophils, are more consistent with chronic inflammation. Inflammation of the lung parenchyma consists predominantly of neutrophils, eosinophils, alveolar macrophages, epithelioid macrophages, or mixed cell population. The type of inflammation may suggest a specific disease process (e.g., large numbers of eosinophils are seen with allergic disease) or cause (e.g., granulomatous inflammation with fungal infection). Increased mucus is a nonspecific finding and may be associated with many pathologic processes of both infectious and non-infectious etiologies.

Chronic Inflammation

There are multiple causes of chronic bronchitis in dogs and cats, including congenital abnormality in structure of the airway or abnormal function of cilia, parasitic infestation, viral or bacterial infection, and inhalation of noxious substances that includes smoke (Padrid and Amis, 1995). In chronic inflammation, macrophages become activated and appear larger with bi- and multinucleated cells frequently observed. Active inflammation is commiserate with the underlying cause, however, suppurative inflammation is the most universal finding. Additional changes are consistent with chronic inflammation (i.e., hyperplastic epithelial cells, goblet cell hyperplasia, and increased mucus). Epithelial hyperplasia is a nonspecific change associated with inflam-

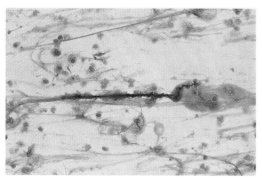

FIGURE 5–30. Curschmann's spiral. TTW.
Lightly basophilic mucus strands and mononuclear cells appear in the background. Inspissated mucus forms a distinct filamentous appearance resembling a bottle washer brush.
These spirals are prominent in cases of chronic
inflammation such as chronic bronchitis.
(Wright-Giemsa; ×25.)

mation, which results in variably sized,
deeply basophilic epithelial cells. Goblet cell
hyperplasia also occurs with inflammation.
Increased mucus is common and may
present as inspissated mucus in a tight spiral coil, also known as a *Curschmann's spiral*, that resembles a bottle washer brush
(Fig. 5–30). These are designative of small
airway disease (see Table 5–3) (Rebar et al.,
1992).

Suppurative Inflammation

Neutrophils are the primary cell seen as
part of a suppurative inflammatory process.
Neutrophils are commonly associated with
both acute and chronic inflammation.
When neutrophils are the predominant cell
type, the sample should be examined closely
for infectious agents, particularly if the neutrophils are degenerate. Degenerate neutrophils, or karyolytic neutrophils, have a
swollen, paler-staining nucleus that has lost
the discrete segmentation of healthy neutro-

phils. Karyolysis is induced by toxic substances or internal enzyme release. If a
sample is not processed immediately, neutrophils can begin to degenerate simply because of poor preservation. These neutrophils will appear karyolytic even in the
absence of bacteria. However, it is still recommended to culture any sample that contains karyolytic neutrophils.

Increased neutrophils may also be observed with noninfectious causes such as
neoplasia or foreign body pneumonia, usually due to an inhaled or aspirated substance (Fig. 5–31A & B). Increased numbers of neutrophils are present in the first
aliquot from a BAL. This is thought to be
due to the relative adhesiveness of cells to
the epithelial lining (Hawkins et al., 1994).
The absolute and relative numbers of neutrophils increase with subsequent BAL or
TTW procedures.

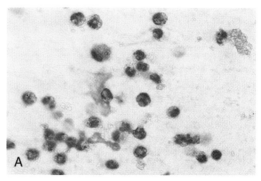

A

**FIGURE 5–31. A, Foreign body reaction
with suppurative inflammation. Sputum
smear. Dog.** Aspiration pneumonia occurred
following a barium study of the digestive tract.
Numerous cells contain yellow-green refractile
crystals and similar material is found in the
background, consistent with the contrast dye.
(Wright-Giemsa; ×250.) (Courtesy of Rose Raskin,
Gainesville, FL.)

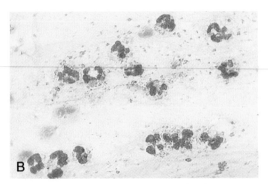

FIGURE 5–31.   B, Barium aspiration. Same case as in Figure 5–31A. Fine yellow-green crystals are seen within degenerate neutrophils. (Wright-Giemsa;   ×250.) (Courtesy of Rose Raskin, Gainesville, FL.)

Macrophagic and Mixed Inflammation

Alveolar macrophages are often seen in either acute or chronic forms of inflammation and may be the predominant cell type

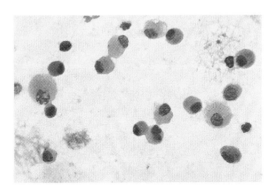

FIGURE 5–32.   Macrophagic inflammation. BAL. Cat. This diagnostic procedure was performed to rule out an active inflammatory condition in the lungs. The cell population consists primarily of alveolar macrophages distinguished by their eccentrically placed nuclei. The cytoplasm is blue-gray with distinct granules noted in some cells. These were later identified as Prussian blue positive for iron and consistent for chronic hemorrhage. (See Figure 5–43B & C.) (Wright-Giemsa;   ×250.) (Courtesy of Rose Raskin, Gainesville, FL.)

(Fig. 5–32). These cells are large, have abundant blue-gray foamy cytoplasm, and are frequently vacuolated and contain phagocytized material. A key feature to aid in the identification of alveolar macrophages is the eccentric position of the nucleus, which is usually round to oval. In chronic disease, binucleate and multinucleate forms may be seen. A mixed inflammatory response composed of nondegenerate neutrophils and macrophages is frequently seen in noninfectious pulmonary disease such as inhalation pneumonia, lung lobe torsion, or necrosis secondary to a neoplastic lesion.

Granulomatous Inflammation

Granulomatous inflammation is characterized by the presence of epithelioid macrophages and multinucleate giant cells. Epithelioid macrophages are blue-gray to pale pink with plump, round, well-defined cytoplasmic borders (Fig. 5–33A). Cells are frequently seen in small aggregates, thus garnering the terminology *epithelioid*. Neu-

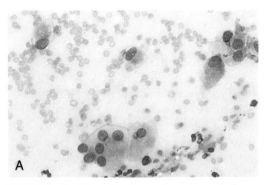

FIGURE 5–33.   A, Granulomatous inflammation. Lung aspirate. Dog. A giant cell with many individualized nuclei is present along with several epithelioid macrophages that have abundant blue-gray cytoplasm and a distinct cytoplasmic outline. (Wright-Giemsa;   ×125.) (Courtesy of Rose Raskin, Gainesville, FL.)

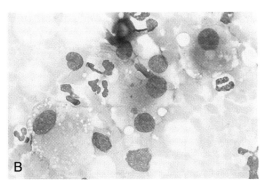

FIGURE 5-33. B, Granulomatous inflammation. Same case as in Figure 5-33A. A tissue aspirate contains epithelioid macrophages along with extracellular yeast forms consistent with *Blastomyces.* (Wright-Giemsa; ×250.) (Courtesy of Rose Raskin, Gainesville, FL.)

trophils may also be present (pyogranulomatous inflammation) as well as lesser numbers of plasma cells, lymphocytes, and eosinophils. Granulomatous or pyogranulomatous inflammation is seen in fungal infections such as blastomycosis (Fig. 5-33B), coccidioidomycosis, and aspergillosis. A foreign body present within the pulmonary parenchyma may provoke the same reaction.

Eosinophilic Inflammation

Clinical signs of allergic bronchitis include coughing, increased tracheal sensitivity, and crackles and wheezes on auscultation of the lung. Cytologically, increased mucus, Curschmann's spirals, and increased numbers of eosinophils characterize this syndrome along with variable numbers of macrophages, neutrophils, and mast cells in TTW and BAL fluids (Fig. 5-34A). Other causes of increased eosinophils in BAL/TTW include eosinophilic granulomas, aspergillosis, paraneoplastic syndromes, and rarely, bacterial pneumonia.

Eosinophils are typically sparse in lung samples (<5%). When eosinophils represent more than 10% of the nucleated cells it suggests a hypersensitivity, parasitic, or infiltrative process (Fig. 5-34B). Eosinophilia in the lung may be seen with or without blood eosinophilia. Other inflammatory cell types may be seen, including small numbers of mast cells, lymphocytes, and plasma cells.

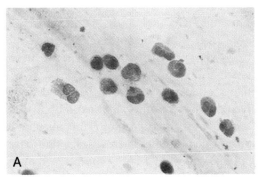

FIGURE 5-34. A, Eosinophilic inflammation. BAL. Cat. Numerous eosinophils accounting for 95% of the cell population were found in this animal with a chronic cough suspected to arise from a hypersensitivity reaction. Eosinophilic amorphous strands consistent with mucus are present in the background. Note the orange to blue-gray color of the eosinophilic granules resulting from altered staining. (Wright-Giemsa; ×250.) (Courtesy of Rose Raskin, Gainesville, FL.)

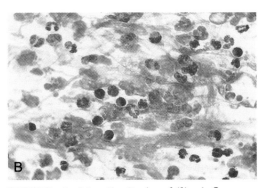

FIGURE 5-34. B, Eosinophilic inflammation. Sputum smear. Dog. Numerous eosinophils are enmeshed in mucus from an animal with heartworm disease that exhibited frequent coughing. (Wright-Giemsa; ×250.) (Courtesy of Rose Raskin, Gainesville, FL.)

Tumor-associated tissue eosinophilia is occasionally seen in dogs and cats and most reports are associated with malignant neoplasia.

Pulmonary eosinophilic granulomatosis is a syndrome identified in dogs characterized by infiltration of the pulmonary parenchyma by eosinophils (Calvert et al., 1988). The cause is unknown but pulmonary eosinophilic granulomatosis is inconsistently associated with *Dirofilaria immitis* infection. Dogs may present with either a diffuse interstitial infiltrate or discrete masses. Cytology is similar in both instances and includes large numbers of eosinophils admixed with variable numbers of macrophages, neutrophils, plasma cells, and basophils (Fig. 5–34C). This condition may be confused cytologically with lymphomatoid granulomatosis, a T-cell lymphoid neoplasm of the lung composed of a similar pleocellular population that is distinguished histologically.

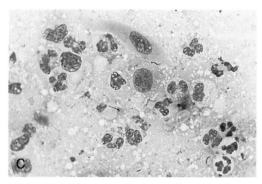

FIGURE 5–34. C, Eosinophilic granulomatosis. Bronchus exudate smear. Dog. Mixed inflammatory cell population consisting of numerous eosinophils and low numbers of neutrophils and mononuclear cells is shown along with a fibroblast (top center). Histopathology of the pulmonary mass confirmed the diagnosis. (Aqueous-based Wright; ×250.) (Glass slide material courtesy of Ruanna Gossett and Jennifer Thomas, Texas A&M University; presented at the 1992 ASVCP case review session.)

Infectious Causes of the Tracheobronchial Tract and Lungs

Neutrophils typically predominate in bacterial, protozoal, viral, and many fungal infections. In addition, macrophages, lymphocytes, and plasma cells may also be present.

Bacterial Pneumonia

Degenerate neutrophils are the most common cell type observed with bacterial pneumonia. Increased mucus and numbers of macrophages are frequently seen also. The presence of intracellular bacteria, in the absence of oropharyngeal contamination, is diagnostic for bacterial pneumonia. Extracellular bacteria are also observed with pneumonia but identification of intracellular bacteria is necessary to confirm the diagnosis. Usually a uniform bacterial population is present, however, a mixed population can be seen with aspiration pneumonia (Rakich and Latimer, 1989).

Bacterial infections may be a primary disease of the lung but are also commonly seen secondary to viral infections, mucosal irritation, decreased mucociliary clearance, fungal infections, and neoplasia. Microbiologic culture and sensitivity is suggested if bacteria are seen since cytologic classification of bacteria based on morphology is frequently unreliable. The presence of filamentous rods is suggestive of infection with either *Nocardia* or *Actinomyces* spp., or rarely *Fusobacterium*. Since these species require special culture techniques, the lab should be alerted if such organisms are suspected.

While *Yersinia pestis* is an uncommon inhabitant of the respiratory tract, the pneumonic form of plague in cats has a high zoonotic potential, thus making identification of the organism crucial. *Yersinia pestis* is a gram-negative bacillus cytologically recognizable as bipolar coccobacilli

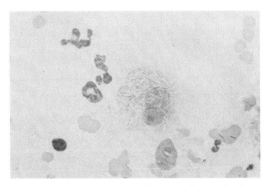

FIGURE 5–35. Mycobacterial infection. Negative staining rod-shaped bacteria located intra- and extracellularly consistent with *Mycobacterium* sp. (Wright-Giemsa; ×250.)

present both intra- and extracellularly with large numbers of degenerate neutrophils. Pneumonic plague accounts for approximately 10% of feline cases and can be seen with or without the classic bubonic presentation (Edison et al., 1991).

While most bacterial pneumonias are associated with suppurative inflammation, mycobacteriosis is typically associated with granulomatous or pyogranulomatous inflammation. In addition to neutrophils, Langhans' multinucleate giant cells and large epithelioid macrophages with ill-defined cytoplasmic borders are seen along with variable numbers of neutrophils. *Mycobacteria* do not stain with routine cytologic stains and can be difficult to visualize. However, careful examination of the cells and background material reveals the presence of distinctive negatively stained thin rod present both intra- and extracellularly (Fig. 5–35). The organisms can be confirmed by acid fast staining. Siamese cats are suggested to have increased susceptibility to mycobacteriosis (Jordan et al., 1994).

Viral Pneumonia

Viral infections are accompanied by neutrophilic inflammation. While this is often due to secondary bacterial infection, BAL samples from cats infected with FIV have been associated with an increase in absolute and relative neutrophil counts. Respiratory viral infections in dogs consist primarily of canine distemper and adenovirus. Rarely, virus inclusion bodies may be seen within the respiratory epithelial cells. In dogs infected with canine distemper virus, finding viral inclusions coincides with systemic signs. Distemper inclusions are eosinophilic, vary in size and can be intranuclear or intracytoplasmic (Fig. 5–36). Inclusions may be observed in multiple cell types, including macrophages, lymphocytes, red blood cells, and epithelial cells. They can persist in lung tissue for more than 6 weeks. Infection with canine adenovirus type-2 results in the presence of large, amphophilic or basophilic intranuclear inclusions, which are most

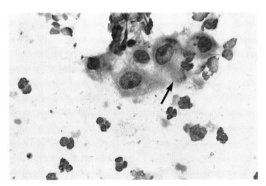

FIGURE 5–36. Distemper inclusions. Lung imprint. Dog. Eosinophilic viral inclusions compatible with canine distemper are present in the macrophage (*arrow*). In the background are several loose crescent-shaped *Toxoplasma* tachyzoites. (Romanowsky stain; ×250.) (Glass slide material courtesy of Ron Tyler and Rick Cowell, Oklahoma State University; presented at the 1982 ASVCP case review session.)

commonly seen in bronchiolar epithelial cells. Acidophilic intranuclear viral inclusions in lung tissue may be seen during the acute infection period in dogs infected with canine herpesvirus, however, these are more commonly demonstrated in nasal respiratory epithelium.

Protozoal Pneumonia

Toxoplasma gondii is a protozoal organism that can cause interstitial pneumonia in the dog and cat. Cytologic examination of TTW or BAL samples reveals an increase in the numbers of nondegenerate neutrophils. *Toxoplasma gondii* tachyzoites are 1 to 4 μm, crescent-shaped bodies with lightly basophilic cytoplasm and a central metachromatic nucleus (Fig. 5–37A & B) (see Table 5–1). Organisms may be found both extracellularly and within macrophages or epithelial cells. These organisms may be retrieved by BAL and rarely by TTW (Hawkins et al., 1996; Bernsteen et al., 1999). However, because toxoplasmosis causes an interstitial pneumonia and these procedures focus on the airways, it may be

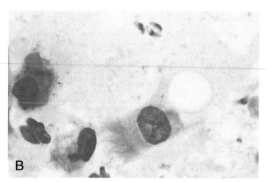

FIGURE 5–37. B, Toxoplasmosis. Same case as in Figure 5–36. Banana-shaped organisms with a metachromatic central nucleus are typical of the tachyzoites of *Toxoplasma gondii*. Similar appearance is found with *Neospora*, which can be distinguished by immunohistochemistry. (Romanowsky stain; ×500.)

difficult to retrieve these organisms unless disease is marked. Absence of organisms in a suspect patient does not negate the possibility of infection. A case of feline toxoplasmosis involving lung aspiration reported the use of immunohistochemical staining for definitive diagnosis (Poitout et al., 1998).

Neospora caninum infection of dogs is usually seen in animals less than 1 year of age and results in progressive, frequently fatal, ascending paralysis. The disease in older dogs is diverse but characterized by systemic involvement, including marked pulmonary infiltration with associated pneumonia (Ruehlmann et al., 1995; Greig et al., 1995). Examination of aspirated samples reveals a mixed inflammatory response composed of neutrophils, macrophages, lymphocytes, plasma cells, and eosinophils with intra- and extracellular tachyzoites indistinguishable from those of *T. gondii*. Tachyzoites are 1 to 5 μm × 5 to 7 μm, oval to crescent-shaped structures with a central metachromatic nucleus and lightly basophilic cytoplasm (see Table 5–1).

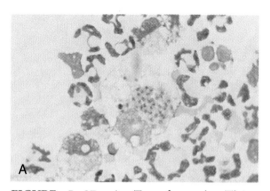

FIGURE 5–37. A, Toxoplasmosis. Tissue aspirate. Mixed inflammation associated with *Toxoplasma gondii* infection. Numerous organisms are seen within the macrophage. Neutrophils show minimal signs of degeneration. (Wright-Giemsa; ×250.)

Fungal Pneumonia

Systemic mycoses spreading to the lungs are more likely to be found in the pulmonary interstitium than in the airways or alveoli. Thus, while mycotic agents may be detected by airway washes (Fig. 5–38A & B) (Hawkins and DeNicola, 1990), fine-needle aspiration of the pulmonary parenchyma has increased sensitivity for detection of these organisms (see Table 5–1).

Blastomyces dermatiditis is a dimorphic fungus that can infect numerous tissues, but the lung is the most frequently involved organ for primary infection. Pulmonary lesions consist of multiple, variably sized nodules dispersed through all lung fields. Infection usually occurs in young, large-breed dogs. The prevalence is less in cats compared to dogs, however, Siamese seem especially susceptible. Organisms can be readily retrieved via TTW/BAL in animals with radiographic evidence of disease (see Table 5–1). Usually, the yeast form of the organism is observed, however, the rare hyphal stage may be seen. The extracellular yeast forms are dark blue, round, and

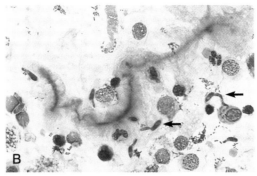

FIGURE 5–38. B, Fungal infection and Curschmann's spiral. Same case as in Figure 5–38A. Tortuous filament of inspissated mucus seen in this chronic fungal infection. Arrows demonstrate short hyphael structures. (Romanowsky stain; ×250.)

5 to 20 μm in diameter with a thick biconcave wall having a granular internal structure (Figs. 5–33 and 5–39). Broad-based budding may be seen. The organisms are likely found in aggregates of mucus and necrotic debris, so that squash preparations are vital for organism identification. Pyogranulomatous or granulomatous inflammation is the rule.

Histoplasma capsulatum is also a dimorphic fungus that infects both cats and dogs.

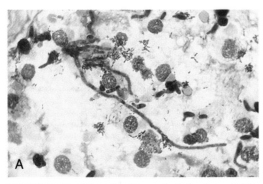

FIGURE 5–38. A, Fungal infection BAL. Dog. Mixed cell inflammation is present along with mixed rod-shaped bacteria and branched, septate hyphae of *Fusarium* sp. (Romanowsky stain; ×250.) (Glass slide material courtesy of Janice Andrews et al., Ohio State University; presented at the 1991 ASVCP case review session.)

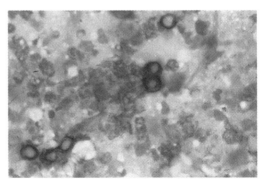

FIGURE 5–39. Blastomycosis. Tissue aspirate. Several large, thick-walled, deeply basophilic yeast forms of *Blastomyces dermatitidis* are present against a necrotic cellular background. (Wright-Giemsa; ×125.)

Pulmonary disease is common in affected cats. In addition to systemic histoplasmosis seen in both species, a self-limiting syndrome of pulmonary histoplasmosis is also seen in dogs. The small yeastlike organisms are round to oval and 1 to 4 μm in diameter with a purple nucleus and lightly basophilic protoplasm surrounded by a thin, clear halo (Fig. 5–40). Organisms are seen within macrophages and neutrophils as well as extracellularly. Macrophages may be packed with organisms. *Histoplasma* induces a mixed to pyogranulomatous reaction.

Coccidioides immitis is primarily a respiratory pathogen found in arid regions. Animals within endemic areas are frequently infected but development of clinical signs is relatively uncommon. Disseminated disease occurs after primary lung infection, especially in dogs. Boxers and Doberman pinschers may be predisposed to disseminated disease. Until recently, cats were thought to be resistant to infection with *Coccidioides,* but more recent cases indicate both susceptibility to infection and development of clinical signs in endemic areas, with respiratory involvement noted in approximately

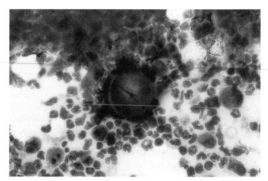

FIGURE 5–41. Coccidioidomycosis. Tissue aspirate. *Coccidioides immitis* spherule with thick, double-contoured wall. (Wright-Giemsa; ×125.)

25% of infected cats (Greene and Troy, 1995). Coccidioidomycosis is associated with pyogranulomatous or granulomatous inflammation. *Coccidioides immitis* spherules (sporangium) are large organisms seen extracellularly (Fig. 5–41). Spherules range in size from 10 to 100 μm in Romanowsky-stained preparations and contain a thick double-contoured wall with finely granular, blue-green protoplasm. Occasionally internal endospores of 2 to 5 μm may be seen. The organism's size and internal structure is easier to appreciate on wet-mount preparations as the fixing and staining process results in shrinkage and distortion of the organism. Organisms are scarce in cytologic preparations and multiple slides may need to be examined to find the organism. TTW or BAL rarely reveals these organisms. Due to the organism's large size, scanning is best done at low magnification (e.g., 10×). Mycelia may rarely be seen in tissue.

Cryptococcosis is frequently associated with the nasal cavity, however, approximately 30% of affected cats also have pulmonary lesions. The capsule material of *Cryptococcus neoformans* can give the sample a mucinous texture. The presence of an inflammatory response varies seemingly re-

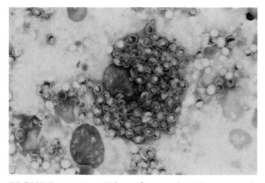

FIGURE 5–40. Histoplasmosis. Tissue aspirate. One macrophage is filled with numerous *Histoplasma capsulatum* organisms as well as many found loose in the background. Note the small size and thin capsule of the yeast form. (Wright-Giemsa; ×250.)

lated to the thickness of the capsule. See Figure 5–10 and the section on nasal cryptococcosis for additional information.

Pneumocystis carinii is most commonly reported in young dogs, primarily miniature dachshunds. Diffuse interstitial pneumonia with abundant foamy fluid present in the alveoli which contain trophozoite and cyst forms. Cysts are extracellular, 5 to 10 μm in diameter, and contain four to eight round, 1- to 2-μm basophilic bodies.

Sporothrix schenckii are uncommonly identified in the pulmonary parenchyma of dogs and cats. When present, large numbers of organisms are seen in infected cats, whereas organisms are relatively rare in other species. Round to oval to cigar-shaped 2×7-μm organisms with a thin, clear halo, slightly eccentric purple nucleus, and lightly basophilic cytoplasm are observed both within macrophages and extracellularly. The presence of cigar-shaped organisms differentiates sporothricosis from histoplasmosis.

Parasitic Infestations

There are numerous parasites capable of infestation of the respiratory tract of dogs and cats. TTW and BAL can be helpful in identifying either the larvae or the egg, however, the etiologic agent is not always present in the sample. An increase in airway eosinophils should be accompanied by heartworm and fecal testing.

Aleurostrongylus abstrusus is a feline metastrongylid lungworm that is generally considered asymptomatic but may induce coughing. Adults live in respiratory bronchioles and alveoli and lay eggs in alveolar spaces, which hatch to release larvae. The ova and larva, not the adults, induce the inflammatory reaction (Rakich and Latimer, 1989). Similar to that seen with *Filaroides* infection, parasitic nodules are more commonly seen in the peripheral lung fields.

Eosinophils and neutrophils found in TTW or BAL samples characterize the early infection associated with the nodules. With time, however, fibromuscular hyperplasia occurs and the reaction appears more fibroblastic. If the organism is observed, it will be the larval stage (Table 5–5). The pale or unstained larvae are usually coiled upon themselves; the tail has a double bend and a dorsal spine.

Paragonimus kellicotti is a trematode primarily seen in cats in North America, while *Paragonimus westermanii* is more common in the orient (Table 5–5). The caudal lung lobes, particularly those of the right side, are frequently affected. This focal location within the caudal lung lobe makes cytologic identification via TTW or BAL difficult, however, the eggs can be readily identified by fecal examination, using either Baermann's apparatus or flotation. Cytologic examination of the inflammatory cysts demonstrates numerous eosinophils with concurrent granulomatous inflammation.

Capillaria aerophila is a parasite of dogs and cats that lives in the trachea and bronchi but also can be found in the nasal passages. Parasite eggs may be observed in bronchial washings (Table 5–5).

Filaroides hirthi is the canine lungworm, which lives in the alveoli and bronchioles (Rebar et al., 1992). Both embryonated ova and larva (Fig. 5–42) can be retrieved by TTW/BAL (Table 5–5) (Rakich and Latimer, 1989). *Filaroides hirthi* and *milksi* can be found in subpleural nodules within the pulmonary parenchyma of dogs (in contrast to *Filaroides osleri,* in tracheal nodules). The adults live in alveoli and respiratory bronchioles. While live worms tend not to generate a significant immune response, dead or dying worms are associated with an eosinophilic granulomatous reaction characterized by variable numbers of eosinophils, macrophages, and fibroblasts. *Filaroides* larvae are more likely to incite a suppurative

TABLE 5–5	Parasites Found in Airway Samples from Dogs and Cats				
Parasite	Species	Location	Adult	Larva	Ova
Filaroides hirthi	Dog	Alveoli Bronchioles	2–3 mm (M) 6–13 mm (F)	240–290 μm	80 × 50 μm Hatch prior to passing in feces
Filaroides osleri	Dog	Trachea Bronchi	5 mm (M) 9–15 mm (F)	232–266 μm S-shaped tail	80 × 50 μm Identical to F. hirthi
Aleurostrongylus abstrusus	Cat	Terminal bronciole Deep lung	7 mm (M) 10 mm (F)	360 μm Notched tail	80 × 70 μm
Paragonimus kellicoti	Cat	Lung parenchyma	7–16 × 4–8 μm red-brown	NA	75–118 × 42–67 μm Single operculum
Capillaria aerophilia	Dog Cat	Trachea Bronchi	15–44 mm	—	58–80 × 30–40 μm Bipolar operculum
Dirofilaria immitis	Dog Cat	Ectopic in lung parenchyma	12–16 cm (M) 25–30 cm (F)	290–330 μm No cephalic hook	—

reaction than an eosinophilic reaction. Cytologic identification of adults or larvae is rare in samples obtained by fine-needle aspiration (Andreasen and Carmichael, 1992). Embryonated ova and larvae are more commonly detected by airway samples (Table 5–5). The ova of *F. osleri* are identical to

those of *F. hirthi*. This parasite is uncommon and causes formation of firm nodules at the tracheal bifurcation (Table 5–5).

Tissue Injury

Hemorrhage

Hemorrhage is characterized cytologically by one or more of several criteria, including erythrophagocytosis, hemosiderin-laden macrophages, and hematoidin crystals (Fig. 5–43A–C). Hemorrhage is a complication of many of the methods used to sample the respiratory tree, so the presence of erythrophagia, preferably with hemosiderin, is important to distinguish pathologic from idiopathic hemorrhage or blood contamination. Hemorrhage is a common sequela to FNA of the pulmonary parenchyma. Increased red blood cells observed in TTW/BAL are observed with congestive heart failure, neoplasia, heartworm emboli, and coagulopathy.

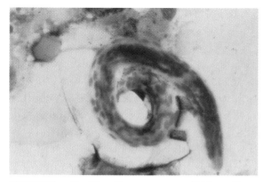

FIGURE 5–42. Lungworm. BAL. Dog. Larva of *Filaroides hirthi* present in an animal with verminous pneumonia. (Wright-Giemsa; ×125.)

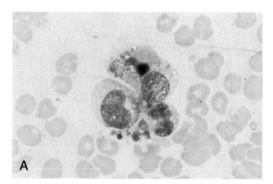

FIGURE 5–43. A, Hemorrhage. Note the macrophage, which has red blood cells as well as hemosiderin within its cytoplasm. Observation of erythrophagia and hemosiderin-laden macrophages is indicative of acute and chronic hemorrhage, respectively. (Wright-Giemsa; ×250.)

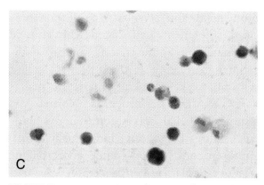

FIGURE 5–43. C, Chronic hemorrhage. BAL. Same case as in Figure 5–43B. Dense blue-black accumulations of iron within the cytoplasm of alveolar macrophages. Nuclear counterstain is red. (Prussian blue; ×250.) (Courtesy of Rose Raskin, Gainesville, FL.)

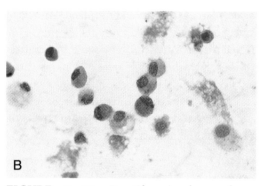

FIGURE 5–43. B, Chronic hemorrhage. BAL. Same case as in Figure 5–32. Alveolar macrophages stain blue-gray and finely granular owing to the presence of hemosiderin, verified in Figure 5–43C. (Wright-Giemsa; ×250.) (Courtesy of Rose Raskin, Gainesville, FL.)

Pulmonary Atelectasis or Collapse

Finding large numbers of respiratory epithelial cells is atypical and suggests pulmonary atelectasis, collapse, or hyperplasia. Respiratory epithelial cells may undergo dysplastic changes (see hyperplasia/dysplasia below) but typically lack sufficient criteria

of malignancy to confirm a diagnosis of neoplasia. Numerous macrophages may also be present.

Necrosis

Necrotic material is frequently aspirated from lungs affected by either inflammatory or neoplastic changes. Necrosis is characterized cytologically by abundant amounts of basophilic granular to amorphous background material. Usually inflammatory or neoplastic cells are admixed within the necrotic debris, however, acellular aspirates or those with only remnant cell membranes or "ghost cells" may occasionally be obtained. In these cases, reaspiration is indicated and particular care should be taken to obtain samples from the periphery of the lesion, while avoiding the necrotic center.

Hyperplasia and Dysplasia of the Lung

Respiratory epithelial cells may undergo hyperplastic or dysplastic changes in non-neoplastic pulmonary disease. Hyperplasia of bronchiolar and alveolar type II pneumo-cytes is frequently associated with chronic inflammation. Epithelial cells appear atypi-cal and share some features with malignant cells but lack sufficient criteria of malig-nancy to diagnose neoplasia. Normal co-lumnar epithelial cells become more cuboi-dal and, when seen individually, may appear round. Nuclei assume a central in-stead of basilar, are increased in size, and contain clumped nuclear chromatin and prominent nucleoli. The cytoplasm stains with an increased basophilia and may con-tain punctate vacuoles.

Increased cell proliferation (*hyperplasia*) and asynchronous cytoplasmic and nuclear maturation (*dysplasia*) can occur secondary to chronic inflammation or tissue necrosis and can be difficult to differentiate cytologi-cally from neoplasia. As a further complica-tion, these cytologic changes may also be seen with preneoplastic changes that can progress to overt neoplasia. Reaspiration at a site more or less affected may be warranted to help characterize the degree of involve-ment or identify an underlying cause. If in-sufficient criteria of malignancy are present cytologically, a lung biopsy is indicated.

Metaplasia of the Lung

Metaplasia is the replacement of normal cells with a secondary, but non-neoplastic, population. Metaplasia can occur in re-sponse to hormonal or growth factor altera-tions or as part of an adaptive response to protect against chronic irritation. Aspirates from areas of squamous metaplasia are moderately cellular, yielding large, round to polygonal squamous epithelial cells that may be seen in sheets or individually (Fig. 5–44). Nuclei are relatively small in com-parison to the cell size (low nuclear-to-cyto-plasmic ratio). Occasional cells may contain pyknotic nuclei as part of the keratinization

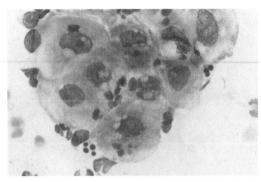

FIGURE 5–44. Squamous metaplasia. In-creased hyalinized cytoplasm associated with squamous metaplasia secondary to chronic in-flammation. (Wright-Giemsa; ×250.)

process. Lightly basophilic cytoplasm is abundant and may become folded or angu-lar as the cells become keratinized. Anuclear superficial cells and keratin flakes may also be seen depending on the degree of keratin-ization. Squamous metaplasia can be diffi-cult to differentiate from squamous neopla-sia. In addition, squamous cell carcinoma of the lung typically originates from areas of squamous metaplasia.

Neoplasia

Primary neoplasia of the lung and respira-tory tree as well as metastatic neoplasia can be diagnosed through bronchial washings and lung aspiration. In dogs and cats, espe-cially young animals, the lung is more often affected by metastatic neoplasia than by pri-mary lung tumors. Both carcinomas and sarcomas may spread to the lung via the blood or lymphatics. Metastatic tumors are more likely to present as multiple nodules scattered throughout all lung lobes, particu-larly the periphery, whereas a solitary lesion is more typical of primary pulmonary neo-plasia. In a study of cats with primary lung tumors, 38 of 45 were identified from cyto-logic samples (Hahn and McEntee, 1997).

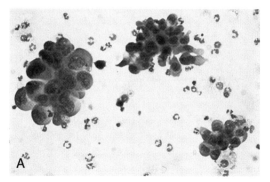

FIGURE 5–45. A, Pulmonary carcinoma. BAL. Dog. Large clusters of pleomorphic epithelium are present along with nonseptic suppurative inflammation. Multinucleated forms are noted. (Romanowsky stain; ×100.) (Courtesy of Robert King, Gainesville, FL.)

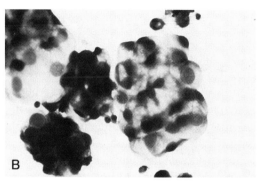

FIGURE 5–45. B, Carcinoma. TTW. Clusters of epithelial cells with pale abundant cytoplasm suggest a secretory function. (Wright-Giemsa; ×50.)

Similarly, cytologic examinations of fine-needle aspirates were helpful in the diagnosis of primary lung tumors in dogs (Ogilvie et al., 1989). The most common neoplasia diagnosed by BAL or TTW is carcinoma, either primary or metastatic (Rebar et al., 1992). Epithelial cells exfoliate readily and can be identified in these samples. It is important to examine cells for criteria of malignancy, specifically variation in cell and nuclear size, prominent nucleoli, multiple nuclei and/or nucleoli, and nuclear molding

(Fig. 5–45A & B). Dysplastic or metaplastic changes to epithelial cells secondary to inflammation can complicate the diagnosis, so the sample should be scrutinized for evidence of inflammation.

Carcinoma

Multiple types of lung carcinomas have been identified in dogs and cats. Adenocarcinomas of bronchogenic or bronchiolar–alveolar origin are most prevalent, however, carcinomas can arise from any level of the respiratory epithelium (Fig. 5–46A & B).

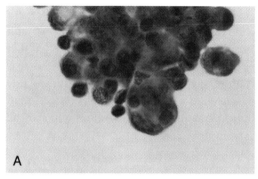

FIGURE 5–46. A, Bronchogenic carcinoma. Note the strongly cohesive arrangement of pleomorphic epithelial cells having high nuclear-to-cytoplasmic ratios. (Wright-Giemsa; ×50.)

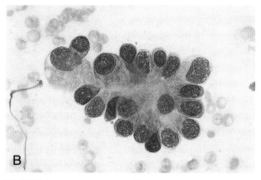

FIGURE 5–46. B, Adenocarcinoma. Lung. Dog. Acinar formation suggesting glandular origin. (Wright-Giemsa; ×250.) (Courtesy of Rose Raskin, Gainesville. FL).

Cytologic differentiation is not possible. Lung carcinomas most typically present as multifocal nodules seen in the periphery of the lung lobes, however, they may involve the entire lung lobe or be present only in the hilar region. Eosinophilic infiltrates may occur in association with bronchoalveolar carcinoma in dogs (Fig. 5–46C).

Numerous carcinomas metastasize to the pulmonary parenchyma, such as mammary carcinomas and carcinomas of the urinary bladder, prostate, and endocrine glands. Cytologic preparations from primary and metastatic carcinomas are similar and the two cannot be definitively differentiated by cytologic evaluation alone (Fig. 5–47).

Aspirates contain moderate numbers of epithelial cells in sheets, aggregates, and clusters with lesser numbers of individualized cells. Individual cells may appear round and can be confused with discrete cell neoplasia but are typically larger than those from discrete cell tumors and can be

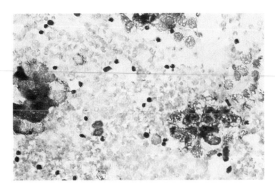

FIGURE 5–47. Metastasis. Lung. Dog. Metastatic lesion suspected to originate from carcinoma affecting the urethra. (Wright-Giemsa; ×125.) (Courtesy of Rose Raskin, Gainesville, FL.)

distinguished by finding cell-to-cell association. Acinar formation indicates glandular origin suggesting an adenocarcinoma. Moderate to marked pleomorphism between clumps of cells as well as within cells of the same cluster is common in pulmonary carcinomas. Nuclei are round and frequently eccentrically placed, and contain coarsely clumped chromatin and prominent, single to multiple nucleoli. Anisokaryosis is common. The cytoplasm is deeply basophilic and punctate vacuolation, particularly in the perinuclear region, is frequently prominent. Other criteria of malignancy that may be seen include nuclear molding, signet ring cell formation, cell or nuclear gigantism, and the presence of binucleate and multinucleate cells.

Only squamous cell carcinoma has distinguishing features that allow for identification during cytologic evaluation. Aspiration of a squamous cell carcinoma tends to yield moderately cellular samples for cytologic evaluation. Cells occur individually, in sheets, and in clusters with moderate to marked variation in cell size, nuclear size, nuclear-to-cytoplasmic ratios, amount of cytoplasm, and degree of keratinization. Indi-

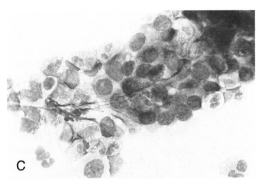

C

FIGURE 5–46. C, Bronchoalveolar carcinoma with eosinophilic infiltrate. Lung mass imprint. Dog. Malignant features present in an epithelial cell cluster along with numerous eosinophils that infiltrate the neoplasm. Suspect a tumor-associated eosinophilic infiltrate. Peripheral eosinophilia was not noted in this case. (Wright-Giemsa; ×250.) (Glass slide material courtesy of Karen Young and Richard Meadows, University of Wisconsin; presented at the 1992 ASVCP case review session.)

vidual cell morphology ranges from basal squamous cells with little or no keratinization to fully keratinized squamous cells. The basal cells are cuboidal to round with deeply basophilic cytoplasm, large central nuclei, coarse chromatin, and prominent nucleoli. Mature squamous cells are large with abundant homogenous cytoplasm and pyknotic or karyorrhectic nuclei. Dysynchrony of cytoplasmic and nuclear maturation is common in squamous cell carcinoma.

Squamous metaplasia may occur with chronic inflammation and caution should be taken when differentiating squamous metaplasia from neoplasia (Fig. 5–44). However, SCC of the lung typically originates from areas of squamous metaplasia of the bronchial epithelium, suggesting that metaplasia may readily proceed to neoplasia in the lower respiratory tract. Bronchogenic tumors frequently contain both glandular and squamous components.

Hemolymphatic Neoplasia

Hemolymphatic neoplasia may disseminate throughout the parenchyma, resulting in diffuse infiltrative disease or as discrete nodules. Several presentations have been identified, including lymphoma, malignant histiocytosis, and lymphomatoid granulomatosis; these are more commonly reported in dogs than in cats.

BAL samples have been shown to be more sensitive than radiographs in diagnosing malignant multicentric lymphoma (Hawkins et al., 1993; Yohn et al., 1994; Hawkins et al., 1995). However, BAL is likely only important for staging this neoplasm, since primary lung lymphoma has not been reported to occur in animals, as it has in humans. The degree of involvement by a monomorphic population of lymphoid cells is helpful in distinguishing between a

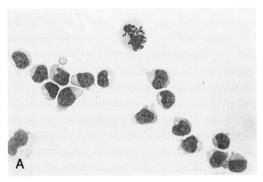

FIGURE 5–48. A, Pulmonary lymphoma. BAL. Dog. Increased fluid cell count (945 cells/μl) with 79% medium-sized lymphocytes having a uniform appearance. Note the atypical mitotic figure in top center. (Wright-Giemsa; ×250.) (Courtesy of Rose Raskin, Gainesville, FL.)

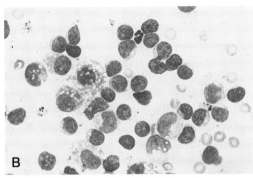

FIGURE 5–48. B, Pulmonary lymphoma. Lung imprint. Same case as in Figure 5–48A. Mixed cell population consisting of activated macrophages and numerous uniform-appearing medium-sized lymphocytes with indistinct nucleoli. Morphology is compatible with the lymphoblastic subtype of lymphoma. (Wright-Giemsa; ×250.) (Courtesy of Rose Raskin, Gainesville, FL.)

reactive population of lymphocytes, especially when malignant features are minimal (Fig. 5–48A & B). Histopathology with immunophenotyping may be helpful in establishing the malignant nature of the lymphoid population (Fig. 5–48C & E).

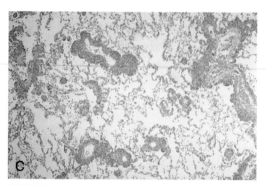

FIGURE 5–48. C, Pulmonary lymphoma. Lung section. Same case as in Figure 5–48B. Neoplastic lymphocytes were present as a cuff around blood vessels and bronchioles primarily. Evidence for vascular invasion and destruction was absent, ruling out lymphomatoid granulomatosis. Dog initially presented with only respiratory signs, suggesting a possible primary pulmonary lymphoma. (H & E; ×25.) (Courtesy of Rose Raskin, Gainesville, FL.)

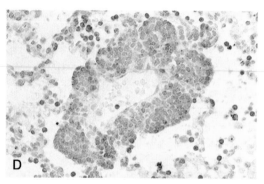

FIGURE 5–48. D, Pulmonary lymphoma. Lung section. Same case as in Figure 5–48C. Positive immunohistochemical staining for T-lymphocytes present around a blood vessel and occasionally within alveolar septa. (CD3 antibody; ×125.) (Courtesy of Rose Raskin, Gainesville, FL.)

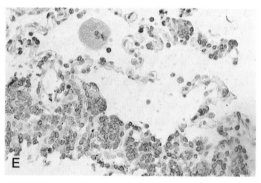

FIGURE 5–48. E, Pulmonary lymphoma. Lung section. Same case as in Figure 5–48D. Dense staining with T-cell markers of cuffed lymphoid cells. Note the negative-stained giant cell with engulfed positive-stained lymphocytes at left of center. (CD3 antibody; ×125.) (Courtesy of Rose Raskin, Gainesville, FL.)

The lung is one of the primary sites of infiltration in canine malignant histiocytosis. Early reports suggested a predisposition in Bernese mountain dogs, golden retrievers, and flat-coated retrievers, however the disease has since been reported in numerous breeds and likely any breed can be affected (Brown et al., 1994). Malignant histiocytosis has also been identified in cats, primarily affecting the liver, spleen, and bone marrow more commonly than the lung (Walton et al., 1997). Malignant histiocytes are large, frequently markedly pleomorphic discrete cells that contain abundant, often vacuolated, deeply basophilic cytoplasm. Nuclei are oval to reniform and contain lacy chromatin and prominent nucleoli (Figure 5–49A–C). A continuum between discrete histiocytic cells and spindled mesenchymal cells may be seen; the appearance frequently varies in masses from the same animal and may even vary from different sites of the same mass. Multinucleated cells are frequently present but the number seen is variable. Cells may also exhibit phagocytosis of erythrocytes and leukocytes, which helps to suggest a histiocytic origin, however, phagocytosis is not a consistent feature. Malignant histiocytosis can be cytologically difficult to differentiate from granulomatous inflammation, large cell anaplastic carci-

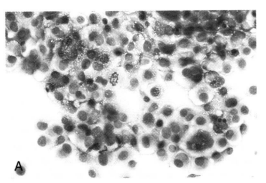

FIGURE 5–49. A, Malignant histiocytosis. Lung imprint. Dog. Highly cellular collection of atypical round cells, many with numerous punctate vacuoles. Note the mitotic figure in the center. (Modified Wright; ×125.) (Glass slide material courtesy of Elizabeth Besteman et al., VA-MD Regional CVM; presented at the 1999 ASVCP case review session.)

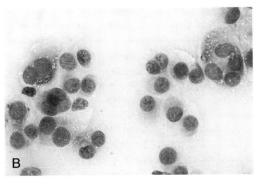

FIGURE 5–49. B, Malignant histiocytosis. Same case as in Figure 5–49A. Binucleate and multinucleate forms are frequent. Cytoplasmic borders range from distinct to indistinct. Immunostaining (not shown) for a histiocytic marker (CD 18) was positive. (Modified Wright; ×250.)

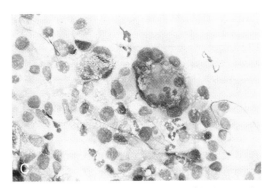

FIGURE 5–49. C, Malignant histiocytosis. Tissue imprint. Numerous vacuolated, pleomorphic histiocytes, including bi-, tri-, and multinucleate cells consistent with malignant histiocytosis. (Wright-Giemsa; ×250.)

noma, large cell T-cell lymphoma, pulmonary lymphomatoid granulomatosis, and plasmacytoma or extramedullary myeloma. Positive immunoreactivity to lysozyme can aid in this differentiation (Brown et al., 1994).

Pulmonary lymphomatoid granulomatosis is an uncommon pleocellular T-cell lymphoid neoplasia that has been recognized primarily in young to middle-aged dogs (Postorino et al., 1989; Fitzgerald et al., 1991; Bain et al., 1997). Typically, extensive infiltration of one or more lung lobes is seen. Pulmonary lymphomatoid granulomatosis is characterized by variable numbers of large pleomorphic mononuclear cells, which range from lymphoid to plasmacytoid to histiocytic in appearance; binucleate cells and mitoses are common (Fig. 5–50A–D). Neoplastic cells may actually compose the minority of the cell population present and are admixed with numerous small lymphocytes, eosinophils, and plasma cells. Peripheral basophilia and canine dirofilariasis have been inconsistently associated with lymphomatoid granulomatous. Grossly and cytolog-

ically, this condition may be confused with eosinophilic granulomatosis, which consists of a pleocellular population of epithelioid cells, macrophages, eosinophils, and lymphocytes. The feature distinguishing them is the presence histologically of vascular and airway invasion and destruction in lymphomatoid granulomatosis that is lacking in eosinophilic granulomatosis.

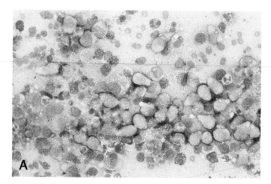

FIGURE 5–50. A, Lymphomatoid granulomatosis. Lung imprint. Dog. Highly cellular sample with many large poorly-differentiated mononuclear cells. (Wright-Giemsa; ×125.) (Courtesy of Rose Raskin, Gainesville, FL.)

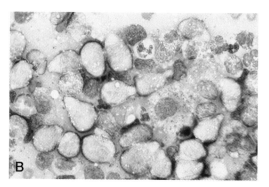

FIGURE 5–50. B, Lymphomatoid granulomatosis. Same case as in Figure 5–50A. Intermixed between the large mononuclear cells are eosinophils, neutrophils, and small lymphocytes. (Wright-Giemsa; ×250.) (Courtesy of Rose Raskin, Gainesville, FL.)

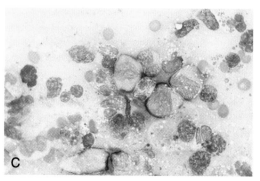

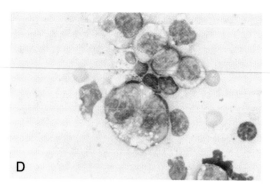

FIGURE 5–50. D, Lymphomatoid granulomatosis. Tissue imprint. Pulmonary lymphomatoid granulomatosis is characterized by the presence of large, discrete, pleomorphic cells such as the one shown here admixed with lymphocytes and eosinophils. (Wright-Giemsa; ×250.)

Mesenchymal Neoplasia

Tumors arising from the pulmonary connective tissue are relatively rare in dogs and cats. These include osteosarcoma, chondrosarcoma, hemangiosarcoma, fibrosarcoma, rhabdomyoma, rhabdomyosarcoma, and schwannoma. When reported, the neoplastic cell population resembles those seen in the more common sites (Fig. 5–51).

Nonrespiratory Aspirate

Occasionally samples are obtained that are not consistent with the lung parenchyma. The two most common nonrespiratory cells seen with lung aspirates are mesothelial cells and hepatocytes. It is important to recognize these cells so as not to mistake them for a neoplastic population. Sheets of mesothelial cells are seen if the lung surface is

FIGURE 5–50. C, Lymphomatoid granulomatosis. Same case as in Figure 5–50A. In some areas, eosinophils are the predominant cell type and normal histiocytes may be found. A malignant T-cell lymphoid population is considered responsible for this neoplasm, as supported by antibody markers. (Wright-Giemsa; ×250.) (Courtesy of Rose Raskin, Gainesville, FL.)

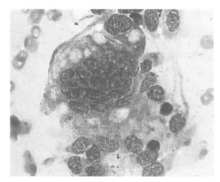

FIGURE 5–51. Giant cell sarcoma. Lung mass. Dog. Multinucleate giant cell and pleomorphic mesenchymal cells from a possible metastatic sarcoma. (Wright-Giemsa; ×250.) (Courtesy of Rick Alleman, Gainesville, FL.)

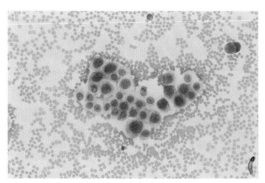

FIGURE 5–52. Mesothelial cells. Lung aspirate. A sheet of mildly pleomorphic mesothelial cells. Presence of mesothelial cells from a lung biopsy indicates sampling of the surface lining only. (Wright-Giemsa; ×50.)

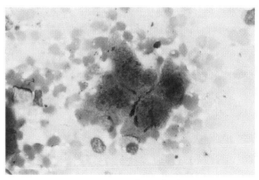

FIGURE 5–53. Accidental liver aspirate. Presence of hepatocytes with prominent canaliculi containing bile, consistent with cholestasis. Liver may be aspirated if the needle is placed too caudally when attempting to sample the lung. (Wright-Giemsa; ×125.)

scraped during the aspiration process. The sheets are comprised of bland, monomorphic cells with angular, cohesive borders resembling fish scales, pale cytoplasm, and small round central nuclei (Fig. 5–52). As the cells begin to exfoliate from the sheets, they round up, become more basophilic, and begin to demonstrate the glycocalyx halo (eosinophilic fringe) associated with more classical mesothelial cells seen commonly in thoracic and abdominal fluids. Aspiration of the liver occurs when the chest is entered too far caudally (Fig. 5–53).

References

Andreasen CB, Carmichael P: What is your diagnosis? Vet Clin Pathol 1992; 21:77–78.

Bain PJ, Alleman AR, Sheppard BJ, et al: What is your diagnosis? An 18-month-old spayed female boxer dog. Vet Clin Pathol 1997; 26:55, 91–92.

Bernsteen L, Gregory CR, Aronson LR, et al: Acute toxoplasmosis following renal transplantation in three cats and a dog. J Am Vet Med Assoc 1999; 215:1123–1126.

Brown DE, Thrall MA, Getzy DM, et al: Cytology of canine malignant histiocytosis. Vet Clin Pathol 1994; 23:118.

Burgener DC, Slocombe RF, Zerbe CA: Lymphoplasmacytic rhinitis in five dogs. J Am Anim Hosp Assoc 1987; 23:565–568.

Burton SA, Honor DJ, Horney BS, et al: What is your diagnosis? Vet Clin Pathol 1992; 21:112–113.

Calderwood-Mays MB: Laryngeal oncocytoma in two dogs. J Am Vet Med Assoc 1984; 184:738–740.

Calvert CA, Mahaffey MB, Lappin MR, et al: Pulmonary and disseminated eosinophilic granulomatosis in dogs. J Am Anim Hosp Assoc 1988; 24:311–320.

Caniatti M, Roccabianca P, Scanziani E, et al: Nasal rhinosporidiosis in dogs: Four cases from Europe and a review of the literature. Vet Rec 1998; 142:334–338.

Clercx C, Wallon J, Gilbert S, et al: Imprint and brush cytology in the diagnosis of canine intranasal tumours. J Sm Anim Pract 1996; 37:423–427.

Dye JA, McKieman BA, Rozanski EA, et al: Bronchopulmonary disease in the cat: Historical, physical, radiographic, clinicopathologic, and pulmonary functional evaluation of 24 affected and 15 healthy cats. J Vet Intern Med 1996; 10:385–400.

Edison M, Thilsted JP, Rollag OJ: Clinical, clinicopathologic, and pathologic features of plague in cats: 119 cases (1977–1988). J Am Vet Med Assoc 1991; 199:1191–1197.

Fitzgerald SD, Wolf DC, Carlton WW: Eight cases of canine lymphomatoid granulomatosis. Vet Pathol 1991; 28:241–245.

Flatland B, Greene RT, Lappin MR: Clinical and serological evaluation of cats with cryptococcosis. J Am Vet Med Assoc 1996; 209:1110–1113.

French TW: The use of cytology in the diagnosis of chronic nasal disorders. Compend Contin Educ Pract Vet 1987; 9:115–121.

Ginel PJ, Molleda JM, Novales M, et al: Primary transmissible venereal tumor in the nasal cavity of a dog. Vet Rec 1995; 136:222–223.

Gori S, Scasso A: Cytologic and differential diagnosis of Rhinosporidiosis. Acta Cytol 1994; 38:361–366.

Greene RT: Cryptococcosis. In Green CE (ed): Infectious Diseases of the Dog and Cat. WB Saunders, Philadelphia, 1998, pp. 383–390.

Greene RT, Troy GC: Coccidioidomycosis in 48 cats: A retrospective study (1984–1993). J Vet Int Med 1995; 9:86–91.

Greig B, Rossow KD, Collins JE, et al: Neospora caninum pneumonia in an adult dog. J Am Vet Med Assoc 1995; 206:1000–1001.

Hahn KA, McEntee MF: Primary lung tumors in cats 86 cases (1979–1994). J Am Vet Med Assoc 1997; 211:1257–1260.

Hawkins EC, Davidson MG, Meuten DJ, et al: Cytologic identification of Toxoplasma gondii in bronchoalveolar lavage fluid of experimentally infected cats. J Am Vet Med Assoc 1996; 210:648–650.

Hawkins EC, DeNicola DB: Cytologic analysis of tracheal wash specimens and bronchoalveolar lavage fluid in the diagnosis of mycotic infections in dogs. J Am Vet Med Assoc 1990; 197:79–83.

Hawkins EC, DeNicola DB, Kuehn NF: Bronchoalveolar lavage in the evaluation of pulmonary disease in the dog and cat. J Vet Intern Med 1990; 4:267–274.

Hawkins EC, DeNicola DB, Plier MC: Cytologic analysis of bronchoalveolar lavage fluid in the diagnosis of spontaneous respiratory tract disease in dogs: A retrospective study. J Vet Intern Med 1995; 9:386–392.

Hawkins EC, Kennedy-Stoskopf S, Levy J, et al: Cytologic characterization of bronchoalveolar lavage fluid collected through an endotracheal tube in cats. Am J Vet Res 1994; 55:795–802.

Hawkins EC, Morrison WB, DeNicola DB, et al: Cytologic analysis of bronchoalveolar lavage fluid from 47 dogs with multicentric malignant lymphoma. J Am Vet Med Assoc 1993; 203:1418–1425.

Jordan HL, Cohn LA, Armstrong PJ: Disseminated Mycobacterium avium complex in three Siamese cats. J Am Vet Med Assoc 1994; 204:90–93.

King RR, Greiner EC, Ackerman N, et al: Nasal capillariasis in a dog. J Am Anim Hosp Assoc 1990; 26:381–385.

Lécuyer M, Dubé P, DuFruscia R, et al: Bronchoalveolar lavage in normal cats. Can Vet J 1995; 36:771–773.

Madewell B, Lund J, Munn R, et al: Canine laryngeal rhabdomyosarcoma: An immunohistochemical and electron microscopic study. Jpn J Vet Sci 1988; 50:1079–1084.

McCauley M, Atwell RB, Sulton RH, et al: Unguided bronchoalveolar lavage techniques and residual effects in dogs. Aust Vet J 1998; 76:161–165.

Medleau L, Barsanti JB: Cryptococcosis. In Green CE (ed): Infectious Diseases of the Dog and Cat. WB Saunders, Philadelphia, 1990, pp. 687–695.

Meuten DJ, Calderwood Mays MB, Dillman RC, Cooper BJ, Valentine BA, Kuhajda FP, Pass DA: Canine laryngeal rhabdomyoma. Vet Pathol 1985; 22:533–539.

Meyer DJ: The management of cytology specimens. Compend Contin Educ Pract Vet 1987; 9:10–16.

Moise NS, Blue JT: Bronchial washings in the cat: Procedure and cytology evaluation. Comp Cont Ed Pract Vet 1983; 5:621–630.

Oakes MG, McCarthy RJ: What's your diagnosis? Granulomatous laryngitis. J Am Vet Med Assoc 1994; 204:1891–1892.

Ogilvie GK, Haschek WM, Withrow SJ, et al: Classification of primary lung tumors in dogs: 210 cases (1975–1985). J Am Vet Med Assoc 1989; 195:106–108.

Padrid P, Amis TC: Chronic tracheobronchial disease in the dog. Vet Clin North Am (Sm Anim) 1995; 22:1203–1222.

Padrid PA, Feldman BF, Funk K, et al: Cytologic, microbiologic and biochemical analysis of bronchoalveolar lavage fluid obtained from 24 healthy cats. Am J Vet Res 1991; 52:1300–1307.

Pass DA, Huxtable CR, Cooper BJ, et al: Canine laryngeal oncocytomas. Vet Pathol 1980; 17: 672–677.

Peréz J, Bautista MJ, Carrasco L, et al: Primary extragenital occurrence of transmissible venereal tumors: Three case reports. Canine Prac 1994; 19:7–10.

Poitout F, Weiss DJ, Dubey JP: Lung aspirate from a cat with respiratory distress. Vet Clin Pathol 1998; 27:10, 21–22.

Postorino NC, Wheeler SL, Park RD, et al: A syndrome resembling lymphomatoid granulomatosis in the dog. J Vet Int Med 1989; 3:15–19.

Rakich PM, Latimer KS: Cytology of the respiratory tract. Vet Clin North Am (Sm Anim) 1989; 19:823–850.

Rebar AH, DeNicola DB, Muggenburg BA: Bronchopulmonary lavage cytology in the dog: Normal findings. Vet Pathol 1980; 17:294–304.

Rebar AH, Hawkins EC, DeNicola DB: Cytologic evaluation of the respiratory tract. Vet Clin North Am (Sm Anim) 1992; 22:1065–1085.

Rudorf H, Brown P: Ultrasonography of laryngeal masses in six cats and one dog. Vet Radiol Ultrasound 1998; 39:430–434.

Ruehlmann D, Podell M, Oglesbee M, et al: Canine neosporosis: A case report and literature review. J Am Anim Hosp Assoc 1995; 31:174–183.

Smallwood CJ, Zenoble RD: Biopsy and cytologic sampling of the respiratory tract. Semin Vet Med Surg 1993; 8:250–257.

Tang KN, Mansell JL, Herron AJ, et al: The histologic, ultrastructural, and immunohistochemical characteristics of a thyroid oncocytoma in a dog. Vet Pathol 1994; 31:269–271.

Teske E, Stokhof AA, van den Ingh TSGAM: Transthoracic needle aspiration biopsy of the lung in dogs with pulmonic diseases. J Am Animal Hosp Assoc 1991; 27:289–294.

Vail DM, Mahler PA, Soergel SA: Differential cell analysis and phenotypic subtyping of lymphocytes in bronchoalveolar lavage fluid from clinically normal dogs. Am J Vet Res 1995; 56:282–285.

Walton RM, Brown DE, Burkhard MJ, et al: Malignant histiocytosis in a domestic cat: Cytomorphologic and immunohistochemical features. Vet Clin Pathol 1997; 26:56–60.

Wood EF, O'Brien RT, Young KM: Ultrasound-guided fine-needle aspiration of focal parenchymal lesions of the lung in dogs and cats. J Vet Intern Med 1998; 12:338–342.

Yohn SE, Hawkins EC, Morrison WB, et al: Confirmation of a pulmonary component of multicentric lymphosarcoma with bronchoalveolar lavage in two dogs. J Am Vet Med Assoc 1994; 204:97–101.

CHAPTER 6

Body Cavity Fluids

Sonjia M. Shelly

Typically there is little fluid present in the peritoneal, pleural, and pericardial cavities. These body cavities are lined by specialized epithelium, termed *mesothelium*. Clinical signs of the presence of fluid include ascites, abdominal pain, dyspnea, muffled heart sounds, and cardiac arrhythmia. Collection and evaluation of fluid from these sites may be therapeutic as well as diagnostic for the presence of inflammatory, hemorrhagic, neoplastic, lymphatic, or bilious conditions. Additionally, further diagnostic tests may be indicated by the cytologic characteristics. Removal and examination of fluid is highly recommended unless anesthetic risks are present or further injury is likely.

COLLECTION TECHNIQUES

Abdominal Fluid

Place the patient in left lateral recumbency and restrain. Clip and surgically prepare an area (e.g., 2 to 3 inches square) between the bladder and umbilicus and just lateral to the midline. The bladder should be emptied prior to performing paracentesis. Infiltrate a small area with local anesthetic. Use an 18- to 20-gauge needle to penetrate the abdomen. For a complete description of the technique see Kirk et al. (1990). Allow the animal to rest quietly while fluid is being removed. Moving the animal or allowing the patient to move while the needle is in the abdomen can result in laceration of the bowel. Some investigators prefer to have the patient standing for fluid removal, however, it is more likely that the omentum will occlude the needle if the patient is in a standing position.

Pleural Fluid

For removal of fluid from the thorax, the patient should be in a standing or comfortable sitting position. Clip the hair and surgically prepare the thoracic wall from the 5th to the 11th intercostal space. Infiltrate a small area at the 7th to 8th intercostal space at the level of the costochondral junction with local anesthetic. It is best to attach extension tubing to the hub of the needle and a three-way stopcock; or use an intravenous Intrafusor system (Sorenson Research Co., Salt Lake City, UT) for removal of pleural fluid. Insert the needle or Intrafusor into the chest wall at the surgically prepared site taking care to avoid the intercostal artery located just caudal to each rib. For a complete description of this technique see Kirk et al. (1990).

Pericardial Fluid

For removal of fluid from the pericardial sac, sedate the patient if necessary. Surgically prepare an area over the lower to mid 4th intercostal space bilaterally. Place the patient in lateral recumbency. Infiltrate an area at the costochondral junction, or approximately where the lower and mid thorax meet, with local anesthetic. Use a venocath or Intrafusor system with a three-way valve to which a 30-ml syringe is attached. Always maintain negative pressure on the syringe as the chest wall is punctured. Carefully advance the needle into the 4th intercostal space in the direction of the heart. Advance the needle until resistance is met (from the pericardium). A release will be felt as the needle enters the pericardial sac. Thread the tubing through the needle so that the tubing is securely within the pericardial sac. For a complete description of this technique, see Kirk et al. (1990).

SAMPLE HANDLING

Note the color and character of the fluid initially upon removal (Fig. 6–1). If the fluid is clear initially then turns red, iatrogenic blood contamination is likely. Fluid should be collected in a lavender-top tube (EDTA anticoagulant). If the fluid appears

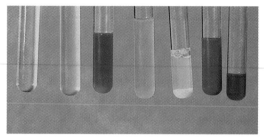

FIGURE 6–1. Gross appearance of various effusions. From left to right these are: (a) clear and colorless—transudate; (b) yellow and slight turbid—modified transudate; (c) red and slightly turbid (likely hemolyzed red blood cells)—hemorrhage; (d) orange and turbid—likely inflammatory fluid with blood; (e) sedimented fluid—note thick pellet of cells on the bottom of the tube; (f) red and turbid—bloody as a result of either hemorrhage or iatrogenic blood contamination; (g) brown and slightly turbid—possible bile or red blood cell breakdown.

turbid or cloudy or colored, place some of the sample in a red-top tube for bacterial culture. Also at collection, make one or two direct unconcentrated smears by a squash or blood smear technique to submit to the laboratory with the fluid sample. This will allow the clinical pathologist evaluating the sample to compare the cellularity of the sample and the appearance of the cells at the time of collection with that submitted in the tube(s).

LABORATORY EVALUATION

Protein Quantitation

Protein quantitation is typically done via refractometry but some institutions will determine protein via spectrophotometry or automated analysis. For cloudy or turbid samples and bloody samples, the fluid should be centrifuged and the protein measured on the supernatant. Turbidity will interfere with evaluation of protein by either refractometry or spectrophotometry. The protein content is used with the nucleated cell count to classify the effusion and help formulate a list of possible causes.

Red Blood Cell and Nucleated Cell Count

Although an initial impression of the cellularity and amount of blood can usually be made by visual inspection of the sample (Fig. 6–1), knowledge of the actual cell counts for erythrocytes and nucleated cells is important for further classification of the type of fluid. With this information one can begin to narrow down the list of possible causes for the abnormal fluid accumulation. For samples being submitted to a reference laboratory, placing some of the sample in a lavender-top tube (EDTA) and some in a red-top tube is recommended. The lavender-top tube contains anticoagulant, which prevents the sample from clotting if there is a high protein content. EDTA is bacteriostatic, however, and is not recommended if a sample is to be cultured. Thus, some of the fluid should also be put into a red-top tube. The cell counts will be done either with a hemacytometer or an automated cell-counting instrument. If the amount of fibrinogen in the fluid sample is high, then the sample in the red-top tube is likely to clot.

Note: Do not use gel-containing serum separator tubes for submission of fluid to a reference laboratory. Cells may bind to the gel in these tubes and result in an artifactually lowered cell count.

Nucleated Cell Differential

Standard procedures for performing a differential of the nucleated cells vary among laboratories. Some laboratories do no differential, others a three-part differential of 100 cells (large and small mononuclear cells and neutrophils), and still others will provide a 100-cell differential of all cell types observed. The differential provides a relative picture of the types and numbers of cells and aids in establishing a list of potential causes for the fluid accumulation. A differential is not a substitute for a cytologic evaluation by a trained clinical pathologist. The cytologic evaluation is then performed to attempt to determine a specific diagnosis.

Cytologic Evaluation and Interpretation

The cytologic evaluation is the most important step for determining whether a fluid contains bacteria, neoplastic cells, erythrophages, or reactive mesothelial cells. A highly skilled cytopathologist or clinical pathologist should perform this evaluation. Although a definitive cause is not always evident with the cytologic evaluation, it is an invaluable step in the overall assessment of an effusion. The reference laboratory will make a series of slides based on the cellularity of the sample and also on the amount of blood that is present. For samples that are very cellular (i.e., $>50,000$ cells/μl) a direct smear is likely to be adequate. For samples of moderate cellularity (i.e., 2000 to 50,000 cells/μl), a direct and a concentrated slide should be prepared. For samples with less than 2000 cells/μl, further concentration (e.g., cytocentrifugation) is helpful. Buffy-coat preparations are recommended for samples that are moderately to very bloody.

ANCILLARY TESTS

In some instances, other laboratory tests on the fluid may be indicated to help determine a specific cause for the fluid accumulation (Table 6–1).

TABLE 6–1	Ancillary Tests Used to Evaluate Effusions	
Test	**Use/Expected Result**	**Effusion**
Creatinine/potassium	Fluid values are higher than those of serum creatinine and/or potassium	Uroperitoneum
Triglycerides	Fluids often contain triglycerides that exceed 100 mg/dl	Chylous
Cholesterol	Fluid level that is higher than that of serum cholesterol	Nonchylous
Bilirubin	Fluid level that is higher than serum bilirubin	Bile peritonitis
Lipase/amylase	Fluid values are higher than those of serum lipase and/or amylase	Pancreatitis
Protein electrophoresis	A:G ratio of <0.8 on the fluid is very suggestive for FIP	FIP infection
Lipoprotein electrophoresis	Presence of chylomicrons in fluid when triglyceride levels are equivocal	Chylous
pH	pH <7.0 suggests benign or non-neoplastic conditions	Pericardial

NORMAL CYTOLOGY AND HYPERPLASIA

Normally, only a very small amount of fluid is found in the peritoneal, pleural, and pericardial spaces, thus cytologic evaluation is not typically performed unless an increased amount of fluid accumulates. Normal fluid is clear and colorless (Fig. 6–1). Several types of cells may be found in body cavity effusions and their relative percentages may vary somewhat depending on the cause of the fluid accumulation. Cells expected to be in normal fluid include mesothelium, mononuclear phagocytes, lymphocytes, and neutrophils. Mesothelium will easily become hyperplastic or reactive when increased body cavity fluid or inflammation is present.

Large Mononuclear Cells

In most cases, the cytologist will find reactive mesothelial cells in body cavity fluids.

Mesothelial cells may be seen as individual cells or in variably sized clusters. They contain a moderate amount of medium-blue cytoplasm. Hyperplastic mesothelial cells are large (12 to 30 μm) with deep-blue cytoplasm and display a pink to red "fringed" cytoplasmic border (Fig. 6–2). This feature

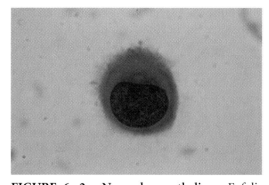

FIGURE 6–2. Normal mesothelium. Exfoliated cell in an effusion with its characteristic pink fringe along the cytoplasmic border. (Wright-Giemsa; ×1000.) (From Meyer DJ, Franks PT: Classification and Cytologic Examination. Compend Contin Educ Pract Vet 9:123–128, 1987.)

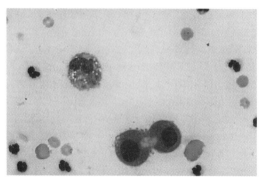

FIGURE 6-3. Reactive mesothelium. Two reactive mesothelial cells (likely just having undergone mitotic division), vacuolated macrophage, neutrophils, and few red blood cells. Reactive mesothelial cells are large with deep-blue cytoplasm. These cells may contain one or more nuclei. Note the presence of the "fringe" (glycocalyx) on the mesothelial cells. (Romanowsky.)

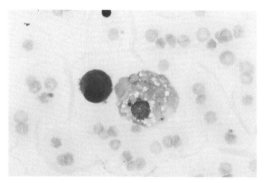

FIGURE 6-5. Reactive mesothelium with acute hemorrhage. Macrophage with phagocytosed red blood cells and reactive mesothelial cell. The erythrophagia indicates pathologic leakage of red blood cells from the vascular space. Also note red blood cells and protein arcs. The degree of hemorrhage cannot be determined from cytologic examination alone. The appearance of the sample and number of red blood cells are also necessary to determine the degree of red cell extravasation. (Romanowsky.)

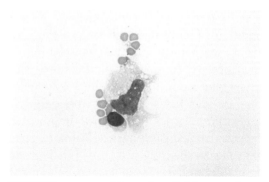

FIGURE 6-4. Normal fluid/transudate. Note the macrophage and small lymphocyte with several erythrocytes. Normal fluid and transudates contain very low nucleated cell counts ($<1000/\mu$l) and low protein content (<2.5 g/dl). (Romanowsky.)

plasm and a round to kidney-bean-shaped nucleus (Fig. 6-4). The nuclear chromatin may be fine and nucleoli may be visible. The macrophage is likely to be the most common cell type in normal or noninflammatory fluids. Macrophages often contain vacuoles or previously phagocytosed cells if there is inflammation or if the fluid has been present for a long time (Figs. 6-4 and 6-5).

Small Mononuclear Cells

Small lymphocytes found in effusions are similar to those found in peripheral blood. These cells are small, nucleated cells with a thin rim of basophilic cytoplasm and a round nucleus. The nucleus nearly fills the cell and the nuclear chromatin is evenly clumped; nucleoli are not visible (Fig. 6-4).

helps identify these cells as mesothelial cells. These cells may contain one or more nuclei of equal size. Nucleoli may be visible and occasional mitotic figures may be evident (Fig. 6-3).

Macrophages are large mononuclear cells with abundant pale-gray to light-blue cyto-

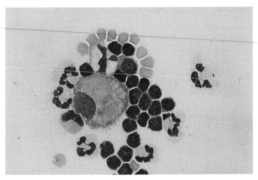

FIGURE 6–6. **Modified transudate. Pleural. Cat.** The effusion cells have been concentrated in this animal with cardiomyopathy. Note large macrophage, many small lymphocytes, and nondegenerate neutrophils. This fluid had a protein of 2.5g/dl and a nucleated cell count of 4000 cells/μl. The macrophage has phagocytized a red blood cell. (Romanowsky; $\times$ 250.)

Neutrophils

Neutrophils are similar to those found in peripheral blood. They are medium-sized cells with pale to clear cytoplasm and a segmented nucleus. Neutrophils should be absent or present in very low numbers in normal fluid but they will be found in increased numbers with chronic fluid accumulation or with inflammation (Fig. 6–6).

GENERAL CLASSIFICATION OF EFFUSIONS

Effusions are usually classified as transudates, modified transudates, and exudates, related to the protein concentration, nucleated cell count, and cell types present (Table 6–2).

Transudate

Fluids are classified as transudates when they have a low protein content and a low cell count (protein $<$ 2.5 g/dl and cells

$<$ 1000/μl). These fluids accumulate in response to physiologic mechanisms, such as increased hydrostatic vascular pressure or decreased colloidal osmotic pressure, that cause the normal homeostatic mechanisms of fluid production and resorption to be overwhelmed. Some causes for transudate accumulation include severe hypoalbuminemia, portal hypertension, hepatic insufficiency, portosystemic shunt, and early myocardial insufficiency. The cells commonly found in transudates are mostly mononuclear cells consisting of macrophages, small lymphocytes, and mesothelial cells. Neutrophils may compose a small percentage of the population.

Modified Transudate

A fluid is classified as a modified transudate when a transudate becomes changed by the addition of nucleated cells or protein. The major mechanism for this transudation is increased venous hydrostatic pressure. The underlying cause for a modified transudate may or may not be evident with cytologic evaluation. Causes of modified transudates include cardiac insufficiency, cardiomyopathy (Fig. 6–6), compression of vessels from neoplasia, vascular insult such as pulmonary thrombosis, inflammation or torsion of an organ, and sterile irritants such as recent urine leakage. Many cases of modified transudate can be further classified based on the types of cells present, the color/turbidity of the sample, the cytologic evaluation, or other ancillary tests where appropriate.

Exudate

Exudates are the result of increased capillary permeability secondary to inflammation or chemotactic stimuli. An exudative fluid contains both increased protein and an increased nucleated cell count. The total pro-

TABLE 6–2	Classification of Common Body Cavity Effusions Based on Fluid Characteristics				
Effusion Type	Color/ Turbidity	Total Protein (g/dl)	Specific Gravity	WBC (# per μl)	Predominant Cell Type(s)
General Conditions					
Transudate	Colorless/clear	<2.5	<1.017	<1000	Mesothelium Mononuclear phagocytes
Modified Transudate	Light yellow to apricot/clear to cloudy	≥2.5	1.017–1.025	>1000	Mononuclear cells
Exudate	Apricot to tan/cloudy	>3.0	>1.025	>5000	Neutrophils *Nonseptic* (nondegenerate) *Septic* (degenerate)
Specific Conditions					
Chylous	White/opaque	>2.5	>1.017	Variable	*Acute:* Small lymphocytes *Chronic:* Mixed population
Neoplastic	Light yellow to apricot/clear to cloudy	>2.5	>1.017	Variable	Reactive mesothelium Neoplastic cells
Hemorrhagic	Pink to red/ cloudy	>3.0	>1.025	>1000	Erythrocytes WBCs similar to blood Macrophages display erythrophagocytosis
Bilious	Dark yellow or brown or green/opaque	>3.0	>1.025	>5000	Mixed population with blue-green, brown, or yellow material phagocytized by macrophages

tein is usually greater than 3.0 g/dl with greater than 5000 cells/μl. Infectious causes for exudates include bacteria (Figs. 6–7 and 6–8), fungi, virus, or protozoa such as *Toxoplasma* (Toomey et al., 1995). Noninfectious causes involve organ inflammation such as pancreatitis (Fig. 6–9), steatitis, inflammatory neoplasia, bowel perforation, pulmonary abscess, and irritants such as bile or urine. Cytologic evaluation is useful to determine an underlying cause in cases of exudative effusions.

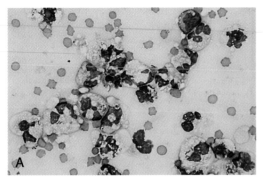

FIGURE 6–7. A, Septic exudate. Pleural. Cat. Note many variably degenerate neutrophils, one macrophage, and red blood cells. Degenerate neutrophils are bloated, with foamy or vacuolated cytoplasm and also swollen lytic nuclei. Note also the presence of small bacterial rods in some of the neutrophils. Aerobic and anaerobic cultures are recommended in cases of pyothorax. This sample contains many nucleated cells (>100, 000 cells/μl) and >3.0 g/dl protein. (Romanowsky; ×160.)

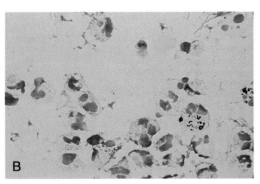

FIGURE 6–7. B, Septic exudate. Same case as in Figure 6–7A. Note presence of small gram-positive, pleomorphic bacterial rods. (Gram; ×250.)

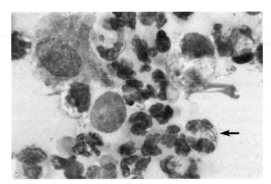

FIGURE 6–8. Septic exudate. Pleural. Cat. Pleomorphic intracellular bacteria identified as *Actinomyces* sp. appear as filamentous forms as well as short rods and cocci within neutrophils (*arrow*) and macrophages. (Wright; ×500.) (Courtesy of Rose Raskin, Gainesville, FL.)

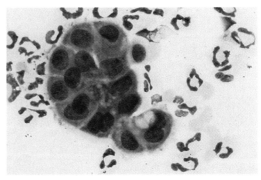

FIGURE 6–9. Nonseptic exudate. Peritoneal. Dog. Concentrated fluid from an animal with pancreatitis showing one cluster of reactive mesothelial cells and neutrophils. The protein content in this sample was 3.0 g/dl with a cell count of 8000 cells/μl. Most of the cells are neutrophils suggesting an underlying inflammatory condition. Further testing (e.g., fluid and serum lipase or ultrasonography) is required to determine the specific cause for the fluid accumulation. (Romanowsky.)

Feline Infectious Peritonitis

Effusions associated with feline infectious peritonitis (FIP) virus infection are inflammatory and therefore properly classified as an exudate. The cellularity of FIP effusions ranges from 1,000 to 30,000 cells/μl (although there are exceptions to this). The protein content is high, often greater than 4.5 g/dl. Electrophoresis of this fluid demonstrates that most of the protein is globulin (beta or gamma). An albumin to globulin ratio of less than 0.8 on the fluid is very suggestive for FIP. Alternatively, if the

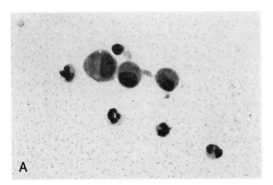

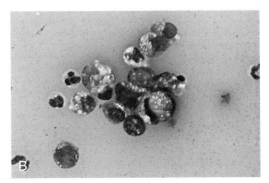

FIGURE 6–10. A, Nonseptic exudate. Peritoneal. Cat. This animal was diagnosed with FIP. Note the presence of neutrophils and macrophages and stippled proteinaceous background throughout. One small lymphocyte is also present. The cell count in cases of FIP are variable (usually 1000 to 30,000 cells/μl). The protein content is usually high (>4.5 g/dl) and often is seen as a granular precipitate throughout the slide. (Romanowsky; ×160.)

FIGURE 6–10. B, Nonseptic exudate. Same case as in Figure 6–10A. FIP fluid showing foamy vacuolated macrophages, mildly degenerate neutrophils, and intermediate to large lymphoid cells. Lymphocytes may be intermediate in size and appear reactive in some cases of FIP. Also note the granular precipitated protein throughout the slide. (Romanowsky; ×250.)

gamma globulin is greater than 32%, the effusion is likely due to FIP (Shelly et al., 1988). Typical cells found in fluid from cases of FIP are macrophages, mildly degenerate neutrophils, lymphocytes, plasma cells, and mesothelial cells (Fig. 6–10). No bacteria are present. There is granular pink stippling to the background of the slides as a result of precipitated protein (Fig. 6–10).

PERICARDIAL EFFUSIONS

Pericardial effusions may also be classified as transudates, modified transudates, or exudates. In many cases, however, the fluid is hemorrhagic. Causes of pericardial effusions include neoplasia, which involves 41% (Kerstetter et al., 1997) to 58% (Dunning, 1997) of canine cases examined. Benign idiopathic pericardial hemorrhage accounted for up to 45% of cases in dogs in one study (Kerstetter et al., 1997). A variety of other infre-

quently seen causes, including infection, cardiac insufficiency, uremia, trauma, foreign body, coagulopathy, pericarditis, hernia, or left atrial rupture, have been reported (Bouvy and Bjorling, 1991; Petrus and Henik, 1999). Pericardial effusions in cats are most often related to congestive heart failure (28%). FIP accounted for 17% as the second most frequent disease causing pericardial effusion in cats (Bouvy and Bjorling, 1991).

Cytologic evaluation of pericardial effusion is challenging, but is most valuable to rule out infection and inflammation. Most often the pericardial effusion is hemorrhagic and in many of these cases the cause cannot be identified by cytological examination (Figs. 6–11 and 6–12). The pericardium is notorious for mesothelial hyperplasia. These mesothelial cells become very large and basophilic with prominent nucleoli and mitotic figures. It is often not possible to distinguish these reactive mesothelial cells from possible neoplastic cells. In addition,

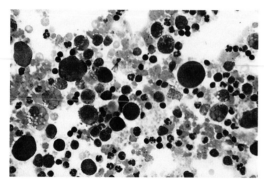

FIGURE 6-11. Hemorrhagic effusion. Pericardial. Dog. Buffy-coat preparation. Note the variety of cells, including neutrophils, lymphocytes, erythrophages, and reactive mesothelial cells. This fluid was red and turbid with 5,000,000 red blood cells/μl, 7000 nucleated cells/μl, and protein of 4.0 g/dl. (Romanowsky.)

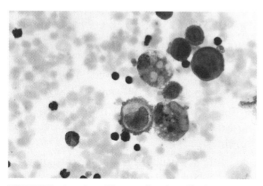

FIGURE 6-12. Hemorrhagic effusion. Pericardial. Dog. Observe the erythrophagia, reactive mesothelial cells, macrophage, and small lymphocytes with many red blood cells. Also note that one macrophage contains brown hemosiderin pigment. One mesothelial cell contains two nuclei. Cytologic evaluation of pericardial fluid is important to rule out infection and some types of neoplasia. Often additional testing is required to determine the cause of hemorrhagic pericardial effusion. (Romanowsky.)

hemangiosarcoma may cause pericardial hemorrhage, but neoplasia of mesenchymal origin typically will not shed neoplastic cells into effusions. In one study (Sisson et al., 1984), 74% of 19 neoplastic effusions were not detected on the basis of cytologic findings and 13% of 31 non-neoplastic effusions were falsely reported as positive, leading the authors to conclude that pericardial fluid analysis did not reliably distinguish neoplastic from non-neoplastic disorders.

Further testing is required (e.g., ultrasonography, coagulation testing, pericardiectomy, finding other evidence of trauma) to determine the underlying cause for the hemorrhage. Recently in a study of 51 dogs with pericardial effusions, the pH of the fluid was examined and compared with a final diagnosis (Edwards, 1996). The pH when measured by precise instrumentation indicated that a reading greater than 7.3 was likely due to noninflammatory conditions, usually neoplasia. Using a less accurate urinary dipstick, pericardial fluid pH $\geq$ 7.0 was associated with neoplasia in 93% of the cases, while <7.0 suggested benign or non-neoplastic conditions. The pH of the fluid needs to be measured shortly after obtaining the sample.

SPECIFIC CLASSIFICATIONS OF EFFUSIONS

A specific classification may be used for those effusions having a distinctive color, cytologic appearance, or positive ancillary test (Table 6-1). The presence of turbidity or color indicates the addition of cells or pigments, respectively, to a fluid. Lipids also will result in increased turbidity.

Chylous Effusion

Chylous effusions contain chyle, which is a mixture of lymph and chylomicrons. Chylo-

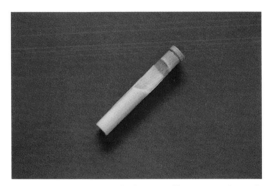

FIGURE 6–13. Chylous effusion. Pleural. Cat. A pink tint is found in this chylous effusion, indicating some degree of hemorrhage is present. The fluid had 13,000/μl nucleated cell count, 267 mg/dl triglycerides, and 169 mg/dl cholesterol. (Courtesy of Rose Raskin, Gainesville, FL.)

microns, derived from dietary lipids processed in the intestine and transported to lymphatics, are primarily composed of triglycerides. These triglycerides provide a "milky" white to pink-white turbid appearance to the fluid (Fig. 6–13). In the past chylous effusions were thought to be solely a result of thoracic duct rupture. At that time other turbid fluids were classified as "pseudochylous." It is now known that there are a variety of causes for chylous effusions and that rupture of the thoracic duct is in fact quite uncommon. It is the experience of this author as well as others (Meadows and MacWilliams, 1994), that most turbid, nonviscid fluids are truly chylous effusions and that pseudochylous effusions are indeed quite rare in veterinary medicine. Pseudochylous fluids contain higher cholesterol content than serum and generally are associated only with very chronic pleuritis or peritonitis, while chylous effusions contain triglycerides at a level higher than that found in serum in a ratio greater than 3:1 (Meadows and Mac-

Williams, 1994). A cholesterol-to-triglyceride (C/T) ratio of less than 1 is generally considered characteristic of a chylous effusion (Fossum et al., 1986b). Based on lipoprotein electrophoretic studies, pleural chylous effusions can be better identified by fluid triglyceride concentrations greater than 100 mg/dl and nonchylous effusions by concentrations less than 100 mg/dl (Waddle and Giger, 1990). In those same studies, C/T ratios were less reliable.

Causes for chylous fluid accumulation in the thoracic cavity mostly involve leakage of lymphatic vessels from trauma or obstruction as a result of cardiovascular disease, neoplasia (e.g., lymphoma, thymoma, lymphangiosarcoma), heartworm disease, diaphragmatic hernia, lung torsion, mediastinal fungal granulomas, chronic coughing, vomiting, or idiopathic (Fossum 1993; Fossum et al., 1986a; Forrester et al., 1991; Waddle and Giger, 1990). In one study (Fossum et al., 1986a) Afghan hounds appeared to have a higher incidence of chylothorax compared with other breeds.

Chylous ascites is less common. Causes for chyle to accumulate in the peritoneal cavity include intra-abdominal neoplasia, steatitis, biliary cirrhosis, lymphatic rupture or leakage, postoperative accumulation following ligation of the thoracic duct, congenital lymphatic abnormalities, and other causes (Fossum et al., 1992; Gores et al., 1994).

Cell counts and protein concentrations are elevated over pure transudate levels and generally fit into modified transudate or exudate categories depending on the degree of chronicity. It is more conventional to term these effusions chylous based on the milky color and elevated triglyceride concentration (Table 6–2).

Cell counts are variable and cell types change from mostly small lymphocytes in early cases to a mixed cell population with

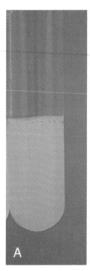

FIGURE 6–14. A, Chylous effusion. Pleural. Cat. Turbid "milky" fluid in most cases, this is due to the presence of chyle. Measurement of high fluid triglyceride levels confirms the diagnosis. The cell count of this sample is <10,000 cells/μl and the protein is 4.0 g/dl.

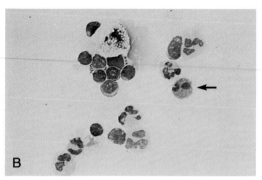

FIGURE 6–14. B, Chylous effusion. Same case as in Figure 6–14A. Note small lymphocytes, neutrophils, one eosinophil (*arrow*), and one large macrophage. Initially chylous effusions contain predominantly small lymphocytes and macrophages. As the duration of fluid presence increases, neutrophils and eosinophils will increase in number. (Romanowsky; ×160.)

many neutrophils and vacuolated macrophages when fluid has been present for a while (Fig. 6–14).

Hemorrhagic Effusion

Red turbid fluids contain many red blood cells and are termed *hemorrhagic* (Table 6–2). These may be a result of pathologic hemorrhage or iatrogenic introduction of red blood cells when obtaining the sample. Pathologic hemorrhage occurs as a result of bleeding (e.g., ruptured or bleeding neoplasm, anticoagulant intoxication, trauma) (Fig. 6–15). Iatrogenic hemorrhage can be distinguished from pathologic hemorrhage in several ways. When blood is introduced at the time of collection, the sample usually changes from clear or yellow to red as the collection procedure progresses. In addition, platelets are evident on cytologic evaluation and there is usually no erythrophagia. If the

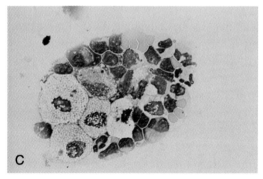

FIGURE 6–14. C, Chylous effusion. Same case as in Figure 6–14B. Concentrated preparation. Note the punctate lipid vacuoles within macrophages along with small lymphocytes, neutrophils, and low number of red blood cells. (Romanowsky; ×250.)

spleen was inadvertently sampled, the sample may clot in the red-top tube, there will be platelets in the smear, and hematopoietic precursors (from extramedullary hematopoiesis) may be evident. In cases of pathologic hemorrhage, the sample usually will not clot even in the clot tube, there should be evidence of erythrophagia (Fig. 6–5), and platelets should not be seen.

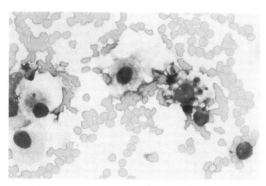

FIGURE 6–15. Hemorrhagic effusion. Peritoneal. Cat. This animal was previously hit by a car. Shown are activated macrophages, a hemosiderophage, two small lymphocytes, and red blood cells. Hemosiderin in macrophages indicates that the hemorrhage occurred more than 2 days prior to collection. (Romanowsky.)

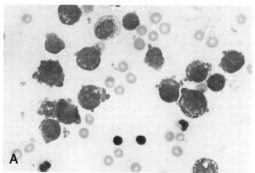

FIGURE 6–16. A, Neoplastic effusion— lymphoma. Pleural. Dog. Note the individual large round cells with high nuclear-to-cytoplasmic ratio and mildly vacuolated cytoplasm. Also evident are two small lymphocytes and one neutrophil. Light-purple, round structures are free nuclei from lysed cells. These cells cannot be evaluated. The cellularity of this sample is 15,000 cells/μl with a protein of 3.4 g/dl. (Romanowsky.)

Neoplastic Effusion

Effusions associated with neoplasia may be classified as modified transudates or exudates and occasionally as a transudate. Cytologic evaluation is most beneficial for determining the presence of neoplastic cells, for example, lymphoma (Figs. 6–16 and 6–17), carcinoma (Figs. 6–18 and 6–19), or mesothelioma (Fig. 6–20). In the case of sarcomas, an effusion may develop but neoplasms of mesenchymal origin seldom shed cells into the effusion. Regardless of the type of neoplasia present, diagnostic cells may or may not be evident in an effusion. If a mass is known to be present, fluid analysis as well as fine-needle aspiration of the mass may be necessary for definitive diagnosis. In one study of the detection of malignant tumors in abdominal and tho-

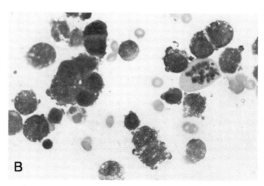

FIGURE 16–16. B, Neoplastic effusion— lymphoma. Same case as in Figure 6–16A. Note individual lymphoblasts, one mitotic figure, two intermediate-size lymphocytes, and one small lymphocyte. A few lysed cells and red blood cells are also present. (Romanowsky.)

racic fluids, sensitivity was low at 64% for dogs and 61% for cats, however, specificity was high at 99% for dogs and 100% for cats (Hirschberger et al., 1999).

Text continued on page 202

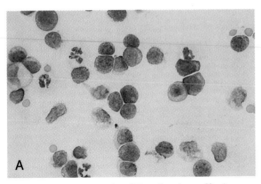

FIGURE 6–17. A, Neoplastic effusion — lymphoma. Pleural. Cat. Note the monomorphic population of large lymphoblasts, few neutrophils, and few lysed cells. The lymphoblasts are larger than neutrophils and contain a small rim of cytoplasm with a large round nucleus. The nuclear chromatin is fine and nucleoli are visible in many of the cells. The nucleated cell count of this fluid is 14,000 cells/μl with increased protein (4.0 g/dl). (Romanowsky; ×200.)

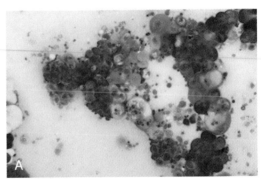

FIGURE 6–18. A, Neoplastic effusion — adenocarcinoma. Pleural. Cat. Note the presence of clusters and sheets of large cells. This fluid is highly cellular (23,000 cells/μl) and has an increased protein content (3.6 g/dl). Inflammatory cells are often found in effusions associated with neoplasia. (Romanowsky; ×63.)

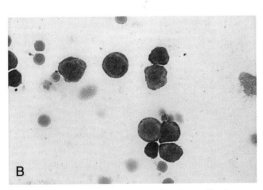

FIGURE 6–17. B, Neoplastic effusion — lymphoma. Same case as in Figure 6–17A. Note monomorphic lymphoblasts and one small lymphocyte with few red blood cells. (Romanowsky; ×250.)

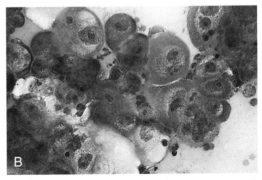

FIGURE 6–18. B, Neoplastic effusion — adenocarcinoma. Same case as in Figure 6–18A. Note that the cells are large with abundant basophilic, lightly vacuolated cytoplasm. The nuclei are round with granular coarse chromatin and a large prominent nucleolus. Neutrophils can be seen within the cytoplasm of some of the neoplastic cells. (Romanowsky; ×160).

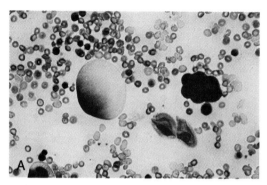

FIGURE 6–19. A, Neoplastic effusion—adenocarcinoma. Pleural. Dog. The neoplastic cells are very large with abundant pale cytoplasm. Tiny vacuoles are present. One of the cells is binucleate. Red blood cells and small lymphocytes are also noted. (Romanowsky; ×160.)

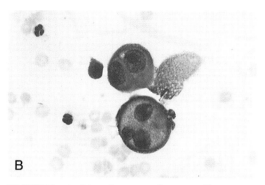

FIGURE 6–20. B, Neoplastic effusion—mesothelioma. Same case as in Figure 6–20A. These cells contain a variable amount of cytoplasm with one or more nuclei. The nuclei may be of odd number and variable size. (Romanowsky; ×160.)

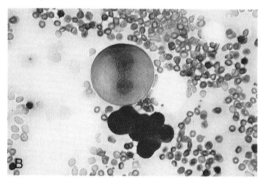

FIGURE 6–19. B, Neoplastic effusion—adenocarcinoma. Same case as in Figure 6–19A. A small cluster of cells likely represents reactive mesothelial cells and these may resemble carcinoma cells. (Romanowsky; ×160.)

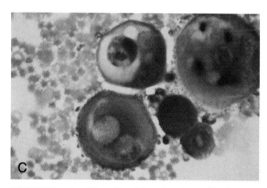

FIGURE 6–20. C, Neoplastic effusion—mesothelioma. Same case as in Figure 6–20A. The nuclear chromatin is coarsely granular and irregularly clumped with large prominent nucleoli. Many cells retain the fringed glycocalyx border. Also present are low number of small lymphocytes, neutrophils, and red blood cells. (Romanowsky; ×160.)

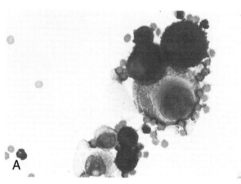

FIGURE 6–20. A, Neoplastic effusion—mesothelioma. Pleural. Dog. The neoplastic cells are present as individual cells and in small clusters. The nucleoli are variably shaped and very prominent. (Romanowsky; ×160.)

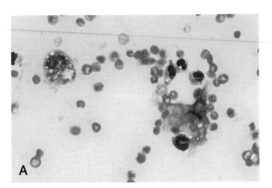

FIGURE 6-21. A, Bilious effusion. Peritoneal. Dog. Note the extracellular gold brown
pigment, neutrophils, red blood cells, and
foamy macrophage. The nucleated cell count
of this fluid is 20,000 cells/μl and the protein
is 3.5 g/dl. (Romanowsky.)

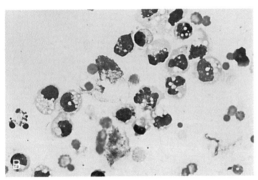

FIGURE 6-21. B, Bilious effusion. Same
case as in Figure 6-21A. Note extracellular
gold-brown pigment, vacuolated neutrophils,
and macrophages. Some of the neutrophils
contain pyknotic nuclei and others contain
karyolytic nuclei. (Romanowsky; $\times$250.)

Bilious Effusion

The presence of bile in the peritoneal cavity
results in an inflammatory response, which
may be sterile initially but later become
septic. This fluid is usually brown to green
to deep yellow (Table 6-2). Bile pigment,
extracellular or intracellular, may be found
on cytologic review of the sample and
ranges in color from yellow to blue-green

(Figs. 6-21 and 6-22). The cells consist of
mildly degenerate neutrophils and macrophages with lower number of other type
cells. Comparison of the bilirubin level in
the fluid with that in the serum can be
helpful in determining if there has been
leakage of bile from the gall bladder or bile
ducts into the peritoneal space (Table 6-1).

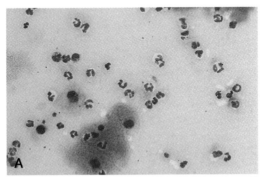

FIGURE 6-22. A, Bilious effusion. Peritoneal. Dog. Large numbers of mostly nondegenerate neutrophils accompany the presence
of amorphous material. The basophilic bile
material is coated by stain precipitate giving a
pink granular appearance. This greenish floc-
culent fluid had a protein of 3.0 g/dl and an
estimated nucleated cell count of greater than
60,000/μl. (Wright-Giemsa; $\times$125.) (Courtesy of
Rose Raskin, Gainesville, FL.)

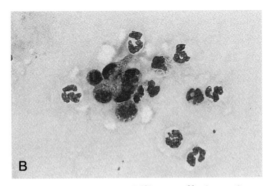

FIGURE 6-22. B, Bilious effusion. Same
case as in Figure 6-22A. Note the phagocytized blue-green granular material by macrophages. (Wright-Giemsa; $\times$250.) (Courtesy of
Rose Raskin, Gainesville, FL.)

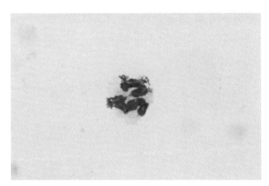

FIGURE 6–23. Uroperitoneum. Dog. The fluid contained a high number of neutrophils and many appeared similar to this "ragged" cell. Urine acts as a chemical irritant causing karyolytic changes to cells. (Wright-Giemsa; ×500.) (Courtesy of Rose Raskin, Gainesville, FL.)

Uroperitoneum

Urine in the peritoneal space results in a chemical irritation. The protein content may be low as a result of dilution from the urine but the cell count and predominant cell type is usually indicative of inflammation or an exudate (Table 6–2). Early in the condition a mononuclear cell population may predominate, suggestive of a modified transudate. Bacteria may or may not be present. Neutrophils exposed to the irritant material may show karyolysis with ragged nuclear borders (Fig. 6–23). In some cases urinary crystals are found on cytologic examination, which leads to a diagnosis of uroperitoneum. In one study in cats, creatinine or potassium is increased in fluid and is a useful predictor for uroperitoneum (Table 6–1), generally in a ratio of 2:1 compared with that in serum (Aumann et al., 1998).

Eosinophilic Effusion

Greater than 10% eosinophils is considered to be a significant increase and fluids with that appearance are termed *eosinophilic effu-sions* regardless of the protein content or cell count. This condition is occasionally seen in veterinary medicine. With large numbers of eosinophils, the fluid grossly may have a green tint. The presence of eosinophils does not provide a specific diagnosis and the cause is often unknown in these cases. Neoplasia such as lymphoma or mastocytosis involved half of the cases in one study (Fossum et al., 1993). Parasitic migration or parasitic disease, immunologic and hypersensitivity conditions, and lymphomatoid granulomatosis are other possibilities (Bauer and Woodfield, 1995; Bounous et al., 2000).

Parasitic Ascites (Abdominal Cestodiasis)

In a small number of dogs with ascites, often from western North America, the cause is aberrant cestodiasis from *Mesocestoides* infection (Stern et al., 1987; Crosbie et al., 1998). Rare reports of infection involve cats. Peritoneal aspirates from anorexic, ascitic dogs are exudates and are granulomatous in nature with the appearance of tapioca pudding or cream of wheat (Fig. 6–24).

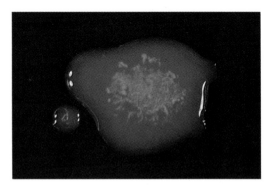

FIGURE 6–24. Cestodiasis. Peritoneal. Dog. The ascitic fluid had a tapioca pudding appearance grossly. Motility of these granules may be observed with the unaided eye. (Courtesy of Jocelyn Johnsrude, IDEXX, West Sacramento, CA.)

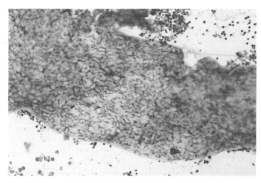

FIGURE 6–25. Cestodiasis. Acoelomic metacestode tissue with amorphous degenerate debris and calcareous corpuscles. Inflammatory cells are also present surrounding the structure. (Romanowsky.)

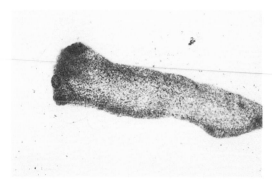

FIGURE 6–26. Cestodiasis. Tetrathyridia larval stage. Same case as in Figure 6–24. Note the oval structures at one end that represent suckers and identify the parasite as *Mesocestoides* spp. (Romanowsky; ×40.)

Motile cestodes can be seen in fluid with the unaided eye. Microscopic examination may show acephalic metacestodes or acoelomic tissue with calcareous corpuscles (Fig. 6–25), which may be seen in nonspecific cestode infections. Less often seen microscopically are metacestodes with visible tetrathyridia, a unique larval form having four suckers that represents the asexual reproductive form of *Mesocestoides* spp. infection (Fig. 6–26). Cestode ova are not usually found in the feces (Crosbie et al., 1998).

References

Aumann M, Worth LT, Drobatz KJ: Uroperitoneum in cats: 26 cases (1986–1995). J Am Anim Hosp Assoc 1998;34:315–324.

Bauer T, Woodfield JA: Mediastinal, pleural and extrapleural diseases. In: Ettinger EJ, Feldman EC (eds): *Textbook of Veterinary Internal Medicine,* 4th ed. WB Saunders, Philadelphia, 1995, pp 819–828.

Bounous DI, Bienzle D, Miller-Liebl, D: Pleural effusion in a dog. Vet Clin Pathol 2000;29:55–58.

Bouvy BM, Bjorling DE. Pericardial effusion in dogs and cats. Part I. Normal pericardium and causes and pathophysiology of pericardial effusion. Compend Contin Educ Pract Vet 1991;13:417–424.

Crosbie PR, Boyce WM, Platzer EG, et al: Diagnostic procedures and treatment of eleven dogs with peritoneal infections caused by *Mesocestoides* spp. J Am Vet Med Assoc 1998;213:1578–1583.

Dunning D: Pericardial effusion. In: Wingfield WE (ed): *Veterinary Emergency Medicine Secrets.* Hanley and Belfus, Philadelphia, 1997, pp 190–193.

Edwards NJ: The diagnostic value of pericardial fluid pH determination. J Am Anim Hosp Assoc 1996;32:63–67.

Forrester SD, Fossum TW, Rogers KS: Diagnosis and treatment of chylothorax associated with lymphoblastic lymphosarcoma in four cats. J Am Vet Med Assoc 1991;198:291–294.

Fossum TW: Feline chylothorax. Compend Contin Educ Pract Vet 1993;15:549–567.

Fossum TW, Birchard SJ, Jacobs RM: Chylothorax in 34 dogs. J Am Vet Med Assoc 1986a;188: 1315–1318.

Fossum TW, Hay WH, Boothe HW, et al: Chylous ascites in three dogs. J Am Vet Med Assoc 1992; 200:70–76.

Fossum TW, Jacobs RM, Birchard SJ: Evaluation of cholesterol and triglyceride concentrations in differentiating chylous and nonchylous pleural effusions in dogs and cats. J Am Vet Med Assoc 1986b; 188:49–51.

Fossum TW, Wellman M, Relford RL, Slater MR: Eosinophilic pleural or peritoneal effusions in dogs and cats: 14 cases (1986–1992). J Am Vet Med Assoc 1993; 202:1873–1876.

Gores BR, Berg J, Carpenter JL, et al: Chylous ascites in cats: Nine cases (1978–1993). J Am Vet Med Assoc 1994; 205:1161–1164.

Hirschberger J, DeNicola DB, Hermanns W, et al: Sensitivity and specificity of cytologic evaluation in the diagnosis of neoplasia in body fluids from dogs and cats. Vet Clin Pathol 1999;28: 142–146.

Kerstetter KK, Krahwinkel DJ, Millis DL, et al: Pericardiectomy in dogs: 22 cases (1978–1994). J Am Vet Med Assoc 1997;211:736–740.

Kirk RW, Bistner SI, Ford RB: Handbook of Veterinary Procedures and Emergency Treatment, 5th ed. WB Saunders, Philadelphia, 1990, pp 447–448;624–625.

Meadows RL, MacWilliams PS: Chylous effusions revisited. Vet Clin Pathol 1994;23:54–62.

Meyer DJ, Franks PT: Effusion: Classification and cytologic examination. Compend Contin Educ Pract Vet 1987;9:123–129.

Petrus DJ, Henik RA: Pericardial effusion and cardiac tamponade secondary to brodifacoum toxicosis in a dog. J Am Vet Med Assoc 1999;215: 647–648.

Shelly SM, Scarlett-Kranz J, Blue JT: Protein electrophoresis on effusions from cats as a diagnostic test for feline infectious peritonitis. J Am Anim Hosp Assoc 1988;24:495–500.

Sisson D, Thomas WP, Ruehl WW, et al: Diagnostic value of pericardial fluid analysis in the dog. J Am Vet Mad Assoc 1984;184:51–55.

Stern A, Walder EJ, Zontine WJ, et al: Canine Mesocestoides infections. Compend Contin Educ Pract Vet 1987;9:223–231.

Toomey JM, Carlisle-Nowak MM, Barr SC, et al: Concurrent toxoplasmosis and feline infectious peritonitis in a cat. J Am Anim Hosp Assoc 1995;31:425–428.

Waddle JR, Giger U: Lipoprotein electrophoresis differentiation of chylous and nonchylous pleural effusions in dogs and cats and its correlation with pleural effusion triglyceride concentration. Vet Clin Pathol 1990;19:80–85.

CHAPTER 7

Oral Cavity, Gastrointestinal Tract, and Associated Structures

CLAIRE B. ANDREASEN
ALBERT E. JERGENS
DENNY J. MEYER

Endoscopy has facilitated increased access to the mucosal surface of the gastrointestinal tract and enhanced the application of diagnostic cytology for its evaluation. It is an especially useful adjunct procedure when combined with the histologic examination of tissue for the complete assessment of gastrointestinal tract. The cytologic and histologic findings tend to be disparate when: (1) the specimens are obtained from different sites, (2) the lesion is deeply located in the lamina propria or submucosa precluding exfoliation, (3) surface-associated findings are lost during processing of the histologic sample, and (4) cell or tissue distortion (artifact) is present in either the cytologic or the histologic specimen.

In our experience, both touch imprint and brush cytologic preparations can provide useful information when concurrently examined with the histologic specimen (Jergens et al., 1998). Brush cytology tends to exfoliate more cells but also has the potential to induce hemorrhage and introduce leukocytes that may be mistaken for inflam-

mation. Brush cytology often represents pathology of the deeper lamina propria compared to touch imprints, which reflect the surface and mucosal changes. The criteria that differentiate benignity and malignancy must be carefully evaluated when examining esophageal and gastrointestinal cytologic specimens since the cellular atypia associated with epithelial hyperplasia and regeneration as a consequence of inflammation can mimic epithelial neoplasia.

ORAL CAVITY

The most common reason for the cytologic examination of the oral cavity is for the evaluation of a mass or an ulcerative lesion. Radiographic findings will indicate if there is bone involvement.

Normal Cytology

Superficial and intermediate squamous epithelial cells are the commonly exfoliated cell type. A variety of oropharyngeal bacteria can be seen in samples from the oral cavity. Noteworthy is *Simonsiella* sp. (Fig. 7–1). Neutrophils are normally lost via transmigration through the mucous membranes into the oral cavity and may be observed in low numbers.

Inflammation

Inflammatory diseases that can affect the oral cavity include immune-mediated diseases such as bullous disease, foreign bodies, dental disease, systemic manifestation of uremia, and bacterial, viral, and fungal infections (Guilford, 1996). The inflammatory exudate can be composed of leukocytes, necrotic debris, and bacterial flora. Additional tests are warranted when the cause is not apparent cytologically.

Neoplasia

Epithelial, mesenchymal, and discrete (round) cell neoplasia can involve the oral cavity. As in other organ systems, the diagnostic sensitivity of cytology is highest for discrete cell neoplasia and lowest for mesenchymal tumors. This is due to reduced exfoliation and the difficulty differentiating neoplastic mesenchymal cells from reactive fibrocytes/fibroblasts that compose inflammatory/reparative lesions. Discrete cell neoplasia includes lymphoma, mast cell tumor, plasmacytoma, transmissible venereal tumor, and histiocytoma (Tyler et al., 1999). The plasmacytoma can involve the oral mucus membranes, tongue, or mucosa of the digestive tract and be difficult to diagnose definitively without immunocytochemical or immunohistochemical characterization (Rakich et al., 1994). The most common epithelial neoplasm is squamous cell carcinoma (Fig. 7–2A & B). Less common is epithelial odontogenic neoplasia (Poulet et al., 1992) (Fig. 7–3A & B). Squamous cell carcinoma can occur anywhere in the oral

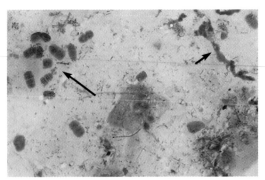

FIGURE 7–1.   Oral cavity. Normal cytologic findings. An angular squamous epithelial cell is covered with *Simonsiella* sp. (rounded rectangular structures with cross striations) (*long arrow*); an angular, partially keratinized squamous epithelial cell is located in the center, and the background is composed of numerous bacteria of varying size and shapes set in a lightly basophilic proteinaceous background. A stream of free nuclear protein from a ruptured cell is present (*short arrow*). (Wright; ×250.)

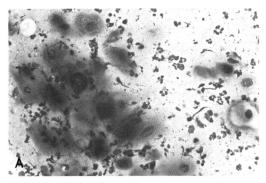

FIGURE 7–2.   A, Oral squamous cell carcinoma. Touch imprint. This specimen is from a mass that extended from the frenulum of the tongue into the mandible of a cat. There are numerous squamous epithelial cells of varying immaturity with shapes that vary from oval to angular. Some of the cells show dyskeratosis (far left). Other abnormal morphologic features include variable nuclear-to-cytoplasmic (N : C) ratios and variable staining. Numerous neutrophils are scattered amongst the neoplastic cells. Many show nuclear degeneration or are ruptured resulting in streaks of free nuclear protein. Squamous cells and keratin often induce neutrophilic inflammation. (Wright; ×250.)

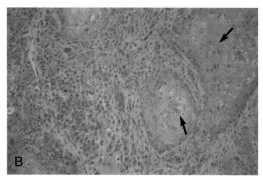

FIGURE 7–2. B, Oral squamous cell carcinoma. Histology. Cords of pleomorphic squamous cells are separated by a fine fibrous stroma. Central cores of keratinocytes (*arrows*) demonstrate dyskeratosis (premature or abnormal keratinization of epithelial cells that have not reached the surface) and stain more intensively eosinophilic. (H & E; ×100.)

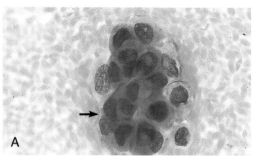

FIGURE 7–3. A, Oral epithelial odontogenic tumor. Touch imprint. A cytologic impression of an epithelial cell neoplasm can be made based on the general morphology of the clustered interdigitating neoplastic epithelial cells. They show mild to moderate anisocytosis and anisokaryosis and the nuclei show mild to moderate shape variation. The lower group appears to be forming a disorganized acinar structure with a central lumen (*arrow*). The morphologic features are suggestive of an epithelial cell malignancy. Numerous erythrocytes surround the neoplastic cell clump. (Wright; ×250.)

cavity but in cats it often occurs in the frenulum of the tongue with early metastasis to the regional lymph nodes. An epulis is a common gingival mass in dogs that can be a developmental, hyperplastic, inflammatory, or neoplastic lesion. These can be confusing lesions to evaluate cytologically because they can be composed of dental epithelial nests enrobed in stromal fibrous tissue. When the diagnosis is in doubt cytologically, it is prudent to pursue an excisional biopsy. Oral melanomas often are malignant and infiltrative, may contain abundant or only minimal pigment (amelanotic melanomas), and rapidly metastasize to the regional lymph nodes (Barker et al., 1993) (Fig. 7–4). Fibrosarcoma, chondrosarcoma, and osteosarcoma (Fig. 7–5) are the mesenchymal tumors that more commonly involve the oral cavity. Fibroma, hemangiosarcoma, and liposarcoma are less frequent (Tyler et al., 1999). Fibrosarcomas of the mandible and maxilla occasionally can have cytologic and histologic benign

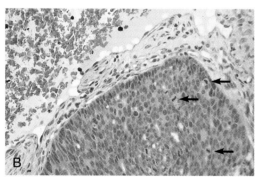

FIGURE 7–3. B, Oral epithelial odontogenic malignancy. Histology. The dense neoplastic epithelial cell population shows mild central swirling with palisading cuboidal to columnar epithelial cells located at the periphery. Mitotic figures are present (*arrows*). The neoplastic cells are surrounded by a less-dense (pale pink) fibrovascular stroma. (H & E; ×100.)

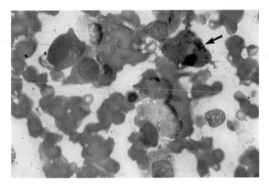

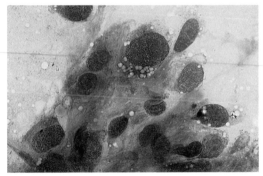

FIGURE 7–4. Oral malignant melanoma. Touch imprint. Pleomorphic polyhedral cells with variable N:C ratios, anisocytosis, and variable staining intensity are indicative of neoplasia. Abundant intracytoplasmic dark pigment (melanin) is noted in one cell (*arrow*). Most of the other cells do not contain obvious pigment (amelanotic) and can be easily confused with neoplastic epithelial cells or anaplastic mesenchymal cancer cells. (Wright; ×250.)

FIGURE 7–5. Oral osteosarcoma. Touch imprint. Pleomorphic mesenchymal cells show marked anisocytosis and anisokaryosis. The nuclei have stippled nuclear chromatin that contains multiple faintly stained variably sized nucleoli and are surrounded by moderately abundant basophilic cytoplasm with indistinct cell borders. The swirls of intercellular eosinophilic matrix produced by the neoplastic cells supports the cytologic impression of a malignant bone tumor. (Wright; ×250.)

morphologic features but demonstrate aggressive biologic behavior (Ciekot et al., 1994). Neoplasia detected in the soft or hard palate may be extensions from the nasal cavity.

SALIVARY GLAND

Normal Cytology

Cytologic evaluation of salivary gland disease is diagnostically rewarding. The salivary gland also may be sampled accidentally when attempting to aspirate the submandibular lymph node. Cytologically, the salivary gland contains uniform secretory epithelial cells that are clustered and/or individual with eccentric, dark basophilic nuclei, and clear, vacuolated to foamy cytoplasm (Fig. 7–6). The cytoplasmic staining of the cells differs between serous cells (distinguishable) and mucous cells (may appear

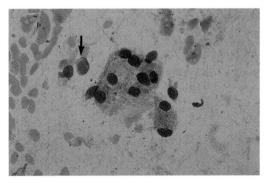

FIGURE 7–6. Salivary gland epithelial cells, normal. Touch imprint. The epithelial cells that compose this small cluster have abundant basophilic, granular-appearing cytoplasm that surrounds a dense, often eccentric nucleus. The morphologic features are consistent with normal secretory epithelium such as salivary gland. A large lymphocyte with a small rim of lightly basophilic cytoplasm (*arrow*) and a free round nucleus are located to the left of center. The surrounding erythrocytes can be used to judge the size of the cells. (Wright; ×125.)

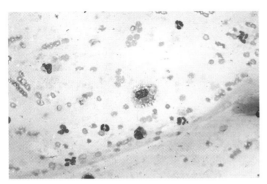

FIGURE 7–7. Sialocele **(salivary mucocele).
Aspirate.** This specimen is an aspirate from a
fluctuant submandibular swelling. The pinkish-
blue mucus (*asterisk*) and occasional foamy
macrophage along with a low number of neutrophils and erythrocytes are indicative of a
sialocele. The rowing of erythrocytes (linear arrangement) suggests the presence of mucus.
(Wright; ×125.)

clear). Individual epithelial cells can be difficult to differentiate from macrophages,
however, they have uniformly clear to finely
vacuolated cytoplasm and do not contain
phagocytic material. Eosinophilic-staining
mucus is commonly observed and when
present may cause erythrocytes to "stream"
or line up in parallel rows (Fig. 7–7).

Hyperplasia

Hyperplasia is suspected when there is glandular enlargement and the epithelial cells
appear relatively normal cytologically. The
cells may be surrounded by abundant mucus. A differential consideration would be a
sialocele.

Inflammation

The most common inflammatory lesion is a
salivary mucocele (sialocele) or ranula. A
ranula is a cystic distension of an epithelial

lined duct in the floor of the mouth. A
sialocele is an accumulation of salivary secretions in nonepithelial lined cavities adjacent to the duct. While the cause is not
known, trauma plus a developmental predisposition is proposed. The accumulated
saliva stimulates an inflammatory reaction.
The initial inflammatory influx is composed
of neutrophils and macrophages along secretory epithelial cells set in an eosinophilic
to basophilic mucus background (Fig. 7–7).
Lymphocytes replace the neutrophil component over time and can be a prominent
feature. Although the foamy macrophages
can appear morphologically similar to the
plump secretory epithelial cells, differentiation is not necessary when formulating the
cytologic impression.

Neoplasia

The salivary adenocarcinoma is uncommon
and demonstrates the general characteristics
of epithelial malignancy that range from
relatively well-differentiated to marked pleomorphism (Spangler and Culbertson, 1991).
The neoplastic epithelial cells can form acinar structures and some of the cells can
have abundant retained cytoplasmic secretions that displace the nucleus to the periphery, forming a cell that appears similar
to a signet ring. Mixed salivary neoplasms
are rare and contain both neoplastic epithelial cell and mesenchymal cell components
that can include bone and cartilage.

PANCREAS

Normal Cytology

The pancreas is not usually sampled unless
a mass is detected. Cellular characteristics
can rapidly deteriorate owing to extracellular pancreatic enzyme activity associated
with pancreatitis.

Inflammation

Pancreatitis may cause focal abdominal fluid accumulations or effusions with the characteristics of a modified transudate or sterile purulent exudate. If a proteinaceous background is present, it can have a "dirty," moderately basophilic appearance that corresponds to saponified fat observed histologically. A hemorrhagic effusion is occasionally noted. Pancreatic cysts or abscesses can be detected as intra-abdominal masses and sampled by ultrasound-guided aspiration. The samples are often sterile and composed of neutrophils embedded in a proteinaceous background (Salisbury et al., 1988).

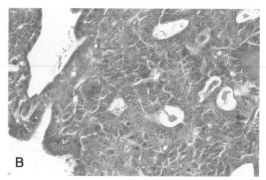

FIGURE 7–8. B, Pancreatic adenocarcinoma (exocrine). Histology. Papillary (elongated clump) and cluster formation of pancreatic exocrine epithelial cells that are forming disorganized glandular and ductular structures. A mitotic figure is located at the top-center. (H & E; ×100.)

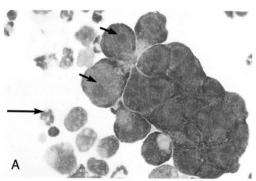

FIGURE 7–8. A, Pancreatic adenocarcinoma (exocrine). Touch imprint. This specimen was taken from a pancreatic mass. There is a dense, slightly elongated basophilic epithelial cell cluster that shows marked anisocytosis and anisokaryosis. The cytoplasm is not easily observed but the N:C ratio is markedly increased. Gigantic nucleoli are observed in some of the cells (*short arrows*). The cells at the upper end of the cluster appear to be forming a disorganized acinar structure. The inappropriately large size of the neoplastic cells can be appreciated by comparison to a neutrophil (*long arrow*). (Wright; ×250.)

Neoplasia-Exocrine Pancreas

Pancreatic adenocarcinoma can be diagnosed directly via ultrasound-guided cytology/biopsy. It is a diagnostic consideration when carcinoma cells are observed in an abdominal effusion or in a thoracic effusion secondary to their metastasis via the diaphragmatic lymphatics. The pancreatic adenocarcinoma has characteristics similar to those of other adenocarcinomas, including a high nuclear-to-cytoplasmic ratio, fine cytoplasmic vacuolization, and cytoplasmic hyperchromatic basophilia (Fig. 7–8A & B).

ESOPHAGUS

Normal Cytology

The mucosal layer of the esophagus has a stratified squamous epithelium that contains openings for the ducts of the esophageal mucus glands. Exfoliated stratified squamous epithelial cells can either appear angular or have the rounded shape of intermediate epithelial cells and basal cells with eccentric nuclei. Large numbers of basal epithelial cells can indicate trauma, inflammation, or erosion (Green, 1992). The stromal cells and glandular cells usually do not exfoliate. Samples from the gastroesophageal region may contain squamous epithelium mixed with gastric columnar epithelium. Ingesta with oropharyngeal flora consisting of a mixed bacterial population of rods, cocci, and *Simonsiella* sp. may be noted in esophageal samples (see Fig. 7–1).

Inflammation

Reflux esophagitis most commonly involves the distal esophagus. It is caused by the action of regurgitated gastric (pepsin and acid) and possibly duodenal (bile acids and pancreatic enzymes) secretions that have a corrosive effect on the stratified squamous epithelium. Esophageal inflammation has a prominent neutrophilic component (Fig. 7–9) and the epithelial cells show reactive hyperchromasia, or nuclear and cytoplasmic degenerative changes. Esophageal inflamma-

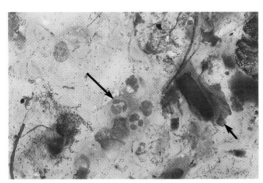

FIGURE 7–9. Esophagitis. Brushing. This specimen was obtained endoscopically from an inflamed site in the esophagus. Esophagitis is indicated by the presence of neutrophils (*long arrow*). Other findings include angular squamous epithelial cells, keratin bar (*short arrow*), and numerous bacteria (oral flora). (Wright; ×250.)

tion is suggested if oropharyngeal contamination is not present and the site sampled appears inflamed endoscopically.

Neoplasia

The differential considerations for esophageal masses include the neoplasia and parasitic granuloma. Squamous cell carcinoma has neoplastic features that vary from relatively well-differentiated to anaplastic. Well-differentiated squamous cell carcinomas can be difficult to differentiate from hyperplasia, but the presence of bizarre cell forms along with variable nuclear-to-cytoplasmic ratios, variable cytoplasmic basophilia, and fine cytoplasmic vacuolization support a neoplastic cell population. An adenocarcinoma of the esophageal glands is a less common epithelial neoplasm. Its location and cytologic features can be similar to a thyroid carcinoma. *Spirocerca lupi* is a spirurid nematode that parasitizes the esophageal wall of dogs in warm climates where the dung beetle serves as the intermediate host. Endoscopically, the mass appears as a smooth, nonulcerated firm tumor. It can be diagnosed by finding embryonated eggs in a fecal flotation. Pleomorphic spindle-shaped cells exfoliated from the granuloma are easily mistaken for sarcoma. In fact, esophageal sarcomas are usually associated with the presence of the parasite (Fox et al., 1988; Barker et al., 1993).

CRITERIA FOR GASTROINTESTINAL CYTOLOGY

Cytologic grading criteria provide guidelines for the uniform evaluation of the gastrointestinal specimen, in which the frequent presence of bacterial flora and cell debris complicates the cytologic interpretation. These criteria ensure that a consistent and

TABLE 7–1	Cytologic Findings That Comprise the Grading System of the Cytologic Specimen of the Gastrointestinal Tract

Inflammatory cells: Neutrophils, lymphocytes, plasma cells, eosinophils, macrophages

Atypical cells

Epithelial cell clusters

Spiral bacteria that resemble gastric spiral organisms

Bacterial flora consisting of rods and cocci

Hemorrhage (recent)

Debris or ingesta consisting of plant or food fiber and dark particulate material

Mucus consisting of diffusely stained secretory product or mucin granules (globules)

quantifiable assessment of the gastrointestinal cytologic specimen is achieved. Fibrosis and lesions deep to the lamina propria usually will not be detected with endoscopic cytology.

Table 7–1 lists the categories developed by Jergens and co-workers (1998) that compose the grading system. A scale of 0 to 7 was applied to all categories. The one used for epithelial cell clusters differs from the others. Tables 7–2 and 7–3 list the definitions of the grading system for the microscopic findings (Jergens et al., 1998). Depending on the location, some categories would be present normally, such as bacterial rods and cocci in colonic or rectal scrapings, yet the complete absence of bacteria may indicate an alteration in flora due to prolonged antibiotic use or sampling technique. Even though bacterial flora is categorized, bacterial overgrowth cannot be diagnosed cytologically.

Knowledge of the patient's history, endoscopic appearance of the lesion, and endoscopic site sampled is vital for formulating an accurate interpretation of gastrointestinal cytologic specimens. Adequate assessment of these cytologic specimens is relatively time consuming and labor intensive. Cytology and histology are complementary processes for the evaluation of gastrointestinal disease.

TABLE 7–2	Definition of Grades Used for the Microscopic Findings Listed in Table 7–1

Inflammatory cells
   Grades 0 to 7 denote the corresponding total number of inflammatory cells per 50x-oil objective (e.g., finding 3 inflammatory cells per 50-oil objective is assigned a grade 3; finding 7 or more inflammatory cells per 50-oil objective is assigned grade 7)

Atypical cells
   Grades 0 to 7 denote the corresponding total number of atypical cells per 50x-oil objective

Spiral bacteria that resemble gastric spiral organisms, bacterial flora, hemorrhage, debris or ingesta, and mucus or mucin granules were each graded as follows:
   Grade 0 = none present
   Grades 1 to 2 = slight
   Grades 3 to 4 = moderate
   Grades 5 to 7 = marked

A minimum of 10 fields should be examined since there often is exfoliation variability among the tissue imprint areas. Because of sampling and exposure to digestive contents, neutrophils may appear slightly degenerate and lymphocytes may exhibit cellular swelling, both morphologic changes resulting in reduced chromatin clumping and staining intensity. For the inflammatory and atypical cell categories, grades of 2 or less are considered of questionable diagnostic importance (i.e., considered within normal variation).

TABLE 7–3	Definition of Grades Used for Epithelial Cell Clusters Per 10x-Objective*	
Grade 0 = 0 cell clusters	Grade 4 = 6 to 7 cell clusters	
Grade 1 = 1 to 2 cell clusters	Grade 5 = 7 to 8 cell clusters	
Grade 2 = 3 to 4 cell clusters	Grade 6 = 9 to 10 cell clusters	
Grade 3 = 4 to 5 cell clusters	Grade 7 = greater than 10 cell clusters	

*Adequate cell clusters are needed for a representative sample. Samples with epithelial clusters of grade 2 or less are not likely to yield diagnostic information.

However, one should not be discouraged if pathology is not detected either cytologically or histologically. In one study, the majority of gastric specimens, 25% of intestinal samples, and 33% of colonic samples were classified as normal even though gastrointestinal disease was suspected (Jergens et al., 1998).

STOMACH

Normal Cytology

Gastric mucosal epithelial cells are columnar and appear as uniform cell clusters with oval to round nuclei and moderate amounts of lightly basophilic to light eosinophilic cytoplasm (Fig. 7–10A & B). There can be a mucin vacuole at the luminal surface of the columnar cells. The columnar morphology is more obvious in large cell clusters. The variable amount of mucus in the cytologic specimen has variable staining characteristics. Fundic glandular epithelium consists of rounded parietal cells (lightly eosinophilic cytoplasm) and chief cells (granular lightly basophilic cytoplasm) and may be seen in oval to elliptical clusters (Fig. 7–11A & B). Mucus neck cells also may be seen in association with parietal cells (Fig. 7–12). The tinctorial characteristic of the cell appears to be affected by the amount of mucus present. Cardiac glands and pyloric glands also secrete mucus, but do not contain parietal and chief cells.

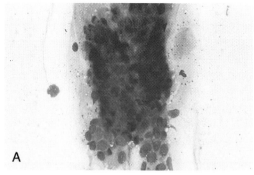

A

FIGURE 7–10. A, Gastric mucosal epithelial cells, normal. Touch imprint. The epithelial cells in this touch imprint are relatively uniform with round to oval nuclei containing dispersed chromatin and moderate amounts of basophilic cytoplasm. The features can be observed at the periphery of the cell cluster where the cells are in a monolayer, emphasizing the importance of proper sample management. (Wright; ×250.)

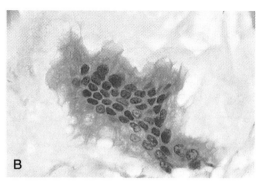

B

FIGURE 7–10. B, Gastric mucosal epithelial cells. Histology. Note the relatively uniform morphologic features and the absence of leukocytes and bacteria. The jagged border of the tissue is an artifact. (H & E; ×250.)

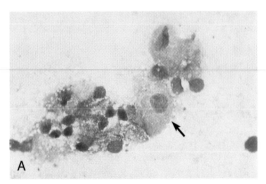

FIGURE 7–11. A, Gastric fundic glandular epithelial cells. Touch imprint. Two epithelial cell populations are present. The larger epithelial cells (*arrow*) with abundant, homogeneous, lightly eosinophilic cytoplasm are consistent with parietal cells. The smaller epithelial cells with granular-like or microvesicular basophilic cytoplasm are consistent with chief cells. Both cell types compose the fundic glands of the stomach. (Wright; ×250.)

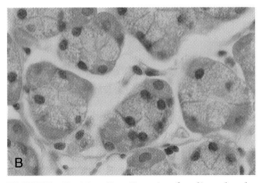

FIGURE 7–11. B, Gastric fundic glands. Histology. The oval-shaped fundic glands are composed of two epithelial cell types. The parietal cells stain intensively eosinophilic and the pale-staining chief cells have microvesicular cytoplasm. (H & E; ×250.)

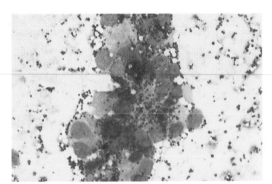

Figure 7–12. Gastric biopsy with mucin granules. Touch imprint. There is a dense cluster of mucin-producing epithelial cells that are identified by the presence of numerous purplish mucin granules (globules) located in their cytoplasm. Many extracellular mucin granules from ruptured cells are observed. The size and morphology of the mucin granules appear similar to bacterial cocci. These cells should not be confused with mast cells that have smaller metachromatic cytoplasmic granules. Contrast to Figure 8–19. (Wright; ×250.)

The presence of oropharyngeal flora such as *Simonsiella* sp., along with mucus, pyknotic neutrophils, mixed bacterial flora, and digesta debris, is a common finding in gastric samples from a nondiseased stomach. These neutrophils probably represent those blood cells that are continually lost through the mucous membranes of the gastrointestinal tract. Neutrophils that are not associated with oropharyngeal or esophageal digesta may represent true gastritis (Fig. 7–13). Again, the endoscopic visualization of an inflamed area corroborates the cytologic impression of gastritis.

Gastric spiral bacteria often are associated with the mucus and are more consistently observed in brush cytology specimens. The organisms may not be observed histologically owing to the loss of the mucus biolayer (Happonen et al., 1996). *Helicobacter felis*-like bacteria and *Gastrospirillum*-like bacteria cannot be differentiated by light microscopy (Fig. 7–14A & B). The experienced cytopathologist can potentially differentiate them from *Helicobacter pylori*-like bacteria because of their smaller size. In 96 gastric samples, 48% contained gastric spiral

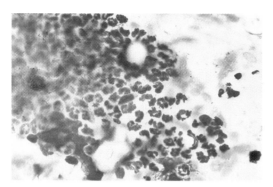

FIGURE 7–13. Neutrophilic gastritis. Brushing. Marked numbers of neutrophils are observed. Ulcerative and erosive lesions were observed endoscopically. (Wright; ×250.)

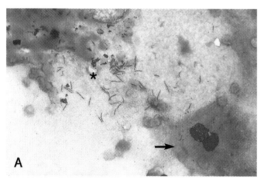

FIGURE 7–14. A, Spiral-shaped bacteria. Touch imprint. Numerous *Helicobacter*-like or *Gastrospirillium*-like spiral-shaped bacteria are embedded in the mucus (*asterisk*). Spiral-shaped organisms are commonly observed cytologically in both nondiseased and diseased stomachs of dogs and cats. An angular squamous epithelial cell is present (*arrow*). (Wright; ×250.)

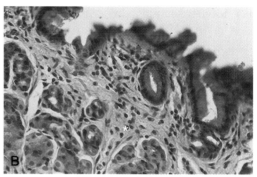

FIGURE 7–14. B, Lymphocytic gastritis. Histology. Although no inflammatory cells were observed in the cytologic specimen, there was mild increase in lymphocytes, stromal fibrosis, and edema around the gastric glands (*asterisk*). Microscopic examination of a biopsy is generally required to determine the presence or absence of inflammation. Only a rare spiral-shaped organism was observed (not shown) on the mucosal surface, probably due to the absence of the mucus layer. A Warthin-Starry stain can be used to identify the organism in tissue. (H & E; ×250.)

organisms (Jergens et al., 1998). The Warthin–Starry stain accentuates the identification of the organism. Culture is needed to identify specific types of spiral bacteria. The importance of spiral bacteria as a cause of gastric disease in dogs and cats requires additional clarification since these organisms are common in animals without clinical disease or histologic abnormalities and do not alter gastric function experimentally

(Eaton, 1999; Jenkins and Bassett, 1997; Happonen et al., 1996; Hermanns et al., 1995; Simpson et al., 1999a, 1999b).

Hyperplasia

The cytologic impression of mucosal and secretory hyperplasia is subjective. Increased numbers of mucosal secretory cells or goblet cells with attendant diffuse mucus granules (globules) may indicate mucosal secretory hyperplasia. A definitive diagnosis requires histology.

Inflammation

Neutrophils along with other inflammatory cells are associated with gastric ulcers (Fig. 7–13). As indicated above, the presence of oropharyngeal flora or digesta admixed with neutrophils tempers the cytologic impression of true inflammation. Mucosal inflammation, per se, is devoid of mixed bacterial flora and digesta. The presence of lympho-

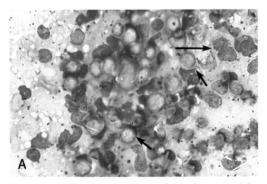

FIGURE 7–15. A, Lymphocytic gastritis. Touch imprint. A dense population of lymphocytes is a notable feature. The predominant cell type is a medium to large lymphocyte with a nucleus that is composed of bland chromatin surrounded by minimal cytoplasm (*short arrows*). There are frequent irregular formations of free nuclear protein from ruptured cells (*long arrow*) and numerous granules that represent mucin granules. The differential considerations include lymphocytic gastritis or gastric lymphoma. (Wright; ×250.)

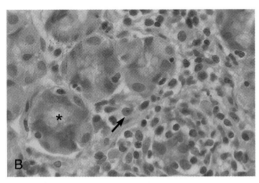

FIGURE 7–15. B, Lymphocytic gastritis. Histology. A heterogeneous population of lymphocytes (*arrow*) surrounds the gastric glands (*asterisk*). A small number of plasma cells were admixed (not shown) resulting in a morphologic diagnosis of lympho-plasmacytic gastritis. (H & E; ×250.)

cytes with or without plasma cells along with macrophages defines chronic inflammation. Lymphocytic or lymphoplasmacytic inflammation is associated with chronic gastritis (Fig. 7–15A & B). *Physaloptera* sp. is one specific cause of chronic inflammation that can be observed endoscopically (Fig. 7–15C). Other parasites that cause gastritis, especially in cats, are *Ollulanus* and *Gnathostoma* (Barker et al., 1993; Guilford and Strombeck, 1996). Parasites or parasite fragments are rarely seen on cytology (Jergens et al., 1998). Gastric nodular lymphocytic inflammation can be associated with *Helicobacter* sp.

Gastric phycomycosis or zygomycosis can be associated with severe gastric inflammation (Miller, 1985). Prolonged treatment with antibiotics or immunosuppression may lead to gastric candidasis (Fig. 7–16). The oral and esophageal mucus membranes are additional sites for candidiasis. Periodic acid-Schiff or Gomori's methenamine silver stains can be used to highlight yeast and fungal organisms.

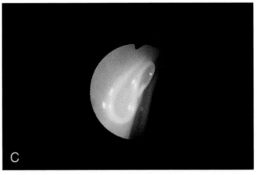

FIGURE 7–15. C, Physaloptera. Gastric endoscopic view. An approximately 2-cm-long white nematode consistent with Physaloptera was endoscopically observed in the fundus of a dog with recurrent vomiting. It is one cause (uncommon) of chronic gastritis. (Barker et al., 1993; Guilford and Strombeck, 1996) (Slide courtesy of Colin Burrows and Denny Meyer.)

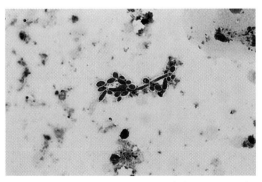

FIGURE 7–16. Gastric candidiasis. Brushing. Numerous basophilic pseudohyphae and blastospores of *Candida* sp. A silver stain (Gomori's methenamine stain) can be used to highlight the organism in tissue. (Wright; ×250.)

Neoplasia

Gastric neoplasms are uncommon and most are malignant. The relatively more common carcinoma/adenocarcinoma is difficult to diagnose cytologically when it is located in the submucosa or muscularis. In addition, the occasional development of reactive fibrosis adds an additional barrier that precludes exfoliation of the neoplastic cells. Malignant cells usually exfoliate readily when gastric ulceration is present.

More commonly, infiltrative lymphoma (lymphosarcoma) can be diagnosed on gastric cytology (refer to Figs. 7–27 and 7–35 for examples). Unless there are large numbers of predominantly immature lymphocytes present cytologically, lymphoma can be difficult to differentiate from severe lymphocytic inflammation. Small cell lymphoma (well-differentiated lymphocytes) usually cannot be confidently diagnosed with cytology and requires the histology.

INTESTINE

Normal Cytology

The intestinal mucosal epithelium is columnar and glands are present. The duodenum is the region most commonly sampled endoscopically. Mucosal cell types that can be observed in cytologic specimens include columnar epithelial cells, mucus-producing goblet cells, and globule leukocytes (Figs. 7–17 to 7–19). The mucosal epithelial cells contain basophilic round to oval nuclei with moderate amounts of light basophilic cytoplasm and chromatin that is smooth to finely stippled (less aggregated than that observed in lymphocytes) and indistinct nucleoli. Mucus may be diffuse or seen as distinct basophilic to purple granules (Fig. 7–20). These structures should not be confused with the irregularly shaped granular magenta-stained particles of gel-type products that are used for lubrication and are common contaminants (Fig. 7–21). Paneth cells contain coarse eosinophilic granular cytoplasm and can be difficult to distinguish from mucus-producing cells.

Aggregated lymphoid follicles (Peyer's patches) are scattered in the mucosa of the antimesenteric wall of the small intestine. Endoscopically they appear as oval to elongated thickenings that are a few millimeters

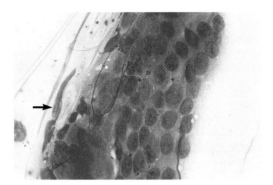

FIGURE 7–17. Intestinal epithelial cells, normal. Touch imprint. Cluster of uniform epithelial cells with round to oval nuclei and confluent basophilic cytoplasm. Streaks of free nuclear protein are noted on the left (*arrow*). (Wright; ×250.)

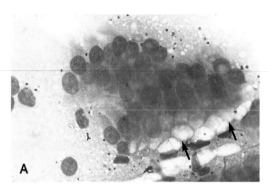

FIGURE 7–18. A, Intestinal mucosal epithelial cells, normal. Touch imprint. The columnar epithelial cells have large clear cytoplasmic vacuoles (*arrows*) that represent apical mucus vacuoles. The cells have indistinct cell borders and a few mucin granules are scattered around them. (Wright; ×250.)

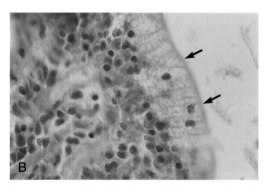

FIGURE 7–18. B, Intestinal mucosal epithelial cells, normal. Histology. The columnar epithelial cells contain basilar nuclei and show cytoplasmic rarefaction (increased lucency) in the apical end (*arrows*) due to their cytoplasmic mucus content. (H & E; ×250.)

to several centimeters in diameter. They may project slightly above the mucosal surface or appear as slight depressions and be mistaken for an ulcerlike lesion. The follicular aggregate of B-lymphocytes is covered by a mixed population of T- and B-lymphocytes extending into the lamina propria in rounded mucosal projections (Barker et al., 1993). An erroneous cytologic impression of lymphocytic inflammation or even

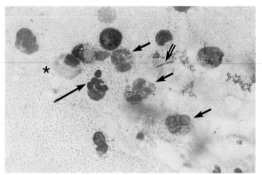

FIGURE 7–19. Globule leukocyte, eosinophilic colitis. Fecal smear. The mononuclear cell left of center (*long arrow*) has a round to oval eccentric nucleus composed of homogeneous chromatin and the light bluish-gray cytoplasm is packed with large, distinct metachromatic cytoplasmic granules. The globule leukocyte is located in the intestinal epithelium of the crypt and lower villus and in the lamina propria. Although controversial, it is probably derived from the mast cell based on cytochemical and ultrastructural findings, may be associated with type-1 hypersensitivity reactions, and is also found in the respiratory tract (Murray et al., 1968; Huntley, 1992; Narama et al., 1999; Breeze and Wheeldon, 1977; Baldwin and Becker, 1993). Intestinal globule leukocyte tumors have been described (Honor et al., 1986). Also present are three eosinophils (*three short arrows*) with poorly stained brownish cytoplasmic granules, a plasma cell with its notable darkly basophilic cytoplasm (top), and another globular leukocyte with an eccentric oval nucleus surrounded by abundant bluish-gray cytoplasm that contains the spherical outlines of globules that did not stain (*asterisk*). A large bacterial rod-shaped bacterium is located to the right of center (*double arrow*). The granules of eosinophils often do not stain intensely in fecal smears. The presence of abundant eosinophils is suggestive of eosinophilic colitis. The morphologic diagnosis from a colonic biopsy was eosinophilic colitis. (Wright; ×250.)

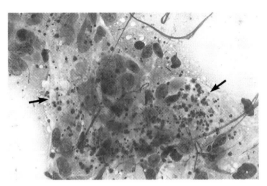

FIGURE 7–20. Intestinal epithelial cells, normal. Touch imprint. Numerous mucus secretory granules cover a dense cluster of uniform intestinal epithelial cells (*arrows*). The cellular distortion is an artifact of the preparation. Streaks of free nuclear protein are present (top). (Wright; ×250.)

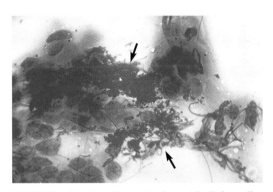

FIGURE 7–21. Intestinal epithelial cells, normal, gel lubricant. Touch imprint. In the center of these dense clumps of intestinal epithelial cells are irregularly shaped homogeneous islands of magenta-stained material that represent the gel used for lubrication of the endoscope (*arrows*). (Wright; ×250.)

lymphoma is possible if a follicle is unknowingly sampled or if the endoscopist does not communicate with the cytopathologist (Fig. 7–22). A heterogeneous lymphocyte population generally comprises a lymphoid follicle or inflammatory reaction and that variability aids in differentiation from the homogeneous lymphocyte population characteristic of lymphoma. Small numbers

of lymphocytes and plasma cells may be seen (grade 0–1) cytologically but they are less frequent than one might anticipate based on the number present histologically in tissue without pathology. Granulated (large granular) lymphocytes may be normally observed in low numbers, especially in cats (Fig. 7–23). Bacteria are usually not

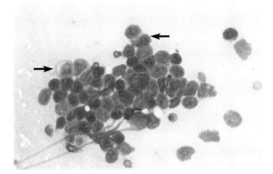

FIGURE 7–22. Intestinal aggregated lymphoid follicle (Peyer's patch). Brushing. This densely packed cluster of lymphocytes is composed of small (darkest stained), medium, and large lymphocytes (lightest stained with visible rim of lightly basophilic cytoplasm, *arrows*). Four free nuclei are located to the far right. (Wright; ×250.)

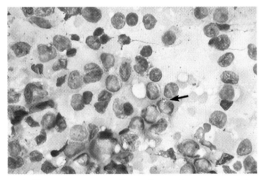

FIGURE 7–23. Lymphocytic enteritis. Grade 6/7, granular lymphocyte. Touch imprint. Medium and large lymphocytes are prominent with scattered small lymphocytes admixed. A granular lymphocyte is located slightly to the right of center (*arrow*). In other areas, occasional neutrophils and macrophages contributed to the inflammatory reaction. (Wright; ×250.)

normally observed or are only present in low numbers (Baker and Lumsden, 2000).

Hyperplasia

A cytologic impression of hyperplasia is based on prominent numbers of mucus-secreting epithelial cells and/or a marked increase in goblet cells. It is important to differentiate changes of epithelial hyperplasia or metaplasia due to reparative lesions from relatively well-differentiated neoplasia. Criteria for hyperplasia include preservation of polarity, uniformity of cell size with minimal anisocytosis, and cohesiveness of cells. Correlation with the histologic findings is recommended when there are problematic cytologic findings.

Inflammation

Inflammatory cells are categorized according to the grading system, with a grade of 2 or more indicating the corresponding degree of significant inflammation (see Table 7–2). The grading system is used to express the presence and magnitude of the neutrophilic (Fig. 7–24) or lymphocytic–plasmacytic inflammatory constituents (Fig. 7–23). Severe lymphocytic enteritis may be difficult to differentiate from malignant lymphoma when medium to large lymphocytes are prominent (see Neoplasia, below). Comparative correlation with the histologic findings is imperative. An increase in the number of granulated lymphocytes appears to be a nonspecific component of enteritis, especially in the cat. Eosinophils, mast cells, Paneth cells, and mucus-secreting cells may be difficult to confidently differentiate cytologically because of altered staining characteristics (Figs. 7–19 and 7–25), moderate to marked cell distortion, rupture, and lysis that accompanies the general morass of inflammation. When inflammation is present, periodic acid-Schiff or Gomori's methenamine silver stains can be used to highlight

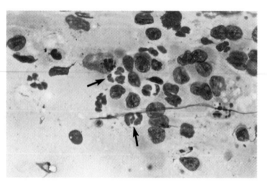

FIGURE 7–24. Purulent enteritis. Grade 5/6. Touch imprint. Numerous neutrophils (*arrows*) are intimately admixed with lightly basophilic-stained intestinal epithelial cells. An occasional eosinophil (not visible) was noted and is a common finding that has no added diagnostic importance. Karyorrhectic debris is located to the lower right. (Wright; ×250.)

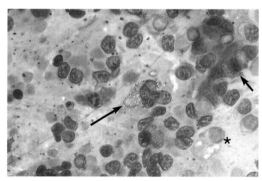

FIGURE 7–25. Intestinal epithelial cells, normal, mast cell. Touch imprint. In the center is a mast cell composed of a distorted oval nucleus with ropy chromatin surrounded by moderately abundant cytoplasm with faint-staining metachromatic granules (*long arrow*). An occasional mast cell is a normal finding in an intestinal cytologic specimen. Basophilic epithelial cells (*short arrow*) and lightly stained medium-sized lymphocytes with round nuclei composed of diffuse chromatin surrounded by a moderate rim of lightly basophilic cytoplasm are present (*asterisk*). Free nuclei that retain moderate chromatin clumping are scattered throughout the specimen. (Wright; ×250.)

fungal and protozoal agents. Giardiasis can be diagnosed by finding the trophozoites in duodenal specimens. They appear as binucleate, pear-shaped organisms with four pairs of flagella (Fig. 7–26).

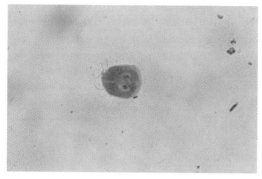

FIGURE 7–26. Giardiasis. Duodenal aspirate. *Giardia intestinalis* (*lamblia* or *duodenalis*) is recognized by its paired metachromatically stained nuclei and multiple eight flagella (two located to the left). A rod-shaped bacterium is on its lower right surface. The diagnosis also can be made by zinc sulfate fecal flotation or ELISA or immunofluoresence fecal tests. (Wright; ×250.) (Slide courtesy of Denny Meyer.)

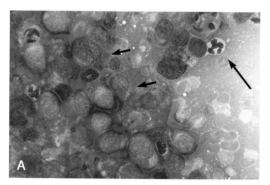

FIGURE 7–27. A, Intestinal lymphoma. Touch imprint. Numerous lymphoblasts are embedded in basophilically stained mucus (*short arrows*). The large immature lymphocytes have an oval to irregularly shaped nucleus composed of homogeneous, pale-staining chromatin surrounded by minimal to moderately abundant lightly basophilic cytoplasm. Their large size can be appreciated by comparison to the neutrophil (*long arrow*). Karyorrhectic debris is located above the neutrophil. (Wright; ×250.) (Slide courtesy of Denny Meyer.)

Neoplasia

The ability to detect intestinal neoplasia cytologically depends on the extent of infiltration and the presence of ulceration. Lymphoma readily exfoliates, which facilitates a cytologic diagnosis (Fig. 7–27A & B). However, it can be missed cytologically because neoplastic lymphocytes often stain less intensively and easily rupture. Occasionally, the differentiation of severe lymphocytic en-

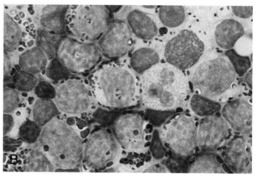

FIGURE 7–27. B, Large granular lymphoma. Fine-needle aspirate of abdominal mass of a cat. This monomorphic population of cells has a round to oval nucleus with ropy chromatin surrounded by a minimal to moderate amount of lightly basophilic cytoplasm and contains prominent variably-sized metachromatically stained granules. Some of the cells have smaller granules that formed a packet in one location of the cytoplasm (not shown). Darkly stained normal small lymphocytes are sandwiched amongst the neoplastic cells and a segmented eosinophil with faintly stained granules is centrally located. At surgery, the confluent mass involved the lymph nodes and small intestine. Franks et al. (1986) published the clinical, histologic, and ultrastructural findings of this case. The neoplasm often involves the intestinal tract and jejunal lymph nodes. (Darbes et al., 1998) One study suggested that these "granulated round cell tumors" have a common cellular origin that may involve cells in transition between mucosal mast cells and globule leukocytes. (Refer to Figure 7–19.) (McEntee et al., 1993) (Wright; ×250.)

teritis from lymphoma is problematic. Also, the reader is referred to the discussion under Normal Cytology, above, regarding the potential misimpression that can occur if an aggregated lymphoid follicle is sampled. Correlation with the histologic findings is

imperative when there are problematic cytologic findings.

The intestinal adenocarcinoma has the general characteristics of neoplastic epithelial cells (Fig. 7–28A & B). In our experience, other intestinal neoplasms (e.g., leiomyosarcomas, leiomyomas, and fibrosarcomas) are difficult to diagnose cytologically because of their deeper location and decreased tendency to exfoliate.

COLON/RECTUM/FECAL

Normal Cytology

Colonic cytologic specimens consist of groups or sheets of uniform columnar epithelial cells with goblet cells that contain mucin and basilar nuclei (Fig. 7–29). A prominent mixed bacterial flora is a common finding. Rectal scrapings contain columnar epithelial clusters and fecal material. Aggregated lymphoid follicles are present in the colon and a mixture of small, medium, and large lymphocytes are observed cytologically. Again the reader is referred to the discussion under Normal Cytology, above,

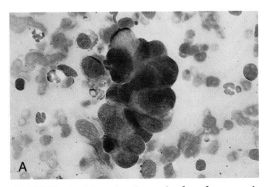

FIGURE 7–28. A, Intestinal adenocarcinoma. Touch imprint. Epithelial cells in this dense cluster demonstrate increased basophilia, marked anisocytosis and anisokaryosis, variable N:C ratios, and overgrowth of neighboring cells. Their abnormally large size is appreciated by comparison to the neutrophils. (Wright; ×250.)

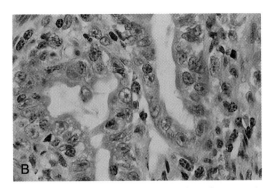

FIGURE 7–28. B, Intestinal adenocarcinoma. Histology. Disorganized epithelial tubules are formed by cells that demonstrate moderate to marked anisocytosis and anisokaryosis, variable nuclear chromatin patterns, prominent nucleoli, variable N:C ratios. (H & E; ×250.)

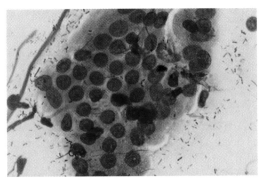

FIGURE 7–29. Normal colonic epithelial cells. Touch imprint. The sheet of epithelial cells demonstrates uniform cytomorphologic features and staining. Numerous bacteria of varying size and shapes are a normal finding. (Wright; ×250.)

regarding the potential misimpression that can occur if an aggregated lymphoid follicle is sampled.

Hyperplasia

Observing a relatively normal-appearing mucosa endoscopically combined with a cytologic finding of a uniform population of epithelial cells supports a diagnosis of mucosal hyperplasia. Hyperplastic epithelial cells can have mild cellular atypia and distinct nucleoli, especially associated with rectal mucosal hyperplasia (Fig. 7–30A & B).

Inflammation

The finding of neutrophils indicates active inflammation involving the colon and/or rectum because neutrophils entering the more proximal intestinal lumen would be rapidly destroyed (Fig. 7–31A). Possible infectious causes of neutrophilic colitis in-

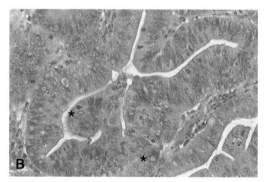

FIGURE 7–30. B, Hyperplastic colonic epithelial cells. Histology. Papillary projections (*asterisks*) are covered by hyperplastic columnar mucosal epithelial cells with basilar nuclei, coarse chromatin, and prominent nucleoli. The tissue architecture is consistent with a benign lesion. (H & E; ×100.)

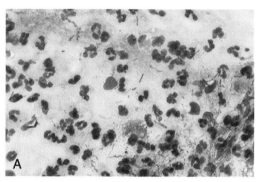

FIGURE 7–31. A, Purulent (neutrophilic) colitis. Scraping. Neutrophils are the prominent abnormal microscopic feature. Colonic bacterial flora is admixed. Differential diagnostic considerations include infections by *Campylobacter, Salmonella, Clostridium,* and *Trichuris.* A cause was not determined in this case. (Wright; ×250.)

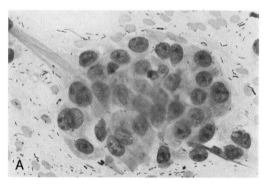

FIGURE 7–30. A, Hyperplastic colonic epithelial cells. Touch imprint. The slightly understained sheet of epithelial cells have nuclei composed of stippled chromatin, contain one to two prominent nucleoli, and show minimal variation in nuclear size and shape. Cytologic differential considerations for this mass lesion are polyp, adenoma, or well-differentiated carcinoma. Numerous bacteria in the background are normal colonic flora. (Wright; ×250.)

clude bacteria (*Clostridium perfringens* [Fig. 7–31B], *Campylobacter jejuni, Salmonella* sp., an enterotoxic strain of *Escherichia coli*) and parasites *(Trichuris vulpis)* (Fig. 7–31C). The presence of small to medium lymphocytes with or without plasma cells is consistent with a generic morphologic impression of chronic colitis (Fig. 7–32A & B). Hemorrhage induced by sampling is

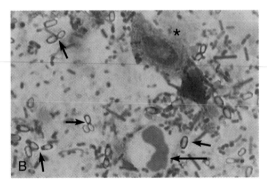

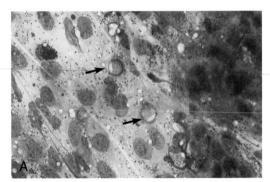

FIGURE 7–31. B, Clostridial colitis. Fecal smear. Numerous neutrophils were present upon scanning of this direct fecal smear. An increased number of large rod-shaped bacterial endospores with a clear center and an increased density predominantly on one end ("safety pin" appearance) are the notable feature (*short arrows*). The bacterial morphology is consistent with *Clostridium perfringens*. Occasional organisms can be normally seen but greater than 5 organisms per 1000× oil field is considered abnormal. (Twedt, 1992) Confirmation was made by measurement of the enterotoxin in the feces. (Twedt, 1992; Marks et al., 1999) A degenerate neutrophil (*long arrow*) and epithelial cell (*asterisk*) are present. (Wright; ×250.) (Slide courtesy of Denny Meyer and Dave Twedt.)

FIGURE 7–32. A, Lymphocytic colitis. Touch imprint. An increased number of small to medium-sized lymphocytes composed of a round to oval nucleus with homogeneous chromatin and a small rim of clear to lightly basophilic cytoplasm are present (*arrows*). Dense basophilic clusters of epithelial cells (far right) and abundant mucus granules suggestive of mucosal hyperplasia are set in a lightly basophilic background of mucus. (Wright; ×250.)

common in colonic and rectal sampling. Leukocytes in the blood can confound the cytologic interpretation, especially if there is a concurrent leukocytosis.

Colonic samples can be used to detect *Prototheca* sp. (rectum), *Histoplasma capsulatum* (intestine, rectum), *Balantidium coli* (rectum), and *Cryptococcus neoformans* (intestine) (Rakich and Latimer, 1999). *Prototheca* sp. is a colorless algae (1.3–13.4 mm wide and 1.3–16.1 mm long) with basophilic granular cytoplasm, a clear cell wall, and a small nucleus (Rakich and Latimer, 1999) (Fig. 7–33). Endosporulation may be noted. Systemic fungal infections can be initially detected by a rectal scraping. These include *H. capsulatum* (2–4 mm) that is often located within macrophages (Fig. 7–34) and *C. neoformans* (yeast, 3.5–7 mm) with its microscopic hallmark of a prominent clear, nonstaining capsule. *B. coli* (40–80 mm × 25–45 mm to 30–300 mm × 30–100 mm) is a ciliated protozoan that infects dogs ingesting pig feces. It is thought

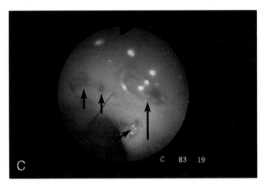

FIGURE 7–31. C, *Trichuris vulpis*-induced colitis. Endoscopic view. *Trichuris vulpis* is attached to a hemorrhagic colonic mucosal site (*long arrow*). Several other areas of mucosal inflammation/hemorrhage are present (*short arrows*). A moderate number of neutrophils were observed in a fecal smear. (Slide courtesy of Colin Burrows and Denny Meyer.)

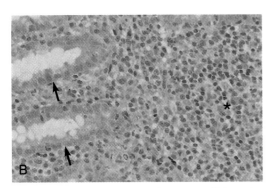

FIGURE 7–32. B, Lymphocytic colitis. Histology. There is a moderate to marked increase in small to medium-sized lymphocytes that invade the deeper mucosal region (*asterisk*). Hypertrophic mucosal glands are lined by prominent goblet cells with large clear mucus-filled vacuoles (*arrows*). (H & E; ×125.)

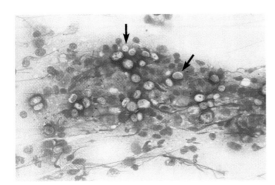

FIGURE 7–33. *Prototheca* sp. Colonic touch imprint. The algae appear as variably sized, oval clear structures with eosinophilic to basophilic stippling (*arrows*). The organisms are embedded in a dense sheet of epithelial cells. (Wright; ×125.)

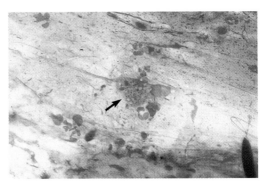

FIGURE 7–34. *Histoplasma capsulatum*. Rectal scraping. The macrophage (*arrow*) is distended with faintly stained oval structures (*H. capsulatum*) giving it a foamy or vacuolated appearance. The organisms almost completely cover the nucleus located at the top of the cell. A neutrophil and a smeared lymphocyte are located beneath and to the right of the macrophage, respectively. Colonic flora and a diffuse, lightly basophilic mucus background are present. (Wright; ×250.)

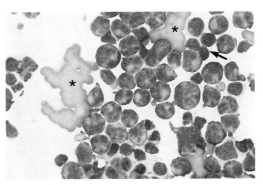

FIGURE 7–35. Colonic lymphoma. Touch imprint. Pleomorphic lymphoblasts composed of irregularly shaped to reniform to convoluted nuclei surrounded by moderately abundant dark basophilic cytoplasm are the notable abnormal microscopic finding. Their anaplastic morphology makes them difficult to recognize as a lymphoid cell type. A few small lymphocytes with dense nuclei and minimal cytoplasm are admixed (*arrow*). Two small islands of yellowish-green erythrocytes are present (*asterisks*). (Wright; ×250.)

that damage to the colonic mucosa by trichuriasis may predispose to *B. coli* infection.

Neoplasia

Colonic carcinoma/adenocarcinoma and lymphoma (Fig. 7–35) are most commonly diagnosed and appear cytologically similar to those described in other parts of the intestinal tract. Plasmacytomas can occur in the colon, as well as other areas of the digestive tract, including the oral cavity (Fig. 7–36).

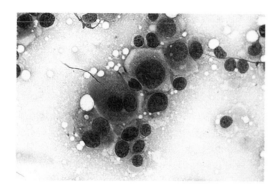

FIGURE 7–36. Colonic plasmacytoma. Touch imprint. These cells demonstrate characteristics of malignancy that include marked anisocytosis and anisokaryosis and variable N : C ratio. While they have morphologic features that are consistent with an anaplastic carcinoma, the eccentric nucleus and basophilic cytoplasm is also suggestive of a plasma cell derivation. Histology along with immunohistochemical staining of the biopsy confirmed a plasmacytoma. (Wright; ×250.)

References/Suggested Reading

Baker R, Lumsden JH: The gastrointestinal tract. In Baker R, Lumsden JH (eds): *Color Atlas of Cytology of the Dog and Cat.* CV Mosby, St. Louis, 2000, pp 177–183.

Baldwin F, Becker AB: Bronchoalveolar eosinophilic cells in a canine model of asthma: Two distinctive populations. Vet Pathol 1993; 30:97–103.

Barker IK, Van Dreumel AA, Palmer N: The alimentary system. In Jubb KVF, Kennedy PC, Palmer N (eds): *Pathology of Domestic Animals,* vol. 2, Academic Press, San Diego, 1993, pp 1–318.

Breeze RB, Wheeldon EB: The cells of the pulmonary airways: State of the art. Am Rev Resp Dis 1977; 116:705–721.

Ciekot PA, Powers BE, Withrow SJ, et al: Histologically low-grade, yet biologically high-grade, fibrosarcomas of the mandible and maxilla in dogs: 25 cases (1982–1991). J Am Vet Med Assoc 1994; 204(4):610–615.

Darbes J, Majoub M, Breuer W, Hermanns W: Large granular lymphocyte leukemia/lymphoma in six cats. Vet Pathol 1998; 35:370–379.

Eaton KA: Editorial: Man bites dog: Helicobacter in the new millennium. J Vet Int Med 1999; 13: 505–596.

Fox SM, Burns J, Hawkins J: Spirocercosis in dogs. Comp Cont Educ Pract Vet 1988; 10:807–822.

Franks PT, Harvey JW, Calderwood-Mays M, et al:

Feline large granular lymphoma. Vet Pathol 1986; 23:200–202.

Green L: Gastrointestinal cytology. In Atkinson BF (ed): *Atlas of Diagnostic Cytopathology.* WB Saunders, Philadelphia, 1992, pp 283–316.

Guilford WG: Diseases of the oral cavity and pharynx. In Guilford WG, Center SA, Strombeck DR, Williams DA, Meyer DJ (eds): *Strombeck's Small Animal Gastroenterology,* 3rd ed. WB Saunders, Philadelphia, 1996, pp 189–201.

Guilford WG, Strombeck DR: Chronic gastric diseases. In Guilford WG, Center SA, Strombeck DR, Williams DA, Meyer DJ (eds): *Strombeck's Small Animal Gastroenterology,* 3rd ed. WB Saunders, Philadelphia, 1996, pp 275–302.

Happonen I, Saari S, Castren L, et al: Comparison of diagnostic methods for detecting gastric *Helicobacter*-like organisms in dogs and cats. J Comp Pathol 1996; 115(2):117–127.

Henry GA, Long PH, Burns JL, et al: Gastric spirillosis in Beagles. Am J Vet Res 1987; 48(5):831–836.

Hermanns W, Kregel K, Breuer W, Lechner J: *Helicobacter*-like organisms: Histopathological examination of gastric biopsies from dogs and cats. J Comp Pathol 1995; 112(3):307–318.

Honor DJ, DeNicola DB, Turek JJ, et al: A neoplasm of globule leukocytes in a cat. Vet Pathol 1986; 23:287–287.

Huntley JF: Mast cells and basophils: A review of

their heterogeneity and function. J Comp Pathol 1992; 107:349–372.

Jenkins CC, Bassett JR: *Helicobacter* infection. Comp Cont Educ Pract Vet 1997; 19(3):267–279.

Jergens AE, Andreasen CB, Hagemoser WA, et al: Cytologic examination of exfoliative specimens obtained during endoscopy for diagnosis of gastrointestinal tract disease in dogs and cats. J Am Vet Med Assoc 1998; 213 (12):1755–1759.

Marks SL, Melli A, Kass PH, et al: Evaluation of methods to diagnose *Clostridium perfringens*-associated diarrhea in dogs. J Am Vet Med Assoc 1999; 214:357–360.

McEntee MF, Horton S, Blue J, Meuten DJ: Granulated round cell tumor of cats. Vet Pathol 1993; 30:195–203.

Miller RI. Gastrointestinal phycomycosis in 63 dogs. J Am Vet Med Assoc 1985; 186(5):473–478.

Murray M, Miller HRP, Jarrett WFH: The globule leukocyte and its derivation from the subepithelial mast cell. Lab Invest 1968; 19:222–234.

Narama I, Ozaki K, Matsushima S, Matsuura T: Eosinophilic gastroenterocolitis in iron lactate-overload rats. Toxicol Pathol 1999; 27:318–324.

Poulet FM, Valentine BA, Summers BA. A survey of epithelial odontogenic tumors and cysts in dogs and cats. Vet Pathol 1992; 29(5):369–380.

Rakich PM, Latimer KS: Rectal mucosal scrapings. In Cowell RL, Tyler RD, Meinkoth JH (eds): *Diagnostic Cytology and Hematology of the Dog and Cat*. CV Mosby, St. Louis, 1999, pp 249–253.

Rakich PM, Latimer KS, Weiss R, et al: Mucocutaneous plasmacytomas in dogs: 75 cases (1980–1987). J Am Vet Med Assoc 1989; 194(6):803–810.

Salisbury SK, Lantz GC, Nelson RW, Kazacos EA: Pancreatic abscess in dogs: six cases (1978–1986). J Am Vet Med Assoc 1988; 193(9):1104–1108.

Simpson KW, Strauss-Ayali D, McDonough PL, et al: Gastric function in dogs with naturally acquired gastric Helicobacter spp. infection. J Vet Int Med 1999a; 13:507–515.

Simpson KW, McDonough PL, Strauss-Ayali D, et al: *Helicobacter felis* infection in dogs: Effects on gastric structure and function. Vet Pathol 1999b; 36:237–248.

Spangler WL, Culbertson MR. Salivary gland disease in dogs and cats: 245 cases (1985–1988). J Vet Med Assoc 1991; 198(3):465–469.

Twedt DC: Clostridium perfringes-associated enterotoxicosis in dogs. In Kirk RW, Bonagura JD (eds): *Current Veterinary Therapy XI–Small Animal Practice*. WB Saunders, Philadelphia, 1992, pp 602–607.

Tyler RD, Cowell RL, Meinkoth JH: The oropharynx and tonsils. In Cowell RL, Tyler RD, Meinkoth JH (eds): *Diagnostic Cytology and Hematology of the Dog and Cat*. CV Mosby, St. Louis, 1999, pp 59–67.

CHAPTER 8

The Liver

DENNY J. MEYER

"The establishment of an accurate diagnosis depends on sampling an adequate amount of tissue and, most important, on a histologic interpretation by someone well versed in liver histopathology."

E. R. Schiff and L. Schiff, 1993

The microscopic examination of hepatic cytology is diagnostically rewarding when applied judiciously. Although fine-needle aspiration biopsy (FNAB) of the liver is practical and economical, it has defined (limited) diagnostic utility and its cavalier use can result in incomplete or inaccurate information. The information cytologically derived from a needle aspirate is often projected to equate with a histologic-based diagnosis. For inflammatory liver disease this is often an erroneous assumption since tissue architecture cannot be assessed and histopathologic findings cannot be quantified. These are critical elements for the microscopic assessment of the hepatic pathology (Ishak, 1994). The ultrasonographic examination of the liver has added another dimension of potential "abnormal" findings that contribute to the complexities of work-ing up patients with abnormal liver tests. It has facilitated the "guided" acquisition of cytologic specimens from focal lesions that can be either diagnostic (e.g., metastatic neoplasia) or descriptively nonspecific (e.g., vacuolar change). The objective of this chapter is to suggest areas of hepatic pathology for which the cytologic interpretation of a FNAB can be diagnostic and to provide histologic comparators that illustrate the limitations of hepatic FNAB as well as provide differential considerations for the descriptive cytologic findings.

SAMPLING THE LIVER

Indications and Contraindications

Hepatic cytology is valuable for the initial evaluation of hepatomegaly. Causes of hepatomegaly include feline hepatic lipidosis syndrome, lymphoma, myeloproliferative neoplasia, mast cell neoplasia, hepatocellular carcinoma, corticosteroid hepatopathy, and amyloidosis. In addition, primary and metastatic neoplasia or a focal infection, identified with ultrasound examination, usually can be further characterized with cytology. However, it is not possible to differentiate benign, focal inflammatory pathology from "chronic" progressive disease or accurately assess the extent of its pathology. It is not possible to make a definitive cytologic diagnosis of nodular regenerative hyperplasia or differentiate its relatively benign inflammatory reaction and hepatocellular cytoplasmic changes from other diseases that cause similar hepatic pathology. For these types of hepatic pathology, histologic examination is required for determining severity, providing a prognosis (e.g., identify bridging necrosis, bridging fibrosis), and directing (and monitor) therapy.

Abnormal hemostasis is a potential contraindication for FNAB of the liver. Since FNAB utilizes either a "capillary" or suction sampling technique, cutting or laceration of the vascular tissue is a relatively lesser risk compared to the use of a cutting needle or wedge biopsy procedure. If one or more of the coagulation tests are abnormal, their temporary correction often can be attained within 12 hours by the subcutaneous administration of vitamin K_1. A reduced platelet count is a greater concern. A value less than 20,000/ul is a contraindication and the sampling procedure should be preceded by the administration of platelet-rich plasma. A platelet count value between 20,000 to 50,000/ul is a relative contraindication. Dependent on the underlying pathology, the sampling procedure can be performed knowing that there is an inherent risk factor with careful monitoring of the patient for 24 hours. Prior to any sampling procedure of a vascular organ, notably liver and spleen, the integrity of platelet function should be assessed. The von Willebrand factor concentration should be measured in breeds at risk (e.g., Doberman pinscher, Airedale terrier, German shepherd, golden retriever) and the history should ascertain if drugs have been recently administered that alter platelet function (e.g., nonsteroidal anti-inflammatory drugs, synthetic penicillins, cephalosporins).

A large cavitational lesion identified by ultrasound examination in an older dog, notably male German shepherd dogs and golden retrievers, is a relative contraindication for FNAB. The probability of a hemangiosarcoma is high, obtaining a definitive cytologic diagnosis is unlikely, and the potential of rupturing a necrotic capsule is a possibility. The spleen should be examined with ultrasound since hepatic metastasis is common. Exploratory surgery should be considered as both a diagnostic and treatment option.

Tumor seeding undoubtedly occurs but the frequency has not been determined (Evans et al., 1987; Navarro et al., 1998; Ishii et al., 1998). However, since treatment options are often limited and long-term survival usually has a poor prognosis, the use of FNAB as a diagnostic tool is a reasonable risk noting the aforementioned caveat pertaining to cavitational lesions.

Technique

Sampling the liver is performed with the patient standing on a nonslippery (e.g., rubber-matted) surface, lying with the right lateral side down, or in dorsal recumbancy. Chemical restraint is dependent on the disposition of the patient. Since the liver moves with the excursions of the diaphram, the needle is directed generally in a craniodorsad direction to reduce the risk of laceration. Choice of needle size ranges from 1- to 2½-inch 20 to 22 gauge depending on the indication and on size of animal. A longer needle is probably of greater value when attempting to sample a focal lesion in a liver that is not enlarged. If a 2½-inch needle is used, the stylet is left in place until the liver is entered to reduce contamination from skin and mesenteric fat as it is penetrated. A 6- to 12-cc syringe can be attached directly to the needle or via an intravenous infusion extension tube to facilitate greater manipulative flexibility if a suction technique is used (see below).

For hepatomegaly, the site of needle entry into the abdominal cavity is at the "triangle" formed by the union of xiphoid and last left rib. Once the needle is within the hepatic parenchyma of the left lobe, it is directed in two or three different planes using a to-and-fro motion. Acquisition of the specimen can be obtained by either aspiration or by nonaspiration ("capillary" action) procedures (see Chapter 1). Generally, the nonaspiration approach should be tried first since it reduces the amount of blood contamination. If the specimen is nondiagnostic, the aspiration technique can be attempted. After collection of the specimen, the tip of the needle is placed over a glass slide and the contents expelled using a syringe filled with several cubic centimeters of air. Often multiple slide preparations can be made from a single sampling procedure by use of the compression method (see Chapter 1). The cytologic slide preparations are air-dried, fixed, and stained. Protection from formalin fumes is critical to preserve morphologic detail (no open formalin containers can be in the room prior to fixation and staining). At least one unfixed cytologic slide preparation should be saved for potential special stains such as a Gram, a copper, iron, Congo red, or immunocytochemical stain.

Occasionally, the gallbladder or large bile duct is penetrated as evidenced by yellow to green to dark green fluid in the syringe.

Aspiration should be continued until no more fluid is obtained. As long as the biliary tissue is healthy, it will heal without side effects, although it is prudent to closely observe the patient for 24 hours for signs of peritonitis. Feeding a small amount of food or the oral administration of corn oil 30 minutes prior to FNAB has been suggested as means of contracting the gallbladder and reducing the risk of penetration. While there is probably no down side, the unpredictability of the canine gallbladder to respond to meal-stimulated contraction (Rothuzien et al., 1990) makes the procedure more palliative for the operator than of precautionary benefit for the patient in most cases. Light-yellow, acellular fluid also can be obtained from cystic lesions, which are especially prominent in cats. These would have been identified as cavitational lesions with ultrasonography and are probably congenital in origin. Obtaining clear to whitish mucinous fluid from a cavitational lesion is suggestive of a cystadenoma.

CYTOLOGIC FINDINGS

Hepatocytes constitute the predominant cell type of a normal liver (Fig. 8–1A–D). An occasional mast cell is a normal finding (Fig. 8–1E). Dense clumps of biliary epithelial cells can be observed occasionally (Fig. 8–2). Sheets of mesothelial cells collected during the sampling procedure can be present and mistaken for biliary epithelium or a neoplastic cell population (Fig. 8–3A & B).

Non-Neoplastic Diseases and Disorders

Cytoplasmic Changes

Hepatocellular cytoplasmic changes are common in association with metabolic disease and secondary to injury. Discrete small

Text continued on page 236

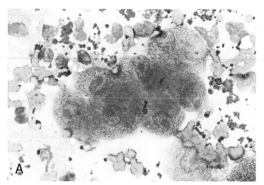

FIGURE 8–1. A, Hepatocytes are slightly oval to polygonal plump cells 25 to 30 μm in diameter (approximately 3 to 4 erythrocyte diameters). They contain a centrally placed, round to slightly oval nucleus composed of a course network of chromatin and a nucleolus that may be prominent. The nucleus is surrounded by abundant moderately bluish to basophilic cytoplasm that is often granular appearing and punctuated by granular pinkish hues because of the varying tinctorial properties of the different organelles. Clumps of greenish-stained erythrocytes and small, irregular clumps of metachromatic-stained gel used for ultrasound examination surround this island of hepatocytes. (Wright; ×250.)

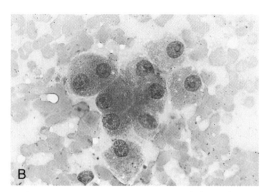

FIGURE 8–1. B, An occasional binucleated hepatocyte (lower left of center) is a normal finding. (Wright; ×250.)

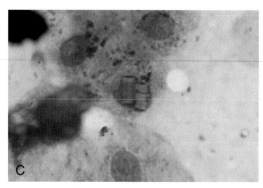

FIGURE 8–1. C, An incidental finding of no known diagnostic importance is a nucleus that contains a crystal-like rectangular structure. The nucleus of the hepatocyte in this image contains two. They are more likely to be found in aged dogs. (Wright; ×500.)

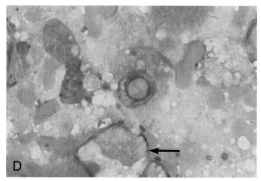

FIGURE 8–1. D, Another type of nuclear inclusion is the hollow globule-like structure that represents a membrane bound, cytoplasmic invagination that contains glycogen and mitochondria (Kelly, 1993). They are more likely to be observed in chronic liver disease and should not be mistaken for a viral inclusion body. In this figure, the spherical structure is located in the nucleus of a poorly stained hepatocyte (cytoplasm out of focus) in an aspirate from a cat that contained a mixture of neutrophils, lymphocytes, and histiocytes (*arrow*) located in a background of proteinaceous debris. Feline infectious peritonitis (FIP) was eventually diagnosed histologically. (Wright; ×500.)

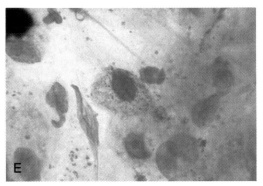

FIGURE 8–1.   E, An occasional mast cell is a normal finding. The granules often do not stain intensively. (Wright; ×500.) Contrast this image to an example of a hepatic mast cell cancer (see Figure 8–19).

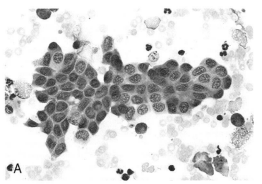

FIGURE 8–3.   A, Their angular shape (fish scale-like) identifies a sheet of mesothelial cells, probably scraped off during the sampling procedure. They should not be mistaken for a metastatic neoplasm. Note that the cell size approximates that of the hepatocyte. Brownish-stained erythrocytes surround the sheet of cells. (Wright; ×150.)

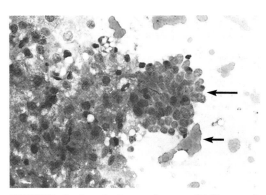

FIGURE 8–2.   A dense cluster of biliary epithelial cells (*long arrow*) is present to the right of a sheet of hepatocytes. The biliary epithelial cells have a scant rim of lightly stained cytoplasm that often appears "invisible." Note that the round nuclei, composed of dense, granular to homogeneous chromatin, are relatively uniform and slightly larger than the nuclei of a hepatocyte. The size relationship is important for the differentiation of normal from neoplastic biliary epithelium—compare to Figure 8–15. Clumps of greenish-stained erythrocytes are also present (*short arrow*). (Wright; ×150.)

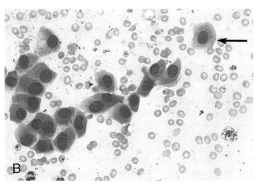

FIGURE 8–3.   B, A discrete mesothelial cell (*arrow*) has an oval appearance that is punctuated by a pinkish "sunburst" effect at the cytoplasmic border. The cell is reminiscent of plasma cell and, along with the eccentric location of the nuclei of other cell constituents, collectively may be mistaken for a plasma cell tumor. Greenish-stained erythrocytes surround the mesothelial cells. (Wright; ×150.)

(microvesicular) or large (macrovesicular) vacuoles in the hepatocyte are representative of lipid that has been cleared during the staining process (Fig. 8–4A & B). Excess accumulation of lipid in the liver is referred to as *lipidosis, fatty liver,* or *steatosis.* The feline hepatic lipidosis syndrome is the most common disease associated with this cytoplasmic alteration. An underlying disease such as cancer in geriatric cats and pancreatitis (identified with ultrasound examination) should always be considered before classifying the lipidosis as idiopathic especially if hepatomegaly is not present. Congenital lipid storage diseases are a cause of hepatomegaly in young animals due to diffuse hepatocyte vacuolar change (Fig. 8–4C & D). Aspiration of mesenteric fat during the collection process is an artifact that can cause a potential misdiagnosis (Fig. 8–4E).

Hepatocellular cytoplasmic rarefaction (lesser cytoplasmic density than normal) that does not form discrete vacuoles can be

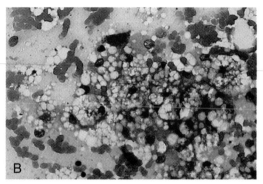

FIGURE 8–4. B, Sometimes the hepatocellular cytoplasm is distended by small, variably sized vacuoles (microvesicular). Both cytomorphologic findings of fatty change are consistent with a diagnosis of the feline hepatic lipidosis syndrome. (Wright; ×150.)

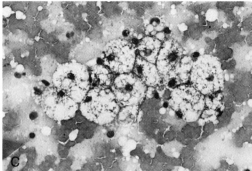

FIGURE 8–4. C, Fine-droplet (microvesicular) lipidosis in an aspirate from a puppy with hepatomegaly and ascites is suggestive of a lipid storage disease. (Wright; ×150.)

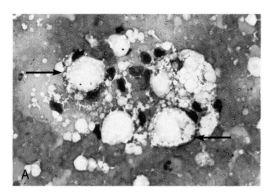

FIGURE 8–4. A, A hepatic aspirate from an icteric 5-year-old cat with a markedly raised serum ALP value and hepatomegaly. The cytoplasm of the hepatocytes is markedly distended by large, clear vacuoles (macrovesicular) that cause nuclear margination (some have a "signet ring" appearance *arrows*) and make the hepatocyte difficult to recognize. (Wright; ×150.)

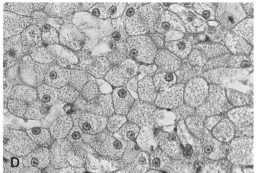

FIGURE 8–4. D, Note the cytologic features observed in Figure 8–4C are similar to a histologic specimen from a kitten with documented lipid storage disease—Niemann–Pick disease type C (Brown et al., 1994). (H & E; ×150.) (Tissue section courtesy of Dr. Diane Brown.)

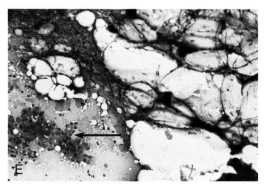

FIGURE 8–4. E, Occasionally mesenteric fat is aspirated which could be confused with hepatic lipidosis. Comparison to a clump of hepatocytes, (*arrow*), is helpful in providing a perspective of the much larger size of the mesenteric adipocyte. (Wright; ×50.)

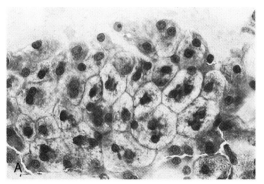

FIGURE 8–5. A, A uniform sheet of hepatocytes with cytoplasmic rarefaction ("vacuolar change") from a dog with hepatomegaly, markedly raised serum ALP activity, and normal serum bilirubin concentration. The finding is consistent with corticosteroid-induced excess glycogen storage (hepatopathy). The hepatic change occurs in association with either hyperadrenocorticism or the administration of corticosteroid medications. Hepatocytes with excess glycogen are swollen, retain a centrally located nucleus, and lack discrete cytoplasmic vacuoles typically associated with lipid accumulation. A periodic acid–Schiff (PAS) staining method, without and with 1% amylase (diastase) digestion for glycogen, is used to identify cytoplasmic glycogen. (Wright; ×150.)

caused by increased glycogen or water content. The latter type of histomorphologic change is also referred to as *hydropic (ballooning) degeneration.* The term *vacuolation* is often used as a nonspecific rubric for cytoplasmic rarefaction. The increased storage of glycogen in response to hypercortisolemia or the administration of exogenous corticosteroids is a common cause of hepatocellular cytoplasmic rarefaction in the canine liver (Fig. 8–5A & B). The unique, robust nature of the canine hepatocyte to store glycogen in response to hypercortisolemia can be sufficiently dramatic to result in generalized hepatomegaly. The volume of the hepatocyte can be increased up to three-fold by excess glycogen accumulation. (Kuhlenschmidt et al., 1991) Various types of hepatocellular injury such as toxic insults and hypoxia will alter the integrity of the cell membrane and cytoplasmic organelles, resulting in increased cellular water content. As a consequence, cytoplasmic rarefaction (hydropic degeneration) is observed morphologically and cannot always be confidently distinguished from the cytoplasmic change associated with increased cytoplasmic

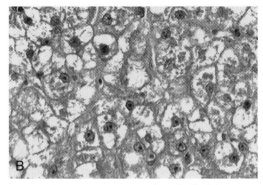

FIGURE 8–5. B, Note the similarities to a histologic specimen from another dog with corticosteroid-induced hepatopathy. (H & E; ×150.)

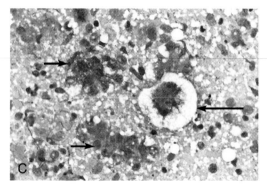

glycogen (Fig. 8–5C–E). In aged dogs, hepatic nodular regenerative hyperplasia is common. The number of nodules ranges from a few to many and are often composed of hepatocytes with cytoplasmic rarefaction and/or vacuolation (Kelly, 1993) (Fig. 8–6A & B).

FIGURE 8–5. **C,** Two markedly swollen hepatocytes demonstrate hydropic (ballooning) degeneration (*long arrow*). Other hepatocytes (*short arrows*) show less cytoplasmic alteration or appear morphologically normal. Also present are a moderate number of inflammatory cells (difficult to recognize as lymphocytes and neutrophils) surrounded by a bluish-gray background ("dirty appearance"), which is suggestive of necrotic debris. (Wright; ×150.)

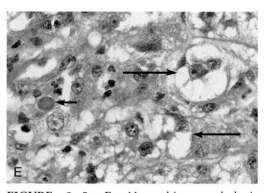

FIGURE 8–5. **E,** Note histomorphologic similarities to a specimen from a dog with acute liver injury associated with the administration of carprofen. (MacPhail et al., 1998) Swollen hepatocytes due to ballooning degeneration (*long arrows*) are admixed with lesser affected hepatocytes. A dense-staining eosinophilic structure (*short arrow*) represents a hepatocyte undergoing apoptotic necrosis. (H & E; ×150.)

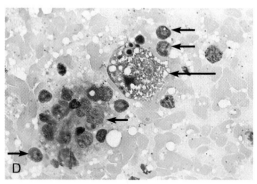

FIGURE 8–5. **D,** In another field a hepatocyte is undergoing degeneration, as illustrated by nuclear condensation and fragmentation within a granular, microvacuolated cytoplasm (*long arrow*). The appearance of its cytoplasm is similar to the "necrotic" background material seen in Figure 8–5C. A few inflammatory lymphocytes are in close proximity (*short arrows*). A small clump of hepatocytes (*thick arrow*) demonstrates regenerative changes consisting of mild anisocytosis and anisokaryosis that were more easily observed in other clumps. The findings along with moderately raised serum ALT and aspartate aminotransferase (AST) values, mild rise in the serum bilirubin concentration, and only a slight rise in the serum ALP value support a morphologic diagnosis of acute liver injury (hepatitis) (e.g., toxin, drug-induced). (Wright; ×150.)

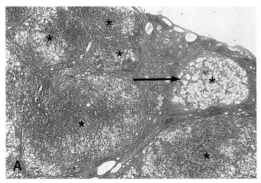

FIGURE 8–6. **A,** Six nodules of varying size (asterisks) can be seen in this low-power wedge biopsy specimen from a clinically healthy 12-year-old mixed-breed dog with mildly raised serum liver enzyme values and numerous hepatic nodules observed at surgery. Note the dramatic variation in hepatocyte morphology among the nodules. If the nodule located to the upper right (*arrow*) was sampled with FNAB or a cutting needle biopsy, the findings would be consistent with "vacuolar hepatopathy," suggestive of a metabolic disease. (Gordon & Sweets reticulin; ×25.)

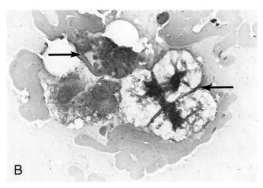

FIGURE 8–6. **B,** A cytologic specimen obtained prior to the aforementioned biopsy shows hepatocytes with morphologic characteristics that range from near normal to marked cytoplasmic rarefaction (*long arrow*). A dense clump of platelets (*short arrow*) is common artifact and should not be confused with a multinucleated cell or infectious agents. (Wright; ×250.)

Neutrophilic (Suppurative), Lymphocytic (Nonsuppurative), and Mixed Cell Inflammation

The assessment of hepatic inflammation by FNAB often provides an incomplete picture of the pathology because of an inability to evaluate the lobular architecture and assess the magnitude of the inflammatory changes. Confounding factors that are problematic for obtaining diagnostically useful information include the common occurrence of reactive neutrophilic and lymphocytic infiltrates that are associated with the relatively benign condition of nodular regenerative hyperplasia in dogs. Marked blood contamination in a hepatic FNAB from a dog or cat with a high neutrophil count or a cat with a mildly raised lymphocyte count can foster an ambivalent cytologic interpretation.

Neutrophilic inflammation is suggested when a high concentration of segmented neutrophils is observed relative to the red blood cell numbers. Finding neutrophils intimately associated with or within hepatocellular clumps is further supportive evidence. The neutrophils and surrounding tissue should be carefully examined for infectious agents (Fig. 8–7A & B). The anatomic location of the neutrophilic infiltration in the lobule cannot be determined cytologically, precluding differentiation between primarily parenchymal inflammation (hepatitis) versus primarily inflammation of the bile ducts (cholangitis). (Fig. 8–7C & D) Linking the morphologic assessment with the biochemical findings can be of value, especially in the dog. Finding a serum alkaline phosphatase (ALP) value that is markedly higher than the serum alanine aminotransferase (ALT) value is supportive of cholangitis/cholangiohepatitis, especially if the serum bilirubin concentration is also raised. This generalization of course does not apply to the differential diagnosis of the

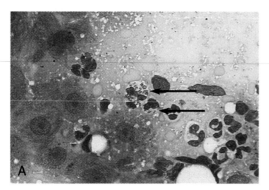

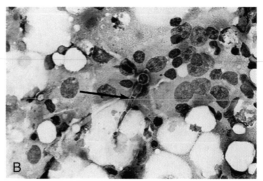

FIGURE 8–7. A, The presence of neutrophils intimately associated with hepatocytes is indicative of suppurative hepatitis. Note the paucity of erythrocytes, which indicates that the majority of the neutrophils are not a component of blood contamination. A careful search for an infectious agent is occasionally rewarding when neutrophils are prominent. Note two neutrophils packed with bacteria (*arrows*). This cat also had moderately raised serum ALT and AST values, a slightly raised serum ALP value, a mild rise in the serum bilirubin concentration, and a mild neutrophilia. (Wright; ×250.)

FIGURE 8–7. B, Neutrophils were prominent in areas (not shown) of this aspirate from a dog with moderately raised liver enzyme tests and hypoechoic foci with ultrasound examination. A mycotic agent (*long arrow*) was discovered after additional searching. A diagnosis of hepatic hyalohyphomycosis, a term applied to opportunistic infections caused by nondematiacious fungi with hyaline hyphal elements as the basic tissue form, was subsequently made based on the culture of *Paecilomyces* species from tissue obtained at surgery. (Wright; ×250.)

feline lipidosis syndrome, primarily a hepatocellular disease, in which the serum ALP activity is often dramatically raised in association with hyperbilirubinemia. Neutrophilic inflammation can be a component of either a sterile inflammatory process (e.g., acute pancreatitis (Fig. 8–7C), feline neutrophilic cholangiohepatitis (Fig. 8–7D), feline infectious peritonitis (FIP) (Fig. 8–7E), or septic inflammation (Fig. 8–7A). Sampling a solitary hypoechoic structure in the hepatic parenchyma in association with neutrophilia and/or fever is a relative contraindication and should be approached with caution because of the potential of rupturing an abscess and inducing peritonitis.

The occurrence of a predominantly uniform population of small lymphocytes with or without a few plasma cells in attendance,

referred to as *lymphocytic portal hepatitis,* is a common finding in older cats (Fig. 8–8A) (Gagne et al., 1999; Weiss et al., 1995). The lymphocytic inflammation is confined to the portal tract and does not demonstrate piecemeal necrosis (lymphocytic inflammation in the portal tract that streams into surrounding parenchyma and is associated with liver cell necrosis) (Fig. 8–8B). The frequency with which the pathology is responsible for illness is not known even when accompanied by raised serum ALT and/or ALP values. The peripheral lymphocyte count is not raised, differentiating it from chronic lymphocytic leukemia with liver involvement. An examination for an extrahepatic disease (e.g., pancreatitis, enteritis, neoplasia) should be thorough before ascribing the illness to primary liver disease. Occasionally the lymphocytic in-

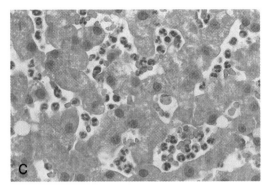

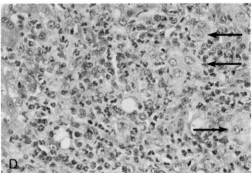

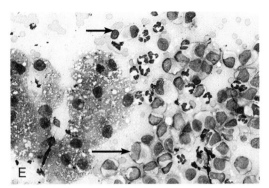

FIGURE 8–7.   E, Neutrophils and histiocytes may be a prominent component of the mixed cell inflammation in cats with FIP involving the liver. This touch imprint is from one of several small white foci on the surface of the liver. The histiocytes are the large mononuclear cells (compare to the size of the neutrophils) with oval to reniform nuclei composed of bland homogenous chromatin surrounded by a moderate amount of bluish-gray cytoplasm (*long arrows*). A lesser number of small mononuclear cells (lymphocytes) are admixed (*short arrows*). Similar lesions were located on the kidney and in the mesentery in this case of noneffusive feline infectious peritonitis confirmed histologically. (Wright; ×150.)

FIGURE 8–7.   C&D, While cytology may be able to identify the predominant inflammatory cell type present in a liver, it cannot determine which component of the hepatic lobule is primarily involved. Contrast the following histologic findings in two icteric cats with moderately raised serum liver enzyme values. The neutrophilic inflammation (**C**) primarily involves the parenchyma (suppurative hepatitis) versus (**D**) primarily bile duct inflammation (suppurative cholangitis). (H & E; ×250, ×150, respectively.) The inflammation in (**C**) was secondary to acute pancreatitis that was diagnosed based on ultrasonographic findings, while severe enteritis was associated with the cholangitis. Arrows identify bile ductular epithelial cells.

---

flammation is dramatic and causes icterus (Fig. 8–8C). It is not known if the pathology is a more severe form of lymphocytic portal hepatitis or another syndrome. The cytologic finding of predominantly small lymphocytes is not common in the dog and should be followed by histologic examina-

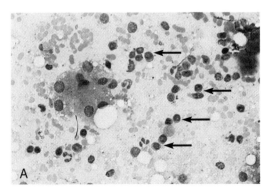

FIGURE 8–8.   A, A predominance of inflammatory (small) lymphocytes (*arrows*) in a liver sample from an aged cat is suggestive of lymphocytic (portal) hepatitis of unknown cause. (Wright; ×150.)

tion for chronic progressive hepatitis (Fig. 8–9A–C).

Relatively equal numbers of lymphocytes and neutrophils in a feline liver cytology specimen is suggestive of feline infectious peritonitis or a chronic form of neutrophilic cholangiohepatitis (Fig. 8–10A & B). If the latter is suspected, a search for an extrahe-

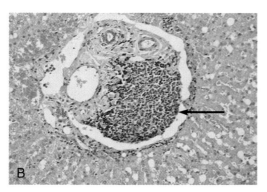

FIGURE 8–8. **B,** The histologic finding in lymphocytic portal hepatitis is a prominent lymphocytic inflammation that is confined to the portal area (*arrow*). (H & E; ×50.) Clinical studies suggest that it may not be associated with any clinical signs, may be associated with a variety of extrahepatic diseases, and may be slowly progressive. (From Weiss DJ, Gagne JM, Armstrong PJ: Characterization of portal lymphocytic infiltrates in feline liver. Vet Clin Pathol 24:91–95, 1995. Reprinted with permission.)

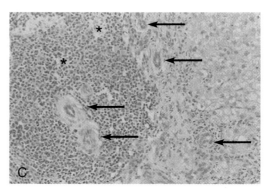

FIGURE 8–8. **C,** Occasionally, extensive lymphocytic infiltration (portal-to-portal bridging) is observed, which results in icterus. In this specimen, there is marked bile duct proliferation (*long arrows*), moderate fibrous tissue, and a dense lymphocytic infiltrate in the portal area that extends upward to connect to another portal tract (*asterisks*). (H & E; ×50.) Microscopic examination of a liver biopsy, preferably a wedge biopsy, is the only way to assess the extent of the disease.

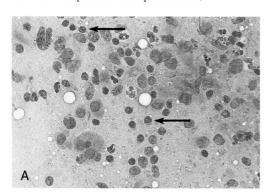

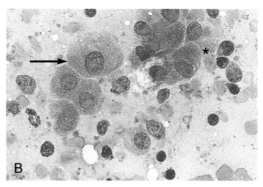

FIGURE 8–9. **A&B,** In the dog, a predominantly lymphocytic inflammation can be associated with chronic progressive hepatitis, a relatively uncommon disease that usually affects middle-aged dogs and has a breed predilection (Guilford, 1995; Sevelius and Jonsson; 1995). **(A)** This cytologic specimen is from a 5-year-old Labrador retriever with clinical lethargy, reduced appetite, and persistent mild to moderate abnormal ALT and AST values documented several times over 6 weeks. Small lymphocytes are the predominant inflammatory cell (*arrows*) and **(B)** are intimately associated with the hepatocytes (*asterisk*). Lesser numbers of neutrophils are also present. The mild to moderate hepatocellular anisocytosis and anisokaryosis (*arrow*) **(B)** is suggestive of a regenerative (or reparative) response. (Wright; ×150, ×250, respectively.)

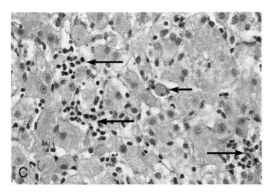

FIGURE 8–9. C, Microscopic examination of a subsequent liver biopsy confirmed the presence of chronic progressive liver disease and defined the extent of the inflammation, bridging necrosis, and fibrotic changes. These are important prognostic criteria that cannot be assessed cytologically. Notable histopathologic findings in this photomicrograph include severe piecemeal necrosis (*long arrows*) (lymphocytes streaming from the portal tracts into the surrounding parenchyma and associated hepatocellular necrosis), increased fibrosis, and apoptotic necrosis (*short arrow*). The dog died of liver failure 7 months later. (H & E; ×150.)

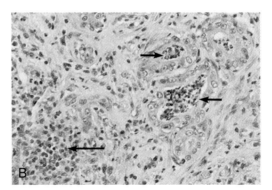

FIGURE 8–10. B, In a subsequent biopsy, the portal tract is markedly distended by a mixed cell inflammation, bile duct proliferation, and periductal fibrosis. A predominance of lymphocytes is observed in the lower left of center (*long arrow*), while neutrophils invade the bile ducts that contain necrotic debris (*short arrows*). (H & E; ×150.) Histology is required to assess the magnitude of the inflammation and degree of fibrosis. The morphologic diagnosis of this specimen is suppurative (neutrophilic) cholangiohepatitis. Studies suggest that the syndrome is initially characterized by a prominent neutrophilic inflammation involving bile ducts with periportal necrosis, as shown in Figure 8–7D, followed by the infiltration of a lymphocytic inflammatory component. The etiopathogenesis of the feline neutrophilic cholangiohepatitis syndrome is not known. Clinical studies suggest that it can be associated with a variety of extrahepatic diseases, notably pancreatitis and inflammatory bowel disease. (From Weiss DJ, Gagne JM, Armstrong PJ: Characterization of portal lymphocytic infiltrates in feline liver. Vet Clin Pathol 24:91–95, 1995. Reprinted with permission.)

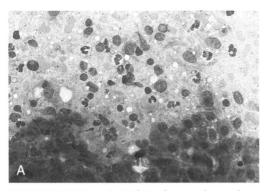

FIGURE 8–10. A, Relatively equal numbers of neutrophils and lymphocytes with an occasional histiocyte were observed in this specimen from a cat with moderately raised serum liver enzyme values. However, the lobular location and the magnitude of the inflammation cannot be determined. (Wright; ×150.)

patic disease such as enteritis or pancreatitis is warranted (Weiss et al., 1996). Mixed cell inflammation (lymphocytes, neutrophils, macrophages) of varying magnitude is a relatively common reaction of the canine liver to both intrahepatic and extrahepatic pathology. In the aged dog, mixed cell inflammation is more likely to be encountered in association with nodular regenerative hyperplasia (see below). If no extrahepatic disease values remain raised on at least three time points over at least 4 weeks, and the patient is clinically ill, histologic examination of preferably a wedge biopsy is required to further characterize the pathology. In both the dog and cat, mixed cell inflammation can be associated with mycotic, protozoal, and mycobacterial infections for which special stains can aid in their recognition. Extra time should be taken to examine the extracellular areas and the cytoplasm of plump macrophages for the presence of these infectious agents. Small numbers of eosinophils may be a constituent of nonspecific mixed inflammatory cell reactions in the dog and cat. A prominent eosinophilic component is observed in cats with the hypereosinophilic syndrome and liver flukes (especially Florida and Hawaii) and in dogs and cats with eosinophilic enteritis (Hendrick, 1981).

Nodular Regenerative Hyperplasia

Nodular regenerative hyperplasia is a common pathology of unknown cause in the older dog, generally older than 8 years of age (Kelly, 1993). The number of nodules ranges from a few to too numerous to count and the nodules range in size from microscopic to macroscopic causing distortion of the hepatic surface (see Fig. 8–6A). Their gross color depends on the tissue constituency—light brown to yellow if the hepatocellular cytoplasm is filled with glycogen or lipid and dark brown if blood is a prominent component. Morphology can vary from nodule to nodule and is probably one of the more common reasons for a histologic diagnosis of "vacuolar hepatopathy" in the aged dog without hyperadrenocorticism or for the administration of corticosteroid medications. Foci of lipid-filled and/or pigment-filled macrophages are common (Fig. 8–11A–C). Inflammatory cells,

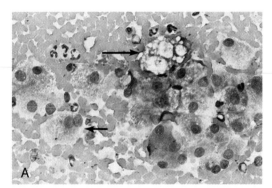

FIGURE 8–11. A, This liver specimen is from a 11-year-old mixed-breed dog with a mildly raised serum ALT value, moderately raised serum ALP value, and variable echogenicity with possible nodules noted with ultrasound. Approximately equal numbers of neutrophils and lymphocytes are scattered amongst the hepatocytes and there is a clump of foamy (vacuolated) macrophages present (*long arrow*). Hepatocytes show mild cytoplasmic rarefaction and some are binucleated (*short arrow*). These findings are nonspecific but compatible with nodular regenerative hyperplasia. In this relatively benign condition, hepatocellular cytoplasmic changes can range from severe rarefaction suggestive of excess glycogen storage or ballooning degeneration to vacuolar change consistent with lipid accumulation (refer to Figure 8–6A). (Wright; ×150.)

neutrophils, and lymphocytes of varying magnitude are often attendant to these foci (Fig. 8–11A). Extramedullary hematopoiesis can be found, most often in the compressed portal areas. Granulopoiesis is most common and is predominantly of segmented and band neutrophils that could easily be mistaken cytologically for neutrophilic inflammation (Fig. 8–11B). Megakaryocytes are the next most common cell type found in these areas of extramedullary hematopoiesis (Fig. 8–11D). Although hematopoietic precursor cells have been demonstrated in the liver of adult animals

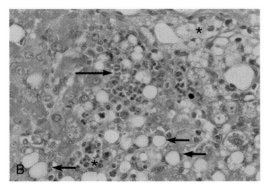

FIGURE 8–11. B, Nodular regenerative hyperplasia was confirmed with a subsequent wedge biopsy. Notable microscopic findings in this specimen include a foci of extramedullary hematopoiesis (granulopoiesis) that is composed of segmented, band, and metamyelocyte neutrophils (*long arrow*), hypertrophy of stellate cells (Ito cell, lipocytes, vitamin A-containing cells) with lipid-filled cytoplasm (*short arrows*), and a foci of yellow-pigmented macrophages (*asterisks*), some of which are vacuolated (upper right) similar to those observed in the cytologic specimen. (H & E; ×150.)

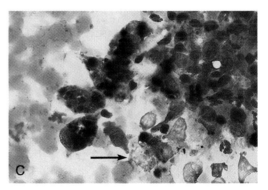

FIGURE 8–11. C, Cytologically, the macrophage foci (*arrow*) can be observed to contain dense, bluish-black material that stains intensively for iron with Prussian blue stain. (Wright; ×150.)

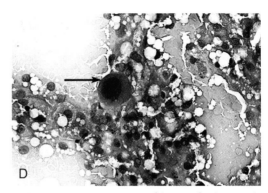

FIGURE 8–11. D, In this cytologic specimen from a 10-year-old Labrador mixed-breed dog with nodular regenerative hyperplasia subsequently confirmed histologically, is a megakaryocyte (*arrow*). Segmented and band neutrophils were associated with hepatocytes in other areas of the cytologic specimen (not shown). Extramedullary hematopoiesis, especially granulopoiesis, is a common finding that can mimic neutrophilic inflammation. Many of the hepatocytes contain variably sized cytoplasmic vacuoles consistent with lipidosis. (Wright; ×150.)

(Crosbie et al., 1999), the mechanism responsible for the formation of the extramedullary hematopoietic tissue is not known.

Amyloidosis

Hepatomegaly can be a consequence of the deposition of amyloid A protein (AA amyloid) and is classified as reactive (secondary) amyloidosis. Amyloid A protein is an amino-terminal fragment of an acute-phase reactant protein, serum amyloid A protein (SAA), that is made by hepatocytes in response to macrophage-derived cytokines interleukin-1, interleukin-6, and tumor necrosis factor. This systemic syndrome develops secondary to chronic extrahepatic inflammation (e.g., osteomyelitis), and is a famil-

ial disease in the Chinese shar-pei dog and Abyssinian cat. The syndrome has also been described in Oriental shorthair and Siamese cats (Loeven, 1994; Zuber, 1993; DiBartola,

1986). Cytologically, serpiginous swirls of eosinophilic material are observed in close approximation of hepatocytes (Fig. 8–12).

Extramedullary Hematopoiesis

The adult liver retains its ability to produce hematopoietic cells (Crosbie et al., 1999). The canine liver appears to occasionally develop extramedullary hematopoiesis, notably granulopoiesis, as a nonspecific reaction to chronic hepatic pathology. Late stages of the erythroid series are the predominant cell type in the liver in association with anemia but both granulocytic and megakaryocytic cell types can be observed. As mentioned previously, segmented and band neutrophils along with lesser numbers of megakaryocytes can be observed in the liver of dogs with nodular regenerative hyperplasia (Fig.

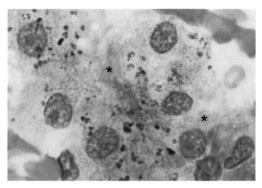

FIGURE 8–12. This FNAB of liver is from a Chinese shar pei dog with dramatic hepatomegaly and minimally raised serum liver enzyme values. Hepatic amyloidosis as a cause of hepatomegaly is indicated cytologically by the presence of ribbons of eosinophilic material that is intimately associated with normal appearing hepatocytes (*asterisks*). Dark-staining cytoplasmic material in hepatocytes is morphologically consistent with bile pigment. (Wright; ×500.) Congo red staining can be used for confirmation.

8–11B & D). A predominance of a uniform population of immature hematopoietic precursors is suggestive of neoplastic disease. The cytologic finding of virtually all bone marrow cellular elements along with adipocytes from a nodular hepatic mass is suggestive of a myelolipoma, a rare tumor.

NEOPLASIA

Hepatocellular Neoplasia

Hepatocellular-derived neoplasia is more common than neoplasia originating from epithelium of the biliary system in the dog (Straw, 1996). The hepatocellular adenoma (hepatoma) is usually a single mass involving one liver lobe and, because it can be as large as 15 cm, is often first detected as an abdominal mass. It is composed of relatively normal-appearing hepatocytes that can demonstrate mild anisocytosis and anisokaryosis. The differentiation of a hepatic adenoma from nodular regeneration is not possible cytologically and is often problematic histologically. The histologic features of no portal tracts or hepatic venules and relatively sharp demarcation support a histologic diagnosis of hepatic adenoma. It has not been shown to progress to a carcinoma. The hepatocellular carcinoma is also usually a single mass that grossly appears to involve only one liver lobe. It can be composed of relatively normal-appearing hepatocytes or obviously malignant ones (Fig. 8–13A & B). When the cell type is relatively well differentiated, histologic features of poor demarcation, metastatic islands surrounding the primary, and vascular invasion are required for differentiation from an adenoma and a definitive diagnosis of malignancy. Hypoglycemia can be a clinicopathologic manifestation of an underlying hepatocellular carcinoma (Strombeck et al., 1976).

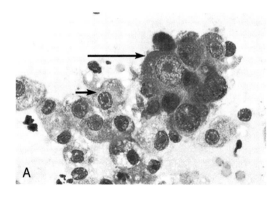

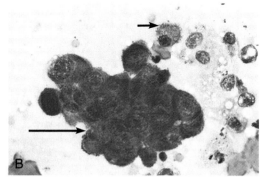

FIGURE 8–13. A&B, Hepatocellular carcinoma may be relatively well differentiated (*long arrow*) (**A**) or can be more poorly differentiated (**B**) (*long arrow*) and mistaken for a metastatic carcinoma (e.g., pancreatic). Normal-sized hepatocytes are located to the left of center for (**A**) (*short arrow*) and at the top of the neoplastic mass for (**B**) (*short arrow*). (Wright; ×250, ×250, respectively.) Both tumors caused asymmetrical hepatomegaly and were confirmed histologically.

Bile Duct Neoplasia

Cholangiocellular neoplasia, originating from epithelium of the biliary system, is the most common nonhematopoietic hepatic neoplasm in cats (Straw, 1996). It usually does not cause hepatic enlargement. Cytologically, both adenomas and carcinomas are composed of relatively normal-appearing bile duct epithelial cells that exfoliate in small sheets, clusters, or in tubular or aci-

nar formations. In contrast to hepatocytes, these cells tend to be more tightly packed with only a minimal amount of relatively clear cytoplasm. Cholangiocellular adenoma is usually confined to one lobe and is an incidental finding. Cystic formation is common and the size varies from small blister-like accumulations to fluid-filled masses as large as a liver lobe. When aspirated, the fluid can either have a bile-like appearance or a mucinous character. Because the cyst has a thin wall, the large ones are especially prone to rupture. A benign variation, the cystadenoma, is usually multilocular and lined by a mucosa that morphologically resembles biliary epithelium (Fig. 8–14). Histologic examination is required for a definitive diagnosis. Cholangiocellular carcinoma is often multiple to diffuse in appearance, involves all lobes of the liver by the time it is detected, and has an umbilicated appearance at the surface of the liver. Because of its invasiveness, it is most likely to cause

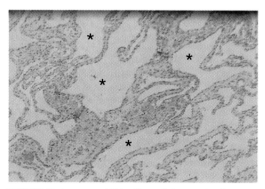

FIGURE 8–14. This liver biopsy is from a 12-year-old cat with oral disease but otherwise clinically healthy. Mildly raised serum liver enzyme tests were noted on a preanesthetic examination. Multiple fluid-filled lesions were noted on ultrasound examination and clear, acellular fluid was obtained via a FNAB. A cystadenoma was diagnosed histologically. Note multiple cystic spaces (*asterisks*). (H & E; ×100.)

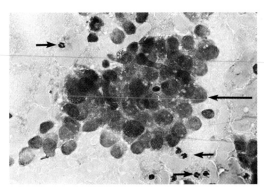

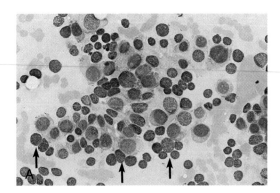

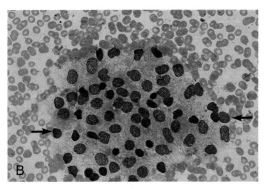

FIGURE 8-15. Cholangiocellular carcinoma appears as a dense pack of large epithelial cells with minimal cytoplasm (*long arrow*). The cells often do not show obvious cytologic criteria of malignancy other than an inappropriate large size and overgrowth of neighboring cells. A metastatic carcinoma of intestinal origin would appear cytologically similar. Several neutrophils (*short arrows*) provide a comparative perspective of the abnormally large size of the neoplastic cells and emphasize the importance of defining size relationships with a "cell micrometer" cytologically. Contrast these findings with normal sized biliary epithelial cells in Figure 8-2. (Wright; ×150.)

FIGURE 8-16. **A&B,** Each cytologic specimen was taken from apparently solitary hepatic masses (based on radiographic and ultrasonographic findings); one from an 8-year-old golden retriever, the other from a 9-year-old chow. The cytologic findings are suggestive of neuroendocrine neoplasia. They have variable amounts of clear to lightly basophilic cytoplasm with indistinct cytoplasmic borders. The round to oval nucleus is composed of bland, homogenous chromatin and **(A)** shows moderate anisokaryosis. Their fragile nature is suggested by frequent free nuclei (examples can be seen at the periphery of the specimen) (*arrows*). The possible tumor types to be considered for both specimens include hepatic carcinoid, metastatic endocrine tumor such as a pancreatic islet cell carcinoma, metastatic gastrinoma, or poorly differentiated plasmacytoma. Microscopic examination of a histologic specimen and immunohistochemical stains would be needed for a definitive diagnosis. Neither patient was available for histologic confirmation. (Wright; ×150, ×150, respectively.)

clinical disease leading to cytologic examination. The sheets or tubular formations of densely packed epithelial cells usually do not demonstrate dramatic characteristics of malignancy cytologically (Fig. 8-15). Malignancy is implicit when combined with either sonographic or visual evidence of diffuse disease involving all lobes of the liver. Histologic examination is required for a definitive diagnosis.

Hepatic Carcinoid

The hepatic carcinoid is highly malignant but is an uncommon tumor in the dog and rare in the cat. The cell type is derived from the scattered argentaffin cells (amine precursor uptake and decarboxylation (APUD) cells) that are found in the walls of intrahepatic bile ducts. Since these cells produce and release biogenic amines and hormones, systemic vasoactive manifestations or endocrine disorders such as hypoglycemia are possible extrahepatic clinical findings. Cytologically, the cell morphology can appear neuroendocrine/endocrine in origin or resemble a hepatocyte (Fig. 8–16A & B). Histologic examination using special stains is necessary for a definitive diagnosis.

Hepatic Lymphoma and Hematopoietic Neoplasia

Hepatic lymphoma is usually a component multicentric lymphoma although occasional apparent primary disease has been diagnosed. (Twedt and Meyer, personal observation) Uniform hepatomegaly is usually present. The diffuse infiltration and noncohesive nature of the cell type affords abundant exfoliation of the immature lymphocyte (Fig. 8–17A & B). Lymphocytic portal hepatitis is a relatively benign common finding in older cats and is composed cytologically of mature small to medium-sized lymphocytes. While cytologic confusion should not commonly occur, indecision should be resolved by the histologic examination of a wedge biopsy (see Fig. 8–8C & D). Finding the same cell population in another organ also supports a lymphoid malignancy (Fig. 8–17C).

Acute myeloid leukemia can involve the liver, resulting in hepatomegaly. An immature cell type of hematopoietic origin can usually be identified in a cytologic specimen from the liver (Fig. 8–18). Additional examination of the peripheral blood cells and/or bone marrow with special stains may be necessary to differentiate myeloid from lymphoid leukemia. In contrast, the invasion of the liver by neoplastic mast cells can be

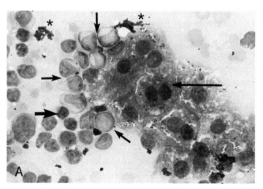

FIGURE 8–17. **A,** This hepatic aspirate was taken from a 3-year-old Labrador retriever with icterus, hepatomegaly, slightly raised liver enzyme test values, and a total bilirubin of 3.1 mg/dl (N < 0.6 mg/dl). Lymphoma (lymphosarcoma) is indicated by the presence of medium to large lymphocytes as the predominant nonhepatocyte cell type (*short arrows*). The binucleated hepatocyte (*long arrow*) contains a small amount of bluish-black granular pigment that is probably bile pigment consistent with intrahepatic cholestasis. A small, darker-staining lymphocyte (left of center) is a useful "micrometer" for assessing size and immature morphologic features of the neoplastic cells (*thick arrow*). Small globs of irregularly shaped, metachromatically stained material represents the gel used for the ultrasound examination (*asterisks*). (Wright; ×250.)

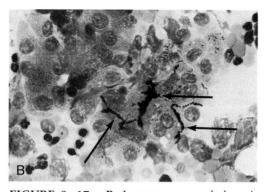

FIGURE 8–17. **B,** In some areas, cholestasis is indicated by black ribbons of inspissated bile that form casts of the bile canaliculi that course along the surface of hepatocytes (*arrows*). (Wright; ×250.)

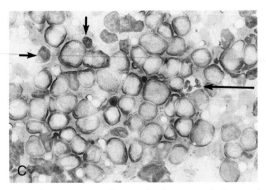

FIGURE 8–17. **C,** A similar population of neoplastic lymphocytes was aspirated from an enlarged spleen. The neutrophil (*long arrow*) and small lymphocyte (*short arrows*) are useful cell micrometers. (Wright; ×250.)

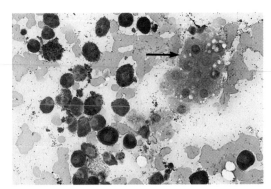

FIGURE 8–19. Marked numbers of mast cells in this hepatic aspirate from a cat with hepatomegaly is indicative of mast cell neoplasia. Hepatocytes (*arrow*) contain a small number of discrete vacuoles compatible with cytoplasmic lipid. (Wright; ×150.)

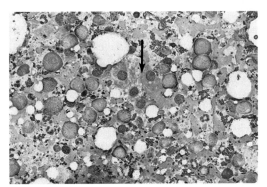

FIGURE 8–18. Large, round to oval, immature discrete cells outnumber hepatocytes (*arrow*) in this liver aspirate from a cat with hepatomegaly, nonregenerative anemia, and neutropenia. The cytologic features are most consistent with an immature cell type of hematopoietic origin. Similar cells were found in the aspirate from the bone marrow and cytochemical stains were used to confirm a diagnosis of acute myelogenous leukemia. A large amount of variably sized, irregular clumps of metachromatic material (ultrasound gel) is located amongst the cells. The large clear spaces are consistent with extracellular lipid that was probably admixed with the specimen from the mesenteric fat during the sampling procedure. (Wright; ×150.)

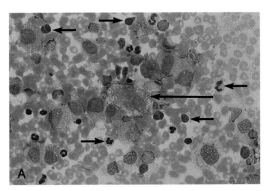

FIGURE 8–20. **A,** Large, variably sized, round to oval, immature discrete cells containing a round to oval to reniform nucleus surrounded by a moderate amount of bluish-gray cytoplasm was the prominent cytologic feature in this liver aspirate from a 5-year-old Rottweiler with hepatomegaly. The cell near the center resembles a macrophage (*long arrow*). Lesser numbers of neutrophils and lymphocytes (*short arrows*), which represent inflammatory cells or a component of blood contamination, are admixed and are useful "micrometers." Greenish-colored erythrocytes are prominent in the background. (Wright; ×150.)

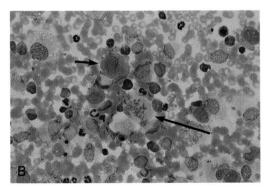

FIGURE 8–20. B, An atypical mitotic figure (*long arrow*) and a gigantic monocytoid cell (*short arrow*) are notable features of this specimen from a rottweiler with hepatomegaly and icterus. (Wright; ×150.) A discrete cell neoplasm, most likely histiocytic, was tentatively diagnosed and a biopsy recommended. Malignant histiocytosis was confirmed with histology and immunohistochemical staining.

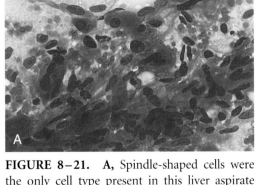

FIGURE 8–21. A, Spindle-shaped cells were the only cell type present in this liver aspirate from a dog with anorexia, weight loss, microcytic anemia, normal serum liver enzyme values, and variable echogenicity on ultrasound examination. A metastatic spindle cell tumor was diagnosed cytologically. (Wright; ×150.) An ulcerated intestinal mass was found at exploratory laparotomy.

readily identified with cytology (Fig. 8–19). Malignant histiocytosis is another discrete cell tumor that can involve both the canine and feline liver (Fig. 8–20A & B). When bizarre cell forms are present, neoplasia is readily recognized but the cell type may be problematic. A more uniform population of malignant histiocytes may resemble an acute myeloid or lymphoid leukemia and require special staining procedures for differentiation.

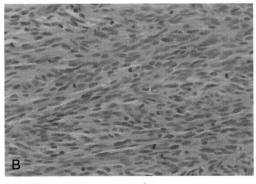

FIGURE 8–21. B, A leiomyosarcoma was diagnosed histologically. Note the histomorphologic similarities with the cytomorphologic features. (H & E; ×100.)

Metastatic Epithelial and Mesenchymal Neoplasia

Metastatic lesions to the liver can be either carcinomas or sarcomas. Because of the vascular and lymphatic relationships, metastasis to the liver is most common from primary cancers involving the pancreas and intestinal tract (Fig. 8–21A & B). Often the cell type present cannot definitively identify the primary neoplastic site cytologically. The

objective of cytology is to identify a neoplastic lesion as part of a staging process or prompt additional diagnostic efforts if the primary lesion is occult.

References and Suggested Reading

Brown DE, Thrall MA, Walkley SU, et al: Feline Niemann–Pick disease type C. Am J Pathol 1994; 144(6):1412–1415.

Crosbie OM, Reynolds M, McEntee G, et al: In vitro evidence for the presence of hematopoietic stem cells in the adult human liver. Hepatology 1999; 29:1193–1198.

DiBartola SP, Tarr MJ, Benson MD: Tissue distribution of amyloid deposits in Abyssinian cats with familial amyloidosis. J Comp Pathol 1986; 96:387–398.

Evans GH, Harries SA, Hobbs KEF: Safety and necessity for needle biopsy of liver tumors. Lancet 1987; 1:620.

Gagne JM, Armstrong PJ, Weiss DJ, et al: Clinical features of inflammatory liver disease in cats: 41 cases (1983–1993). J Am Vet Med Assoc 1999; 214:513–516.

Gagne JM, Weiss, DJ, Armstrong PJ: Histopathologic evaluation of feline inflammatory liver disease. Vet Pathol 1996; 33:521–526.

Guilford WG: Breed associated gastrointestinal disease. In Bonagura J, Kirk RW (eds): Kirk's Current Veterinary Therapy XII, WB Saunders, Philadelphia, 1995, pp 695–697.

Hendrick M: A spectrum of hypereosinophilic syndromes exemplified by six cats with eosinophilic enteritis. Vet Pathol 1981; 18:188–200.

Ishak K: Chronic hepatitis: Morphology and nomenclature. Mod Pathol, 1994; 7:690–713.

Ishii H, Okada S, Okusaka T, et al: Needle tract implantation of hepatocellular carcinoma after percutaneous ethanol injection. Cancer 1998; 82:1638–1642.

Kelly WR: The liver and biliary system. In Jubb KVF, Kennedy PC, Palmer N (eds): Pathology of Domestic Animals, 4th ed, vol 2, Academic Press, San Diego, 1993, pp 319–406.

Kuhlenschmidt MS, Hoffmann WE, Rippy MK: Glucocorticoid hepatopathy: Effect on receptor-mediated endocytosis of asialoglycoproteins. Biochem Med Metab Biol 1991; 46:152–168.

Lefkowitch JH: Pathologic diagnosis of liver disease. In Zakim D, Boyer TD (eds): Hepatology: A Textbook of Liver Disease, 3rd ed, vol 1, WB Saunders, Philadelphia, 1996, pp 844–871.

Loeven KO: Hepatic amyloidosis in two Chinese shar pei dogs. J Am Vet Med Assoc 1994; 204: 1212–1216.

MacPhail CM, Lappin MR, Meyer DJ, et al: Hepatocellular toxicosis associated with administration of carprofen in 21 dogs. J Am Vet Med Assoc 1998; 212:1895–1900.

Meyer DJ: Hepatic pathology. In Guilford WG, Center SA, Strombeck DR, et al (eds): Strombeck's Small Animal Gastroenterology, 3rd ed, WB Saunders, Philadelphia, 1996, pp 633–653.

Navarro F, Taourel P, Michel J, et al: Diaphragmatic and subcutaneous seeding of hepatocellular carcinoma following fine-needle aspiration biopsy. Liver 1998; 18:251–254.

Rothuizen R, de Vries-Chalmers Hoynck van Papendrecht R, van den Brom WE: Postprandial and cholecystokinin-induced emptying of the gallbladder in dogs. Vet Rec 1990; 126:505–507.

Schiff ER, Schiff L: Needle biopsy of the liver. In Schiff L, Schiff ER (eds): Diseases of the Liver, 7th ed. JB Lippincott, Philadelphia, 1993, pp 216–225.

Sevelius E, Jonsson LH: Pathogenic aspects of chronic liver disease in the dog. In Bonagura J, Kirk RW (eds): Kirk's Current Veterinary Therapy XII, WB Saunders, Philadelphia, 1995, pp 740–742.

Straw RC: Hepatic tumors. In Withrow SJ, EacEwen EG (eds): Small Animal Clinical Oncology, 2nd ed., WB Saunders, Philadelphia, 1996, pp 248–252.

Strombeck DR, Guilford WG: Hepatic neoplasms. In Guilford WG, Center SA, Strombeck DR, Williams DA, Meyer DJ (eds): Strombeck's Small Animal Gastroenterology, 3rd ed, WB Saunders, Philadelphia, 1996, pp 847–859.

Strombeck DR, Krum SH, Meyer DJ, et al: Hypoglycemia and hypoinsulinemia associated with hepatoma in a dog. J Am Vet Med Assoc 1976; 169:811–812.

Weiss DJ, Gagne JM, Armstrong PJ: Relationship between inflammatory hepatic disease and inflammatory bowel disease, pancreatitis, and nephritis in cats. J Am Vet Med Assoc 1996; 209: 1114–1116.

Weiss DJ, Gagne JM, Armstrong PJ: Characterization of portal lymphocytic infiltrates in feline liver. Vet Clin Pathol 1995; 24:91–95.

Zuber RM: Systemic amyloidosis in Oriental and Siamese cats. Aust Vet Pract 1993; 23:66–70.

CHAPTER 9

Urinary Tract

Dori Borjesson

The primary indications for cytologic examination of the urinary tract system include unilateral or bilateral renomegaly, focal or generalized prostatic enlargement, discrete bladder masses or bladder wall thickening, and urethral masses. Sampling method depends on lesion location but may involve either direct mass aspiration (frequently with ultrasound guidance) or traumatic catheterization in the case of a urethral mass or bladder mass in the area of the trigone. Prostatic lesions may be alternatively sampled via massage, brush, or urethral wash techniques. Lesions in the urinary tract system generally exfoliate well for cytologic examination; therefore use of these relatively noninvasive techniques frequently allows for differentiation among inflammation/infection, hyperplasia, neoplasia, and benign cystic lesions. Photomicrographs within this chapter will cover all these processes at least once in an area where these lesions are common. Recognize that these are general processes that can, of course, occur in nearly any location within the urinary system. Also, algal and fungal orga-

nisms such as *Prototheca zopfii*, *Cryptococcus neoformans*, and *Aspergillus* sp., although rarely noted, are significant findings when present in any location within the urinary tract system.

Renal aspirates are typically of low cellularity and usually contain small clusters of renal tubular cells admixed with blood. As the kidneys are highly vascular, blood is generally due to iatrogenic hemorrhage at the time of sampling. Renal aspiration is most frequently utilized to rule out lymphoma, especially in cats. Additionally, cytologic evaluation of renal aspirates may reveal other neoplastic lesions, such as transitional cell carcinoma, renal carcinoma, or metastatic neoplasia, as well as septic inflammation (secondary to pyelonephritis), nonseptic inflammation (such as the pyogranulomatous inflammation associated with feline infectious peritonitis), fungal infection, and benign cystic or hemorrhagic lesions.

Bladder and urethral masses are readily accessible using ultrasound and direct fine-needle aspiration or blind traumatic catheterization. The most common neoplastic lesion affecting both these locations is transitional cell carcinoma. Squamous cell carcinomas, malignant tumors of smooth muscle origin (leiomyosarcoma), and metastatic disease are less frequently encountered. Transitional cell carcinoma must be distinguished from transitional cell hyperplasia and benign transitional cell polyps based on cytologic features of malignancy. Aspiration of bladder wall thickenings may reveal reactive transitional cells and concurrent inflammation indicating chronic cystitis rather than neoplasia. Similarly, septic inflammation can be readily identified on cytologic exam.

The most common prostatic lesion identified cytologically is benign prostatic hyperplasia in older, intact male dogs. Squamous metaplasia of prostatic epithelial cells can also be noted. An important differential diagnosis is prostatic carcinoma, usually transitional cell carcinoma, or, less commonly, prostatic adenocarcinoma. Careful evaluation of cytologic criteria of malignancy, including cellular pleomorphism and both nuclear and nucleolar morphology, is important in making this distinction. Fluid-filled prostatic cysts, hematomas, and abscesses are also commonly encountered and readily identified by cytologic examination.

PROSTATE

See Figures 9–1 to 9–5.

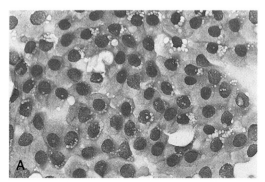 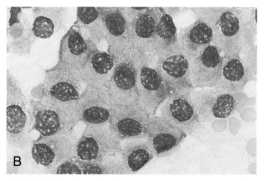

FIGURE 9–1.   A, Benign prostatic hyperplasia. Prostatic cells are cuboidal to columnar in shape and are found in sheets or clusters. Aspirates from hyperplastic lesions are generally of high cellularity and contain cells that are uniform in appearance. Occasional cells have granular or deeply basophilic cytoplasm. There is frequent perinuclear vacuolization in this sheet of cells that is of no diagnostic importance. Marked variation in cell or nuclear size is not noted. Similarly, nucleoli and mitotic figures are infrequent to absent. (Wright-Giemsa; ×187.)

FIGURE 9–1.   B, Benign prostatic hyperplasia. Note the uniform size and shape of the cells as well as the inconspicuous, fine, punctate cytoplasmic vacuolization. Nuclear chromatin can be dispersed and ragged appearing in cells taken from the urothelial system as demonstrated in these cells. (Wright-Giemsa; ×312.)

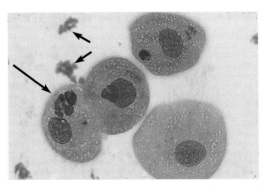

FIGURE 9–2. Squamous metaplasia of prostatic epithelial cells. With chronic irritation or inflammation, prostatic cells can undergo metastatic transformation from normal columnar and cuboidal cell morphology to a more squamous appearance. These cells have abundant basophilic "sky-blue" cytoplasm with fine, punctate cytoplasmic vacuoles. The cytoplasm of one cell contains a neutrophil undergoing emperipolesis (*long arrow*) (a physiologic curiosity in which there is receptor-mediated transport through the cytoplasm of another cell). The background contains irregular, pink clumps of material consistent with ultrasound gel artifact (*short arrows*). (Wright-Giemsa; ×312.)

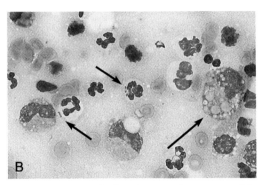

FIGURE 9–3. B, Septic, purulent prostatitis and hemorrhage. Bipolar rod-shaped bacteria have been phagocytized by neutrophils (*short arrows*). Neutrophil morphology varies from nondegenerate to moderately degenerate (reduced chromatin clumping and nuclear segmentation). A large activated (foamy) macrophage (*long arrow*) has several large beige-colored vacuoles that may represent partially digested erythrocytes (see below). *Escherichia coli* was cultured. (Wright-Giemsa; ×312.)

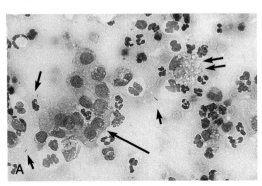

FIGURE 9–3. A. Septic, purulent prostatitis with epithelial reactivity and hemorrhage. Note the small cohesive cluster of basophilic epithelial cells (*long arrow*) admixed with a population of both moderately degenerate (karyolytic) neutrophils as well as nondegenerate neutrophils. Extracellular rod-shaped bacterial organisms are present (*short arrows*). A large activated (foamy) macrophage (*double arrow*) contains intracytoplasmic pale blue material consistent with hemosiderin that is an indication of concomitant chronic hemorrhage. *Escherichia coli* was cultured. (Wright-Giemsa; ×187.)

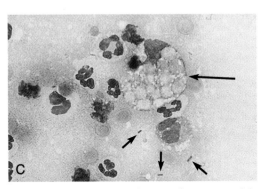

FIGURE 9–3. C, Septic, purulent prostatitis and hemorrhage. Note the marked erythrophagia (*long arrow*). The partially digested erythrocytes appear as beige-colored spheres. There are several extracellular rod-shaped bacteria present (*short arrows*). (Wright-Giemsa; ×312.)

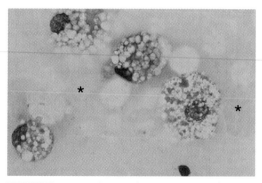

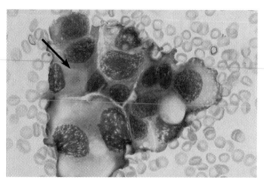

FIGURE 9–4.   Prostatic cyst. Prostatic cysts are characterized by a high protein background that microscopically looks like pink stippling or has areas of variable pink to blue shades. Cystic fluid typically has low cellularity and contains cells composed predominantly of activated macrophages along with an occasional small lymphocyte. Hemorrhage can be a prominent feature. This aspirate is characterized by activated (vacuolated and phagocytic) macrophages that are surrounded by a proteinaceous background that stains with pinkish to bluish hues (*asterisks*). Some of the cytoplasmic vacuoles overlie the nucleus when the cell is flattened giving it a "moth-eaten" appearance. (Wright-Giemsa; ×312.)

FIGURE 9–5.   Prostatic transitional cell carcinoma. Malignant prostatic epithelial neoplasia can arise from the epithelial glandular cells (therefore termed an *adenocarcinoma*) or, more commonly, from the transitional cells lining the prostatic urethra (therefore termed a *transitional cell carcinoma*). The morphologic differentiation is made histologically. Cytologically, an epithelial malignancy is denoted by the pleomorphic characteristics of this transitional cell cluster. The cytologic criteria of malignancy include marked anisokaryosis and anisocytosis, nuclear crowding, variable nuclear-to-cytoplasmic ratio, and prominent variably sized nucleoli. The intracytoplasmic pink material (*arrow*) is probably a secretory product that is normally produced by epithelial cells. The large size of the cancer cells is apparent by comparison to the surrounding erythrocytes. (Wright-Giemsa; ×312.)

BLADDER

See Figures 9–6 to 9–8.

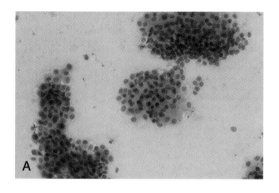

FIGURE 9–6.   A, Transitional cell hyperplasia or benign polyps. Epithelial hyperplasia or polyp formation is distinguished from malignant epithelial neoplasia by the distinctive clustering and uniform appearance of the epithelial cells. (Wright-Giemsa; ×63.)

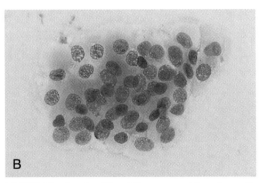

FIGURE 9–6. B, The transitional cells within this hyperplastic epithelial cell cluster have round to oval uniform nuclei. The chromatin is coarse (a common cytomorphologic feature of the urothelial system) without obvious nucleoli. Cell–cell borders are often readily observed and there is only mild pleomorphism. Contrast the features of this cell cluster to the one in Figure 9–5. (Wright-Giemsa; ×187.)

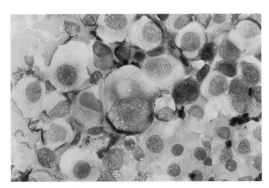

FIGURE 9–7. Transitional cell carcinoma. This sheet of transitional cells shows numerous criteria of malignancy, including marked anisocytosis and anisokaryosis, variable nuclear-to-cytoplasmic ratio, pleomorphic nuclei, cellular encroachment, and variably staining intensity. Malignant cells in other clusters also displayed prominent variably sized nucleoli. Note the cytomorphologic similarities to the cell cluster in Figure 9–5. Contrast these cellular features of malignancy to the benign characteristics of the cell cluster in Figure 9–6B. (Wright-Giemsa; ×187.)

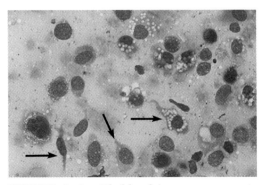

FIGURE 9–8. Bladder leiomyosarcoma. As in other organ systems, cells of mesenchymal neoplasia tend to stingily exfoliate as single cells or small aggregates rather than in cohesive clusters. Cell shape varies from round to oval to spindle shaped, as demonstrated by these malignant cells that were derived from the neoplastic smooth muscle of the bladder wall. A cytologic impression of mesenchymal derivation is endorsed by finding cells with wispy tails (*arrows*). Cytologically, malignancy is characterized by moderate anisokaryosis, anisocytosis, cellular and nuclear pleomorphism, variably staining intensity, and variable nuclear-to-cytoplasmic ratios. The pink to blue proteinaceous background littered with variably sized pink to more basophilic stained pieces of nuclear material ("dirty appearance") is consistent with necrotic debris. Malignant cells derived from mesenchymal tissue can show uniform punctate cytoplasmic vacuolation, as illustrated by some of these cells. (Wright-Giemsa; ×187.)

KIDNEY

See Figures 9–9 to 9–11.

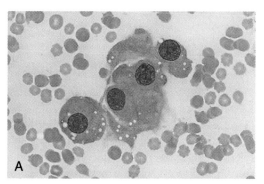

FIGURE 9–9. A, Renal tubular epithelial cells. This is a small cluster of round to oval to columnar renal tubular cells. They have abundant basophilic, occasionally vacuolated cytoplasm that surrounds a uniform, round nuclei. In this setting they have a plasma cell-like appearance. The greenish erythrocytes provide a perspective on cell size. (Wright-Giemsa; ×187.)

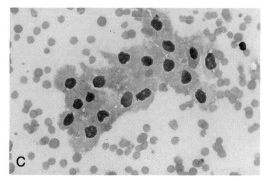

FIGURE 9–9. C, Degenerate renal tubular epithelial cells. Tubular cells often have a bland, ragged appearance that is probably due to urine-induced degenerative changes. (Wright-Giemsa; ×187.)

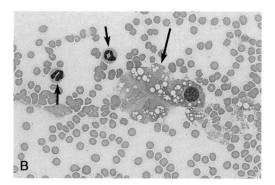

FIGURE 9–9. B, Feline renal tubular epithelial cell. Notable intracytoplasmic variably sized lipid droplets that appear as clear, punctate vacuoles are an added feature of these cells from a feline kidney aspirate. Free vacuolated cytoplasm from a ruptured cell is also present (*long arrow*). Note the size of the tubular cells in comparison to the neutrophils present (*short arrows*). (Wright-Giemsa; ×187.)

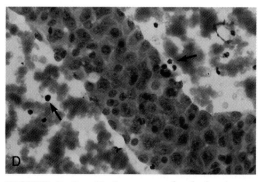

FIGURE 9–9. D, Intact renal tubule. A segment of the tubule occasionally will be aspirated. Cell nuclei are round and uniform with small, regular nucleoli. The large size is suggestive of a collecting duct or distal tubule. Leukocytes provide a perspective of size (*arrows*). (Wright-Giemsa; ×125.)

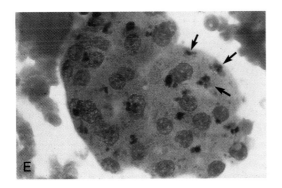

FIGURE 9–9. E, Intact renal tubule. The dark, intracytoplasmic granules (*arrows*) of the cells composing this segment of a tubule are indicative of the ascending loop of Henle or distal tubule as the site of origin. The possibility of a well-differentiated melanocyte tumor could be an initial misleading impression. (Wright-Giemsa; ×250.)

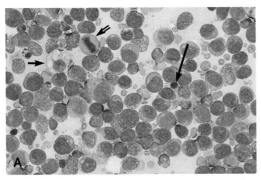

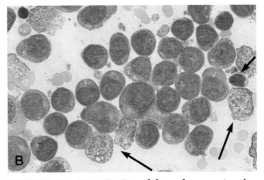

FIGURE 9–10. A, Renal lymphoma. This sample contains a dense population of discrete cells with cytomorphologic features consistent with large, immature lymphocytes. The neoplastic lymphocytes show moderate to marked pleomorphism, have a nucleus composed of homogeneous, smooth chromatin, and have relatively abundant, moderately basophilic cytoplasm compared to a normal lymphocyte (*long arrow*). A less common feature of lymphoma present here is the presence of pink-staining cytoplasmic granules. An activated (vacuolated) macrophage (*short arrow*) and a mitotic figure (*double arrow*) are located in the upper left-hand corner. These cells are differentiated from renal tubular cells by their abundance and the high nuclear-to-cytoplasmic ratio. (Wright-Giemsa; ×187.)

FIGURE 9–10. B, Renal lymphoma. A relatively normal appearing small lymphocyte (*arrow*) accentuates the immature features of the neoplastic lymphocytes. In addition to the above features described in Figure 9–10A, prominent nucleoli can be seen in some of the malignant cells. The cytoplasmic granules are more readily observed. Five or six lacy pink ovoid formations, sometimes referred to as "basket cells" or "smudge cells," represent free nuclear chromatin from lysed cells (*arrow*). It is a frequent finding in aspirates from tissue comprised of fragile cells such as lymphoma. (Wright-Giemsa; ×187.)

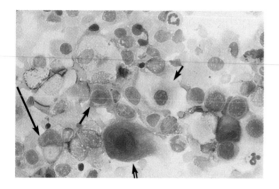

FIGURE 9–11.   Renal transitional cell carcinoma. This cellular renal aspirate is also composed of apparently discrete cells. The marked pleomorphism with a highly variable nuclear-to-cytoplasm ratio and an occasional cell having an epithelial appearance (*short arrows*) supports an epithelial malignancy. The large bizarre cell (*double arrow*) is a very helpful feature in support of a carcinoma. Marked anisocytosis and anisokaryosis as well as prominent and multiple, variably sized, angular nucleoli are noted (*long arrow*). (Wright-Giemsa; ×187.)

Suggested Readings

Batamuzi EK, Kristensen F: Diagnostic importance of urothelial cells of the dog and cat. J Sm Anim Pract 1995; 36(1):17–21.

Biberstein EL, Hirsh DC: The urinary tract as a microbial habitat; urinary tract infections. In Hirsh DC, Zee YC (eds): *Veterinary Microbiology*. Blackwell Science, Malden, MA, 1999, pp. 178–184.

Burkhard MJ, Meyer DJ: Invasive cytology of internal organs. Cytology of the thorax and abdomen. Vet Clin North Am Small Ani Prac 1996; 26(5):1203–1222.

Coffey DS, Walsh PC: Clinical and experimental studies of benign prostatic hyperplasia. Urol Clin North Am 1990; 17(3):461–475.

Jones TC, Hunt RD, King NW: The urinary system. In *Veterinary Pathology*, 6th ed. Williams & Wilkins, Baltimore, 1997, pp. 1111–1147.

Norris AM, Laing EJ, Valli VE, et al: Canine bladder and urethral tumors: A retrospective study of 115 cases (1980–1985). J Vet Intern Med 1992; 6(3):145–153.

Peter AT, Steiner JM, Adams LG: Diagnosis and medical management of prostate disease in the dog. Semin Vet Med Surg (Sm Anim) 1995; 10(1):35–42.

Senior DF, deMan P, Svanborg C: Serotype, hemolysin production, and adherence characteristics of strains of *Escherichia coli* causing urinary tract infection in dogs. Am J Vet Res 1992; 53(4):494–498.

Valli VE, Norris A, Jacobs RM, et al: Pathology of canine bladder and urethral cancer and correlation with tumour progression and survival. J Comp Pathol 1995; 113(2):113–130.

Waters DJ: High-grade prostatic intraepithelial neoplasia in dogs. Euro Urol 1999; 35(5-6):456–458.

CHAPTER 10

Microscopic Examination of the Urinary Sediment

DENNY J. MEYER

"One can obtain considerable information concerning the general trends by examining the urine."

Hippocrates, 5th Century B.C.

The urine specimen has been referred to as a liquid tissue biopsy of the urinary tract—painlessly obtained (Haber, 1988). The routine urinalysis is composed of two major components—the macroscopic and the microscopic evaluations. The chapter will focus on findings that can be microscopically observed in the urinary sediment. The evaluation of the physical characteristics and interpretation of alterations detected by reagent test-strip methodologies can be found elsewhere (Meyer and Harvey, 1998). Microscopic examination of urine sediment should be conducted on every urinalysis even if no abnormalities are detected by the reagent test-strip. Studies indicate that up to 16% of urine samples with unremarkable reagent test-strip findings can have positive microscopic findings, notably pyuria and bacteriuria (Barlough et al., 1981; Fettman, 1987). The findings of an-

other study support the recommendation to routinely examine microscopically and culture the urine of dogs with hyperadrenocorticism and diabetes mellitus since clinical signs of bacterial cystitis often are not present (approximately 95% of the cases) and bacteriuria and pyuria may not be observed (approximately 19% of the cases) (Forrester et al., 1999).

Free catch, catheterization, and percutaneous cystocentesis are the techniques used to obtain urine. The latter method is the surest way to avoid contamination. The specimen should be processed and examined within minutes of collection for the most accurate semiquantitative assessment of the findings. Casts are the most labile constituent and begin to lyse within 2 hours. Cells loose their integrity within 2 to 4 hours depending on the osmolality of the urine. Refrigeration of the urine specimen

TABLE 10–1	Normal Number of Cells Per HPF* in a Urine Sediment and the Interpretation of Increased Numbers

Erythrocytes (RBCs)

<5; varying degrees of crenation are often observed due to the physiochemical environment of the urine (Fig. 10–1A). Increased numbers indicate bleeding associated with (1) renal pathology: glomerular or tubulointerstitial disease, calculus, renal vein thrombosis, vascular dyplasia, trauma—an erythrocyte cast is indicative of intrarenal pathology (Fig. 10–10); (2) lower urinary tract disease: acute and chronic infection, calculus, neoplasia, hemorrhagic cystitis; or (3) contamination from the genital tract—collect urine via percutaneous cystocentesis.

Leukocytes (WBCs)

<5; the neutrophil is the most common leukocyte. Its nuclear segmentation may be lost as a result of the physiochemical environment of the urine and appear round to oval, resulting in an epithelial cell-like appearance but with less cytoplasm (Fig. 10–2B). However, they have less cytoplasm compared to an epithelial cell. Increased numbers are associated with (1) renal disease: pyelonephritis—leukocyte cast may be found (Fig. 10–9A)—calculus; (2) lower urinary tract disease: acute and chronic cystitis, calculus, neoplasia; and (3) contamination from the genital tract—collect urine via percutaneous cystocentesis.

Transitional epithelial cells

<2; mild size variation is normal, with the larger ones located in the urinary bladder and urethra and the smaller ones located in the renal pelvis and tubules. Epithelial cells with "tails" (cytoplasmic projection) are called *caudate epithelial cells* and have been associated with an origin from the renal pelvis. However, size and shape do not reliably indicate the anatomic site of origin. Transitional cell hyperplasia (Fig. 10–4B) is readily stimulated by inflammation (e.g., secondary to infection), irritation, and cyclophosphamide.

Squamous epithelial cells

0; these large polygonal, angular cells are often present in free-catch and catheterized specimens and may be prominent during estrus (Fig. 10–3). Finding bacteria along with squamous epithelial cells is suggestive of contamination and the examination of a specimen collected via cystocentesis is prudent.

*HPF, high-power field = 40×, high dry objective.

(for up to 6 hours) is a good way to preserve the physiochemical properties and crystals and delay cellular degeneration. Lowering the temperature of urine enhances crystal formation, resulting in an inaccurate semiquantitative assessment of their true numbers physiologically. A consistent volume of urine, generally 5 cc, should be routinely assessed so that the findings can be semiquantitated and compared to reference values as well as followed in a patient under treatment. Cells and casts are expressed as the number observed per high-power field (HPF, 40× objective) (Table 10–1). Crystals are expressed as few (occasional), moderate, or many per low-power field (LPF, 10× objective). The urine pH, temperature, and specific gravity affect the solubility of crystals. Ammonium urate (also referred to as *ammonium biurate*), amorphous phosphate, calcium phosphate, calcium carbonate, and struvite (magnesium ammonium phosphate, triple phosphates is a misnomer) have propensity to form in neutral pH or alkaline urine. Urine with a neutral or acidic pH tends to favor the formation amorphous urate, bilirubin, calcium oxalate, cystine, sodium urate, sulfa, and uric acid.

Following centrifugation of the urine specimen in a conical-tipped tube, most of the supernatant is decanted to leave an equal amount of sediment and urine. The sediment is resuspended by flicking the tube several times with the finger. One unstained drop is placed on a clean glass slide with a pipette, a coverslip is applied, and the specimen is examined. Subdued microscopic lighting is required to accentuate the elements in the sediment. The microscope's

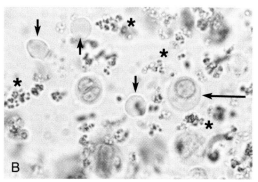

FIGURE 10–1. B, Specimen stained with Sedistain. Applying Sedistain to the specimen highlights cellular detail. An epithelial cell (*long arrow*) and erythrocytes are present (*short arrows*). The stain must be kept free of stain precipitate. As illustrated in this photomicrograph, the stain particles are distracting and give the misleading impression of bacteria (*asterisks*). (Sedistain; ×500.)

condenser must be lowered and the iris diaphram partially closed in order for the constituents to be most conspicuous (Fig. 10–1A). Phase-contrast microscopy accentuates the outline of even the most translucent constituents, simplifying the detection of casts and bacteria. Polarized microscopy is used to enhance the identification of crystals.

A water-based stain (Sedistain, Becton Dickinson, Rutherford, NJ, or 0.5% new methylene blue) can be used to accentuate cellular detail. One drop of stain is added to the resuspended sediment, mixed by flicking the tube with the finger, allowed to incubate for 2 to 3 minutes, and one drop of the stained sediment placed on a clean glass slide with a pipette. Stain precipitate will develop over time in the bottle and microscopically appear similar to bacteria (Fig. 10–1B). When precipitate is observed, new stain must be employed or the current

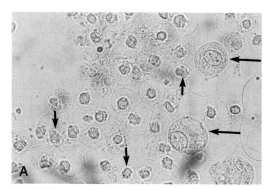

FIGURE 10–1. A, Unstained specimen. This unstained urine sediment illustrates the enhanced contrast of the cellular constituents when the microscope's condenser is lowered. Crenated erythrocytes are predominant (*short arrows*) and two plump epithelial cells with granular-appearing cytoplasm are present (*long arrows*). (Unstained; ×500.)

stain passed through a filter. It is good practice to initially examine an unstained specimen followed by the examination of a stained preparation when there are findings that require additional definition or as a learning tool (Fig. 10–9C). A cytology preparation of the sediment is another approach to characterize cells, organisms, or the composition of casts that are not readily recognized in an unstained preparation (Fig. 10–4A & B). One drop of *unstained*, resuspended sediment is placed near the frosted end of the slide and spread with another slide or a compression (squash) preparation is made, air-dried, and stained (refer to Fig.

1–2 and 1–4). Often the constituents will wash off during the staining process because of the low protein nature of the specimen. Serum-coated slides should be used to "glue" the constituents in the sediment to the surface of the slide (refer to Chapter 1, Key Point).

KEY POINT: To accentuate the constituents in the unstained urine sediment, the iris diaphram is partially closed and the substage condenser of the microscope is lowered. This is a dynamic process conducted while viewing the specimen to determine the most advantageous contrast.

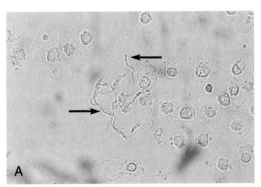

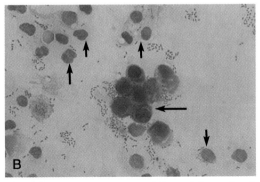

FIGURE 10–2. A, Bacterial cystitis, unstained. Chains of bacteria (*arrows*) and unidentified cells (probably degenerate neutrophils with a mononuclear cell appearance and crenated erythrocytes) are observed in this unstained urine sediment obtained by percutaneous cystocentesis. Bacteria are never considered a normal finding in urine collected by percutaneous cystocentesis even when clinical signs of cystitis are absent (Forrester et al., 1999). Identification of the cell type is not important in this setting and, in fact, may be impossible owing to changes induced by the physiochemical nature of the urine. (Unstained; ×500.)

FIGURE 10–2. B, Bacterial cystitis, stained. A Wright-stained cytologic preparation of an infected urine specimen highlights the bacteria and a clump of uniform epithelial cells (*long arrow*). The majority of the cells, presumably neutrophils, have swollen, rounded nuclei or have lysed owing to the hostile environment and cannot be identified (*short arrows*). In other fields, some of these cells retained slight segmentation and many were observed to contain bacteria supporting their classification as a neutrophil. Again, identification of the cell type is not important in this setting. (Wright; ×500.)

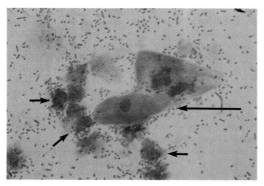

FIGURE 10–3. Contaminated urine specimen, free catch, stained. The presence of mature squamous epithelial cells (*long arrow*) suggest the probability of bacterial contamination. Six or seven distorted nuclei, presumably neutrophils, are also observed (*short arrows*). No bacteria or neutrophils were observed in a second specimen obtained via percutaneous cystocentesis. (Wright; ×500.)

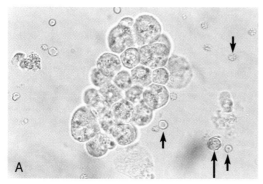

FIGURE 10–4. A, A clump of epithelial cells demonstrate mild to moderate anisocytosis (20 to 40 μm in diameter). Erythrocytes (approximately 5 to 7 μm in diameter, *short arrows*), some with a smooth surface and some with a crenated appearance and a neutrophil (approximately 10 to 12 μm in diameter, *long arrow*) are observed. The cytoplasmic granules of the neutrophil were in random motion (Brownian movement); sometimes referred to as a "glitter cell." These granules should not be mistaken for bacteria. Note the size relationship of the erythrocyte vs. the neutrophilic leukocyte vs. the epithelial cells. (Unstained; ×500.)

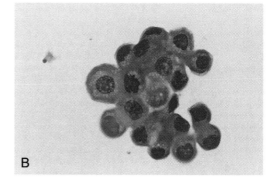

FIGURE 10–4. B, Cytology preparation, hyperplastic epithelial cells. A drop of the sediment was placed on a glass slide (the surface of which was first coated with a thin layer of serum and air-dried), spread, air dried, and stained as a routine cytologic preparation. The stained preparation facilitates the cytologic assessment for criteria of malignancy. The mild to moderate anisocytosis, anisokaryosis, and variable nuclear-to-cytoplasm ratio were considered to be consistent with hyperplasia of transitional epithelial cells. (Wright; ×500.)

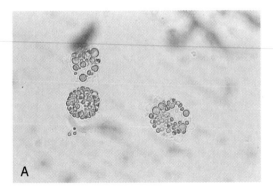

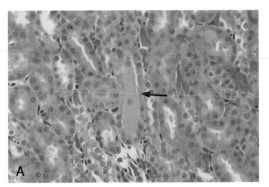

FIGURE 10–6. A, Hyalin cast, H & E. Casts form in the renal tubules (*arrow*) (ascending limb of the loop of Henle and distal tubule) and reflect their shape. Acidity, solute concentration, and flow rate facilitate the precipitation of protein, resulting in the formation of a cast. The matrix of all casts is formed by Tamm-Horsfall protein, a glycoprotein secreted by the ascending loop of Henle and possibly the distal tubule. See Meyer and Harvey (1998) for a more detailed discussion of Tamm-Horsfall protein. (H & E; ×400.)

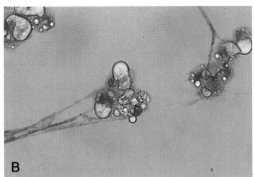

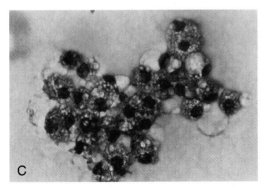

FIGURE 10–5. Lipid droplets in epithelial cells may be a prominent cytomorphologic feature in feline urine sediments. They are identified by their size variation and refractile nature when focusing up and down. (**A**) Unstained; ×500; (**B**) New methylene blue; ×500; (**C**) Wright (the alcohol-based stain that dissolves the lipid droplets, resulting in punctate holes in the cytoplasm of the cells); ×500.

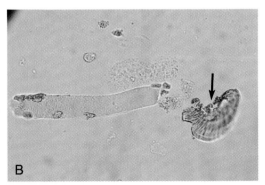

FIGURE 10–6. B, Hyalin cast, unstained; glass chip. Hyalin casts are clear and colorless. They rapidly dissolve, especially in alkaline urine. An occasional cast per 10× field is normal. Cast formation is increased when abnormal amounts of protein enter the tubules, most often excess albumin. Increased numbers are associated with strenuous exercise, fever, congestive heart failure, diuretic treatment, glomerulonephritis, and amyloidosis. A chip of glass is present (*arrow*). (Unstained; ×500.)

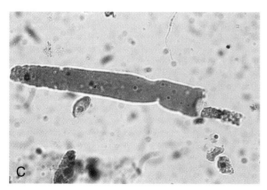

FIGURE 10–6. C, Hyalin cast, stained. (Sedistain; ×500.)

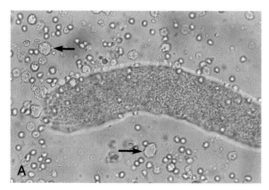

FIGURE 10–7. A, Granular cast, unstained. Granular casts represent degraded cellular material from injured renal tubular epithelial cells or, less often, inflammatory cells, embedded in a protein matrix. The granularity is sometimes further categorized as fine or coarse but the type of granularity is not of diagnostic importance. Nephrotoxins (e.g., gentamicin sulfate, amphotericin B), nephritis, and ischemia are pathologic events that result in their formation. Moderate numbers of epithelial cells (*arrows*), leukocytes, and erythrocytes (inconspicuous) are present. Marked numbers of brightly refractile lipid droplets are prominent in this specimen. The lipiduria was attributed to the lubricant used to facilitate catheterization. (Unstained; ×500.)

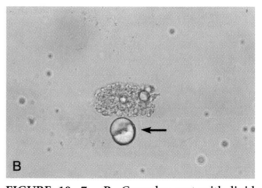

FIGURE 10–7. B, Granular cast with lipid droplets (fatty cast), unstained. This cast was present in the urine of a dog with the nephrotic syndrome. They can be seen in association with diabetes mellitus and in cats with renal tubular injury. A moderate number of lipid droplets (out of focus) are present. A starch granule (glove powder) is located beneath the cast (*arrow*). An "x" with a central depression can be observed by focusing up and down. (Unstained; ×500.)

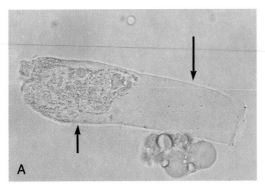

FIGURE 10–8. A, Granular/waxy cast, un-stained. Waxy casts develop from granular casts as illustrated by this cast that has granular cast (*short arrow*) and waxy cast (*long arrow*) characteristics. (Unstained; ×500.)

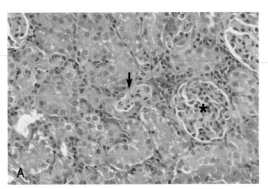

FIGURE 10–9. A, Cellular cast, H & E. Pyelonephritis has resulted in the formation of cellular cast (*arrow*). The pinkish protein matrix contains dark-staining neutrophil nuclei and unidentified nuclear debris. A glomerulus is present (*asterisk*). (H & E; ×400.)

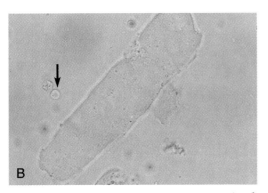

FIGURE 10–8. B, Waxy cast, unstained. These casts indicate chronic tubular pathology since additional time is required for their formation. Implicit in the pathogenesis of their formation is localized tubular obstruction. One sequela is dilation of the tubular lumen, resulting in a wide cast. The term "broad" is sometimes added as a descriptive adjective when the width is two to four times that of a hyalin or granular cast. The magnitude of its width is apparent when contrasted to an erythrocyte (*arrow*). A "fissure" or crack is often observed (top right). (Unstained; ×500.)

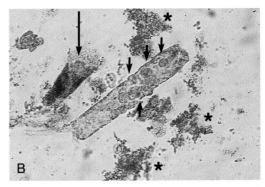

FIGURE 10–9. B, Cellular cast, unstained. Cells, most consistent morphologically with epithelial cells, can be seen embedded in the cast matrix (*short arrows*). The finding is suggestive of acute tubular necrosis. A fragmented granular cast (*long arrow*) and amorphous debris (unrecognizable granular material) (*asterisks*) is observed. (Unstained; ×400.)

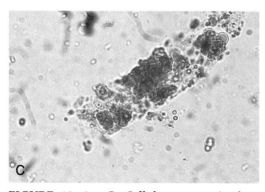

FIGURE 10–9. C, Cellular cast, stained. A specimen stained with Sedistain further supports the identity of cells in the cast as epithelial cells (when focused up and down). A few lipid droplets are observed. (Sedistain; ×500.)

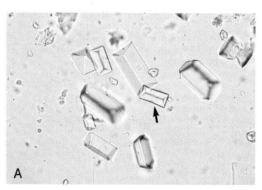

FIGURE 10–11. A, Magnesium ammonium phosphate crystaluria (struvite, misnamed triple phosphates). The small crystal in the center (*arrow*) illustrates the form that has been referred to as a "coffin lid" appearance (closed casket as viewed from the top). They can be a normal finding in dogs and cats or be associated with struvite uroliths (sterile and infected). They tend to be found in urine with a pH > 7. (Unstained; ×600)

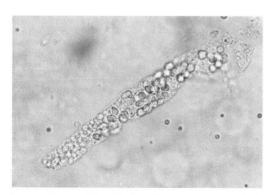

FIGURE 10–10. Red cell cast, unstained. A fragile and uncommon finding, they indicate acute intrarenal injury. The urine specimen is from a dog that had been traumatized (hit by car). A few lipid droplets are present. Note that they are more refractile than erythrocytes and vary in size. (Unstained; ×500.)

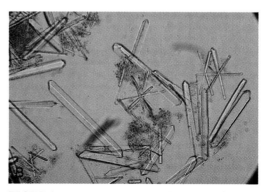

FIGURE 10–11. B, Struvite crystals can form in a variety of shapes, including rod-like in this specimen and a "fern leaf" appearance (not shown). Small islands of reddish-stained amorphous phosphates are present. (Sedistain; ×500.)

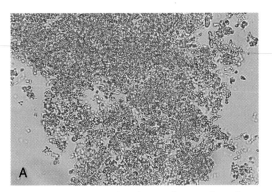

FIGURE 10–12. A, Amorphous phosphate crystals. They have no known diagnostic importance but should not be mistaken for bacterial colonies. They are distinguished from amorphous urate crystals by their lack of color, formation in alkaline urine, and solubility in acetic acid. (Unstained; ×500.)

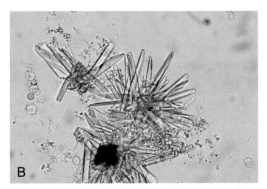

FIGURE 10–12. B, Calcium phosphate (bushite) crystals. These crystals are observed in urine specimens from apparently healthy dogs and in association with calcium phosphate uroliths and calcium phosphate/calcium oxalate uroliths. They tend to form in urine with an acid pH. (Unstained; ×500.)

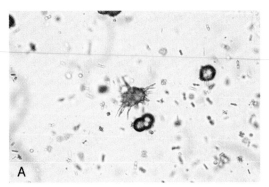

FIGURE 10–13. A, Ammonium urate crystals (also referred to as **ammonium biurate**), **dog.** These crystals are light yellow to yellowish-brown and tend to form sphere-like aggregates with smooth surfaces or with long projections of varying length (referred to as the "thorn apple" form). They are uncommon in healthy dogs and cats. An exception is ammonium urate crystalluria in apparently healthy dalmatians and English bulldogs. Dalmatians have an in-born error of uric acid metabolism in which uric acid is not changed to allantoin and results in hyperuricosuria and the predisposition to ammonium urate crystalluria. In other breeds, the water-soluble allantoin that is formed is excreted in the urine. Ammonium urate crystalluria is associated with congenital portosystemic vascular anomalies (shunts) and with liver insufficiency secondary to reduced hepatocellular mass (e.g., cirrhosis). Many smaller ammonium urate crystals of various shapes, including a dumbbell form, are present and some mimic bipolar rod-shaped bacteria. (Unstained; ×500.)

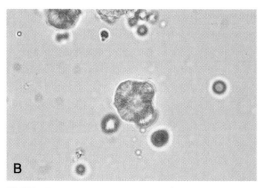

FIGURE 10–13. B, Ammonium urate crystals, cat. The cat tends to form spheroid aggregates of crystals with smooth surfaces as seen in this urine specimen from a cat with a single extrahepatic congenital portosystemic shunt. A few out-of-focus lipid droplets are observed. (Unstained; ×1000.)

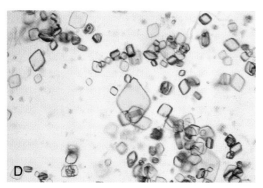

FIGURE 10–13. D, Uric acid crystals. These crystals are uncommonly observed in the dog and cat (although common in humans owing to the difference in purine metabolism). They have the same associations as listed for ammonium urate crystals.

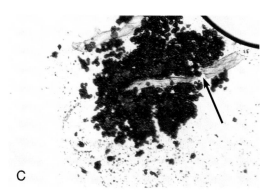

FIGURE 10–13. C, Amorphous urate crystals; cotton fiber. Sodium, potassium, magnesium, and calcium urate salts form a granular precipitate that is yellowish to dark brown. They can appear similar to amorphous phosphate crystal precipitates. A congenital portosystemic shunt was diagnosed (markedly abnormal serum bile acids concentration; portogram) in the Yorkshire terrier from which this specimen was obtained. A cotton fiber is trapped within the crystals (arrow). (Unstained; ×500.)

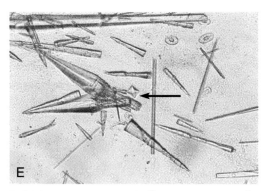

FIGURE 10–13. E, Sodium urate crystals. These crystals were observed in association with ammonium urate uroliths in an English bulldog. A calcium oxalate dihydrate crystal is also observed (arrow). (Unstained; ×500.)

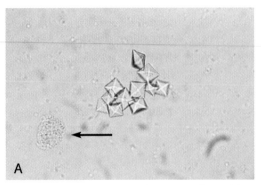

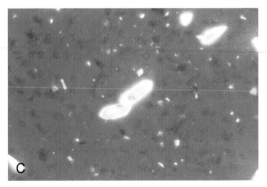

FIGURE 10–14. A, Calcium oxalate dihy-drate crystals, dog, apparently healthy. This photomicrograph illustrates the classical "Maltese cross" form. They can be found in the urine of apparently healthy dogs and cats, and in association with calcium oxalate urolithiasis and ethylene glycol toxicity. The latter should be promptly considered in a dog or cat with acute renal failure. A fragment of a granular cast is located to the lower left (*arrow*). (Unstained; ×500.)

FIGURE 10–14. C, Calcium oxalate mono-hydrate crystals, polarized, dog, same specimen as in Figure 10–14B. Polarization accentuates the "raised lid"-type projection noted on one end of the crystal.

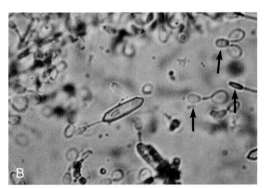

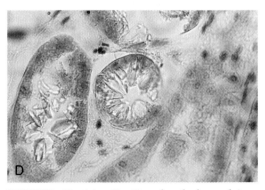

FIGURE 10–14. B, Calcium oxalate mono-hydrate crystals; spermatozoa, dog, ethylene glycol toxicity (erroneously referred to as hippuric acid). These crystals, alone or in combination with the dihydrate form, are observed in association with ethylene glycol toxicity. They have pointed ends (hippuric acid-like appearance) and often a small projection ("raised lid") is observed on one end. Numerous spermatozoa are observed (*arrows*). Spermatozoa can be observed in the urine of male dogs collected by cystocentesis. (Unstained; ×1000.)

FIGURE 10–14. D, Renal tubular calcium oxalate monohydrate crystals in situ, H & E. Calcium oxalate monohydrate crystals are imbedded in two renal tubules in this histologic section obtained from the dog in Figure 10–14B after it died. (H & E; ×1000.)

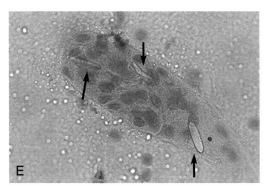

FIGURE 10–14.   E, Renal tubular calcium oxalate monohydrate crystals *in situ*, touch imprint. Calcium oxalate monohydrate crystals are imbedded in the renal tubules (*arrows*) in this touch imprint obtained from the specimen in Figure 10–14D. (New methylene blue; ×500.)

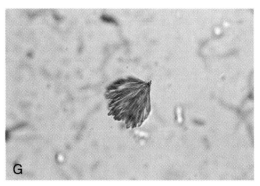

FIGURE 10–14.   G, Calcium oxalate monohydrate crystals, dog. Fan-shaped aggregate of calcium oxalate monohydrate crystals associated with calcium oxalate uroliths. Fan-shaped crystals are also associated with the use of sulfa-containing antibacterials. (Unstained; ×500.)

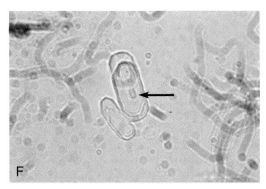

FIGURE 10–14.   F, Calcium oxalate monohydrate crystals, cat, ethylene glycol toxicity. The calcium oxalate monohydrate in the cat is wider than the canine counterpart and has (*arrow*) rounded ends. The "raised lid" effect on one end is apparent on the larger of the two crystals. The out-of-focus elongated material is artifact (dust in the camera optics).

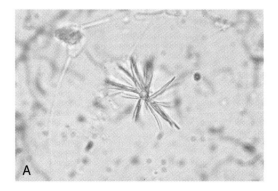

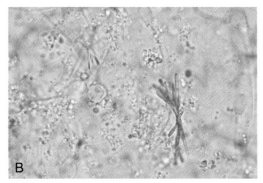

FIGURE 10–15.   A&B, Bilirubin crystals. Bilirubin can crystallize in association with bilirubinuria. The causes of bilirubinuria should be explored. (Unstained; ×1000.)

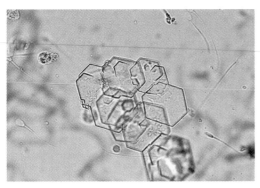

FIGURE 10–16. Cystine crystals. Cystine crystaluria is always an abnormal finding and indicative of the metabolic disorder of cystinuria. Cystine crystaluria may or may not be associated with cystine uroliths. (Unstained; ×500.)

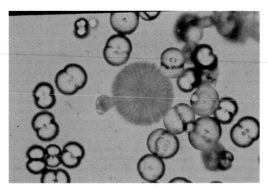

FIGURE 10–18. Calcium carbonate crystals. Calcium carbonate crystals are not observed in dog or cat urine but are observed in the urine of horses, rabbits, and guinea pigs. (Unstained; ×500.)

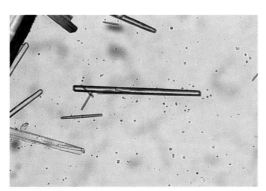

FIGURE 10–17. Needle-shaped crystals. These crystals were observed in association with the use of an iodinated radiopaque contrast agent used for an excretory urogram. (Unstained; ×500.)

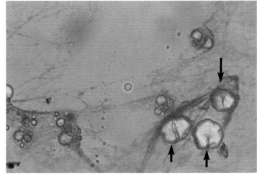

FIGURE 10–19. Starch granules (glove powder) (*arrows*). These structures are contaminants. Poorly formed wisps of mucus stain but variably sized refractile lipid droplets do not stain with the water-based stain. (New methylene blue; ×500.)

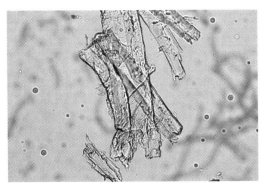

FIGURE 10–20. Cotton fibers. Cotton fibers from clothing or gauze pads can mimic hyalin/granular casts or crystals. (Unstained; ×500.)

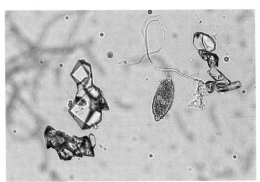

FIGURE 10–21. *Capillaria* plica ovum. The ovum of the bladder worm of dogs and cats has bipolar plugs and a granular appearance. These features help distinguish it from pollen grain contaminants. Aggregates of magnesium ammonium phosphates crystals are also observed. (Unstained; ×400.)

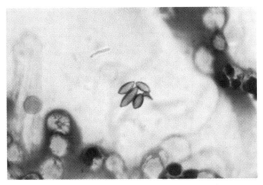

FIGURE 10–22. Pollen grains. Pollen grains of various sizes can contaminate urine. They are often ovoid. (New methylene blue; ×500.)

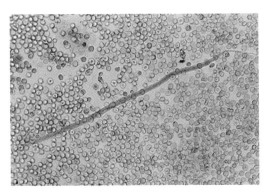

FIGURE 10–23. Microfilaria of *Dirofilaria* **immitis.** An incidental finding in this dog with hemorrhagic cystitis. Numerous erythrocytes are observed. (New methylene blue; ×200.)

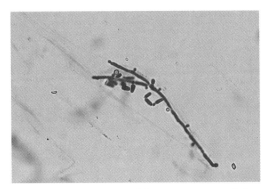

FIGURE 10–24. Budding yeast pseudohyphae. A pseudohyphal form of yeast is suggested by the lack of distinct segmentation. Other forms of yeast can appear morphologically similar to lipid droplets or erythrocytes (not shown). Both yeast and fungi in urine sediments usually represent contaminants. If a stain is used, it should be also examined for fungal growth. Systemic mycosis can result in the shedding of fungal elements in the urine. A urine specimen obtained via percutaneous cystocentesis should be used to confirm the finding. A positive finding should be related to the clinical presentation (e.g., spondylitis, long-term corticosteroids treatment, diabetes mellitus). (New methylene blue; ×500.)

References and Suggested Reading

Barlough JE, Osborne CA, Steven JB: Canine and feline urinalysis: Value of macroscopic and microscopic examinations. J Am Vet Med Assoc 1981; 184:61–63.

Fettman MJ: Evaluation of the usefulness of routine microscopy in canine urinalysis. J Am Vet Med Assoc 1987; 190:892–896.

Forrester SD, Troy GC, Dalton MN, et al: Retrospective evaluation of urinary tract infection in 42 dogs with hyperadrenocorticism or diabetes mellitus or both. J Vet Intern Med 1999; 13: 557–560.

Graff SL: *A Handbook of Routine Urinalysis*. JB Lippincott, Philadelphia, 1983.

Haber MH: Pisse prophesy: A brief history of urinalysis. In Haber MH, Corwin HL (eds): *Clinics in Laboratory Medicine*. WB Saunders, Philadelphia, 1988, pp 415–426.

Meyer DJ, Harvey JW: Assessment of renal function, urinalysis, and water balance. In *Veterinary Laboratory Medicine: Interpretation and Diagnosis*. WB Saunders, Philadelphia, 1998, 221–235.

Osborne CA, Stevens JB: *Handbook of Canine and Feline Urinalysis*. Ralston Purina Co, St. Louis, 1981.

CHAPTER 11

Reproductive System

KRISTIN L. HENSON

FEMALE REPRODUCTIVE SYSTEM: MAMMARY GLANDS AND VAGINA

Mammary Glands

Mammary gland lesions are common in female dogs and cats. Mammary gland enlargement may be related to a wide variety of disease processes, including cysts, inflammation, hyperplasia, and benign or malignant neoplasia. History, age, whether intact or older when neutered, date of last estrus, pregnancy, hormone therapy, size, number, and consistency of lesion(s), attachment to underlying tissue, rate of growth, presence of ulceration, and evidence of metastasis are important information in the investigation of mammary gland disease (Baker and Lumsden, 1999a). Ancillary diagnostic tests used to evaluate mammary lesions include radiography, histopathology, and cytology.

While histopathology and, more recently, cytology have been used to accurately classify mammary lesions as cysts, inflammation, or hyperplasia/neoplasia, determination of the malignant potential of mammary neoplasia can be difficult. Histopathology may often show poor correlation between histologic diagnosis of malignant neoplasia and biologic behavior. While a few studies have compared cytologic evaluation of mammary neoplasms with histologic analysis, no reports have related biologic behavior with cytologic diagnosis. However, the ease of obtaining cytologic specimens from mammary lesions, the low invasive nature, and relatively small expense make exfoliative cytology a useful diagnostic tool in the evaluation of mammary disease. With an understanding of the potential difficulties of mammary cytology, the cytopathologist can provide useful diagnostic information concerning mammary gland disease.

Special Collection Techniques

Cytologic samples from mammary lesions may be obtained by expressing material from the gland or, more commonly, fine-needle aspiration (FNA) of the affected area. FNA is performed similarly as in other body sites. A 22-gauge needle is attached to 12-cc syringe and directed into the lesion. Several aspirations are made and multiple areas of the lesion are sampled. Aspiration of the periphery of a large mass is preferred as the center of such a mass may consist only of necrotic material. The aspirated material is then placed onto a clean microscope slide, lightly smeared, and allowed to air-dry. The slide may be stained with a variety of stains, however, Romanowsky-type stains or modified Romanowsky stains are most commonly used for cytologic evaluation. If the sample is to be sent to a referral laboratory for examination by a pathologist, an unstained slide should be sent along with any stained specimens. The unstained slide may be dipped several times in a fixative solution of 95% or 100% methanol to preserve the cells. A complete history, signalment, and clinical findings should also accompany the submitted sample.

Normal Anatomy and Histology

Mammary glands are compound tubuloalveolar glands that are believed to be extensively modified sweat glands (Banks, 1986a). In dogs and cats, five pairs of mammary glands are arranged as bilaterally symmetrical rows extending from the ventral thorax to the inguinal region. During pregnancy and lactation, the mammary glands undergo marked hypertrophy and hyperplasia to produce immunoglobulin-containing colostrum followed by milk.

Histologically, mammary glands are composed of a secretory component consisting of alveolar secretory epithelial cells and the initial portion of the intralobular ducts (Banks, 1986a) (Figs. 11–1 to 11–3) The secretory portion of the glands are drained

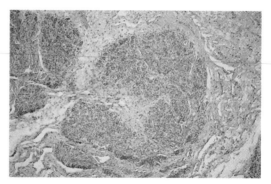

FIGURE 11–1. Tissue section of normal, inactive mammary gland. Lobules of glandular tissue are surrounded by abundant interlobular connective tissue. Canine. (H & E; ×25.)

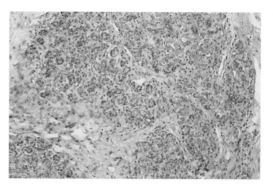

FIGURE 11–2. The glandular portion of mammary tissue is composed of alveoli (acini) and intralobular ducts, which are lined by cuboidal to columnar epithelium. The interlobular ducts, composed of nonsecretory columnar and cuboidal epithelium, drain the alveoli. Reticular connective tissue supports the alveoli and smaller ducts. Bundles of smooth muscle and elastic fibers surround the large ducts. Canine (inactive gland). (H & E; ×50.)

by the ductular system, composed of nonsecretory columnar and cuboidal epithelium. Reticular connective tissue supports the alveoli and smaller ducts. Bundles of smooth muscle and elastic fibers surround the large ducts. Myoepithelial cells can be found between the alveolar epithelial cells and the underlying basement membrane.

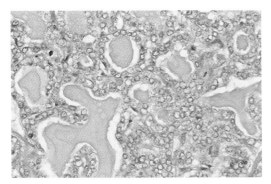

FIGURE 11–3. In this section of an active, lactational mammary gland, the secretory portion of the gland is well-developed and connective tissue elements are decreased. The alveolar lumens contain bright-pink secretory material. Canine. (H & E; ×125.)

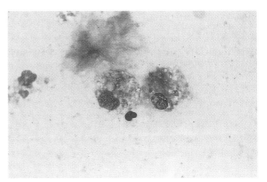

FIGURE 11–4. Two foam cells from a mammary aspirate. The cells have eccentrically located nuclei, low nuclear-to-cytoplasmic ratios, clear cytoplasmic vacuoles, and abundant amounts of basophilic secretory material. The background has a lightly basophilic, proteinaceous appearance consistent with normal mammary aspirates. Feline. (Wright-Giemsa; ×250.)

Normal Cytology

Normal mammary secretions are characterized cytologically by low numbers of sloughed secretory epithelial cells known as foam cells as well as macrophages and occasional neutrophils on an eosinophilic to basophilic proteinaceous background. Foam cells are large, individualized cells characterized by round to oval, eccentrically located nuclei and abundant amounts of vacuolated cytoplasm (Shull, 1999). These cells may also contain amorphous, basophilic secretory material (Fig. 11–4). Foam cells resemble and can be difficult to distinguish from reactive macrophages. FNA cytology of normal mammary tissue usually reveals small amounts of blood with no to low numbers of nucleated cells and moderate to large amounts of basophilic, proteinaceous material, clear lipid droplets, and adipocytes (Shull and Maddux, 1999; Allen et al., 1986). Small sheets and clusters of mammary secretory epithelial cells that are uniform in size and shape may be seen occasionally in aspirates of normal mammary tissue. Secretory epithelial cells exhibit round, dark nuclei and moderate amounts of basophilic cytoplasm. Acinar formations may be noted. Ductular epithelial cells are characterized by oval, basal nuclei with scant amounts of cytoplasm (Shull and Maddux, 1999). Myoepithelial cells may be seen as darkly staining oval free nuclei or as spindle-shaped cells (Shull and Maddux, 1999).

Mammary Cysts

Mammary cysts or fibrocystic disease (FCD), also known as blue dome cyst or polycystic mastopathy, is a form of mammary dysplasia in which dilated ducts expand to form cavitary lesions (Brodey et al., 1983; Shull and Maddux, 1999). FCD generally occurs in middle-aged to older animals, although the disease has been reported in dogs of 1 year of age (Brodey et al., 1983). Formation of FCD may have a hormonal component as administration of medroxyprogesterone has been associated with development of FCD in dogs (Brodey et al., 1983). In dogs, rapid growth during estrus and regression during metestrus has been noted (Brodey et al., 1983). The rapid growth of cysts during estrus may be associated with rupture of the cysts. Ovariohysterectomy should be considered when mammary cysts grow and regress in association with the estrous cycle, particularly if multiple glands are involved (Brodey et al., 1983). FCD is considered a benign lesion in dogs; however, the disease has been associated with development of mammary gland carcinoma (Brodey et al., 1983).

Mammary cysts may present as a well-circumscribed, single cystic nodule or as a flat, rubbery, multinodular mass (Brodey et al., 1983). The nodule(s) exhibit slow expansile growth and the overlying skin may develop a blue color, hence the term *blue dome cyst* (Brodey et al., 1983). Mammary cysts may be classified as simple cysts characterized by a single layer of flattened lining epithelium or papillary cysts containing papillary outgrowths of the lining epithelial cells (Brodey et al., 1983). Aspiration of mammary cysts typically yields a green-brown or blood-tinged fluid containing low numbers of foam cells and pigment-laden macrophages (Brodey et al., 1983; Shull and Maddux, 1999). Neutrophils may be increased if inflammation is also present (Brodey et al., 1983; Shull and Maddux, 1999). Cholesterol crystals, which appear as large, rectangular crystalline structures often with a notched corner, may be present as a result of breakdown of cellular membranes within the cyst (Fig. 11–5). Epithelial cells derived from the cystic lining may be noted, particularly if the cyst has a papillary component (Shull and Maddux, 1999). These cells tend to occur in dense sheets and clusters and may display some mild variation in nuclear size and shape (Shull and Maddux, 1999). Mammary cysts may

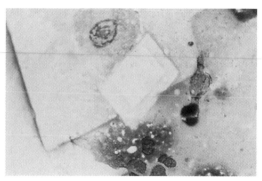

FIGURE 11–5. Cholesterol crystals from an aspirate of a mammary cyst. The clear, rectangular crystals are of varying size. Two foam cells are adjacent to the crystals. Feline. (Wright-Giemsa; ×250.)

coexist with benign and/or malignant mammary tumors (Brodey et al., 1983). Therefore, aspiration or biopsy of solid areas of a mass associated with a cyst or other mammary masses should be performed to rule out the presence of concurrent mammary neoplasia.

Mammary Gland Hyperplasia

Hyperplastic and dysplastic lesions of mammary glands include unilobular and multilobular hyperplasia, adenosis, and epitheliosis (Moulton, 1990; Brodey et al., 1983). These lesions occur in dogs and less commonly in cats (Yager et al., 1993). Mammary hyperplasia is characterized by proliferations of secretory or ductular epithelium or myoepithelial cells resembling the physiologic hyperplasia of pregnancy with some mild histologic atypia (Moulton, 1990). Cytologically, these lesions may be difficult to distinguish from each other and from benign neoplasms such as adenomas or papillomas. Moderate to large numbers of epithelial cells arranged in sheets and clusters can be aspirated from hyperplastic mammary tissue. These cells, which are similar in appearance to normal mammary epithelial cells, display round nuclei of uniform size and shape and scant to moderate amounts of basophilic cytoplasm. Foam cells and macrophages may also be noted.

In cats, a form of mammary hyperplasia occurs that has been variously identified as fibroepithelial hyperplasia, feline mammary hypertrophy, mammary fibroadenomatous hyperplasia, or feline mammary hypertrophy/fibroadenomatous complex. Feline mammary fibroepithelial hyperplasia (MFH) is a clinically benign, fairly common condition affecting estrous-cycling or pregnant female cats usually less than 2 years of age (Hayden et al., 1981; Mesher, 1997). MFH has also been reported in older intact and neutered cats of either gender receiving progesterone-containing compounds, such as megestrol acetate (Hayden et al., 1981; Hayden et al., 1989). MFH is considered a form of mammary dysplasia characterized by a rapid, abnormal growth of one or more mammary glands (Hayden et al., 1981). In contrast to a neoplastic process, paired glands often exhibit a similar degree of enlargement (Moulton, 1990). MFH is notable for a marked intralobular ductular proliferation identical to the ductular proliferation seen during the progesterone-influenced early stages of pregnancy (Moulton, 1990). This typical histologic appearance, occurrence in cycling females or cats administered progesterone, and identification of progesterone receptors in MFH lesions from female and male cats has led to the belief that development of MFH involves endogenous or exogenous progesterone (Hayden et al., 1981; Moulton, 1990). MFH usually regresses over time without treatment, although secondary infections may require appropriate antibiotic therapy (MacEwen and Withrow, 1996). Ovariohysterectomy, performed via a flank incision if the glands are greatly enlarged, will often result in re-

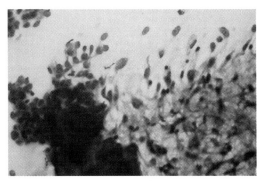

FIGURE 11–6. Sheet of epithelial cells and spindle cells in pink extracellular material from an aspirate of fibroepithelial hyperplasia. The epithelial cells are uniform in size and shape and the spindle cells display some mild anisokaryosis. Feline. (Wright; ×160.) (From Mesher CI: What is your diagnosis? A 14-month old domestic cat. Vet Clin Pathol 1997; 26:4, 13. Reprinted with permission.)

gression of lesions and will prevent future recurrences (MacEwen and Withrow, 1996).

The cytologic appearance of MFH has been recently reported (Mesher, 1997) (Fig. 11–6). Aspirated material of a histologically confirmed MFH lesion consisted of a very uniform population of cuboidal epithelial cells arranged in thick clusters. The cuboidal epithelial cells were characterized by dense, round nuclei with small nucleoli and scant amounts of basophilic cytoplasm. A mesenchymal population of spindle-shaped cells with narrow oval nuclei, one to two nucleoli, and tapering cytoplasm was also present. The mesenchymal cells displayed moderate variation in nuclear size (anisokaryosis) and cellular size (anisocytosis). Moderate amounts of pink extracellular matrix were associated with the mesenchymal cells. These cytologic findings correlated with the histologic findings of hyperplastic ductular epithelium (cuboidal epithelial population) and proliferation of edematous stroma (mesenchymal cells with extracellular matrix). The presence of abundant stromal elements helps to differentiate MFH from mammary neoplasia, which generally contains scant stromal material. Cytologic recognition of the characteristic cell types from mammary masses in a cat with appropriate signalment and clinical history can be considered highly suggestive of MFH, thus eliminating the need for mammary gland excision and allowing for appropriate medical and/or surgical management (Mesher, 1997).

Mammary Gland Inflammation/ Infection

Inflammation of the mammary glands is referred to as *mastitis* and may present as a focal lesion or may involve one or more glands. Mastitis is most often associated with postparturient lactation or pseudopregnancy and is thought to result from entry of infectious organisms through the teat orifice or damaged overlying skin (Gruffyd-Jones, 1980). Mastitis may infrequently occur from hematogenous spread of organisms, nonlactation-associated trauma, fight wounds, or infected neoplasms (Roudebush and Wheeler, 1979). Neonatal morbidity or mortality may be the first indication of mastitis (Gruffydd-Jones, 1980). Clinical signs associated with mastitis include swollen, painful glands that result in discomfort while nursing. The glands may become abscessed or gangrenous with necrosis of overlying skin. The bitch or queen may also present with symptoms of systemic illness such as anorexia, fever, vomiting, or diarrhea (Roudebush and Wheeler, 1979). A complete blood count may reveal an inflammatory leukogram characterized by either an increase in segmented and nonsegmented (band) neutrophils or a degenerative left shift with a predominance of immature neutrophils, especially if gangrenous mastitis is present (Roudebush and Wheeler, 1979).

Cytologic examination of secretions from inflamed and/or infected mammary glands is usually diagnostic; however, FNA may be needed for focal lesions (Shull and Maddux, 1999). Large numbers of neutrophils are present, which may exhibit degenerative changes of karyolysis and karyorrhexis. Reactive macrophages, small lymphocytes, and plasma cells may also be seen, particularly with more chronic lesions. Infectious organisms may be visualized within neutrophils and, less commonly, macrophages, indicating a septic process. The most frequently cultured organisms are streptococcal, staphylococcal, and coliform bacteria, although other types of bacteria and fungi can be isolated (Shull and Maddux, 1999). Culture and sensitivity of inflammatory mammary secretions or aspirated material are warranted to determine appropriate antibiotic therapy.

Treatment of septic mastitis will be dependent on the severity of the lesions. Systemic antibiotic therapy based upon culture and sensitivity results should be administered (Roudebush and Wheeler, 1979). Abscessed glands will need to be surgically debrided or drained. Warm moist topical packs may be used for gangrenous mastitis and the necrotic tissue can be excised or allowed to slough (Roudebush and Wheeler, 1979). Supportive care, including intravenous fluid therapy, may be necessary for the bitch or queen as well as nursing puppies or kittens. Also, puppies or kittens may require appropriate antibiotic therapy and should be weaned and reared by hand (Roudebush and Wheeler, 1979).

Some noninfectious inflammatory conditions of mammary glands have been described. Focal mastitic lesions may leave residual fibrotic nodules consisting of epithelial cell metaplasia, pigment-laden macrophages, nondegenerate neutrophils, small lymphocytes and plasma cells (Brodey et al., 1983; Shull and Maddux, 1999). Unlike mammary gland tumors, fibrotic nodules tend to occur in young dogs, do not increase in size, and are usually associated with a previous history of mastitis (Brodey et al., 1993).

Neoplasia

Canine Mammary Gland Tumors

Following skin tumors, mammary neoplasms are the second most common tumor in dogs and the most commonly seen tumor in bitches (MacVean et al., 1978; Priester and Mamel, 1971; Dorn et al., 1968). Mammary gland tumors (MGT) rarely occur in male dogs, with a reported incidence of less than 1% (based upon a literature survey of studies involving 1954 dogs) (Brodey et al., 1983). Many of the MGT reported in male dogs have been associated with hormonal abnormalities, such as estrogen-secreting Sertoli cell tumors (Moulton, 1990). The median age for development of canine mammary gland tumors is 10 to 11 years of age. MGT are considered rare in dogs less than 5 years of age (MacEwen and Withrow, 1996). Breed tendencies for MGT have been reported, however, breeds vary in the different reports, suggesting that breed predisposition may not be present (Hahn et al., 1992). Recently, a heritable, familial tendency for development of mammary neoplasms in beagles has been suggested (Benjamin et al., 1999). Development of MGT appears to have a hormonal component as evidenced by the sparing effect of ovariohysterectomy and association of MGT with administration of progesterone (MacEwen and Withrow, 1996; Misdorp, 1991). Estrogen and progesterone receptors have been identified in normal mammary tissue and a majority of mammary neoplasms (Donnay et al., 1995; Inaba et al., 1984; Rutteman et al., 1988). Interestingly, hormone receptor expression, which is a characteristic feature

of mature mammary epithelial cells, tends to be decreased or absent in poorly differentiated tumors and metastatic lesions (Donnay et al., 1995; Rutteman et al., 1988). Canine mammary tumorigenesis may involve the progesterone-mediated stimulation of growth hormone production by mammary epithelial cells (van Garderen et al., 1997). Acting in an autocrine or paracrine manner, growth hormone may increase proliferation of susceptible or transformed mammary epithelial cells, resulting in neoplasia (van Garderen et al., 1997).

Mammary tumors can present as single, firm, well-circumscribed masses to multiple, infiltrative nodules involving one or more glands. Clinical findings associated with malignant neoplasms include a tumor diameter greater than 5 cm, recent rapid, growth, infiltration of surrounding tissue, erythema, and edema (Allen et al., 1986). However, most canine mammary tumors, both benign and malignant, exhibit none of these signs (Allen et al., 1986). The majority of mammary neoplasms occur primarily in the caudal glands, presumably because of the larger amount of glandular tissue present (MacEwen and Withrow, 1996). Multiple mammary neoplasms are common, with 50% to 60% of dogs presenting with more than one mammary tumor. Multiple MGT in a dog are often not of the same histologic type and may exhibit differing biologic behaviors (MacEwen and Withrow, 1996; Benjamin et al., 1999). Thus, a thorough search for additional tumors should be undertaken if a mammary mass is found, and separate cytologic and/or histologic analyses should be performed on each mammary tumor.

The ultimate goal of clinical, histologic, and cytologic evaluation of mammary gland neoplasms is to accurately predict the biologic behavior of the tumor. About 50% of canine MGT have been classified as malignant based upon histologic appearance (MacVean et al., 1978; Priester and Mamel,

1971; Brodey et al., 1983). While some classifications of mammary gland tumors, such as carcinosarcomas or sarcomas, have a consistently poor prognosis, histologic evidence of malignancy does not always imply a malignant course (MacEwen and Withrow, 1996). In fact, only 50% of histologically diagnosed mammary carcinomas result in tumor-associated deaths (Brodey et al., 1983). Recent evidence indicates that morphologic criteria of malignancy, such as cellular pleomorphism, are not sufficient criteria for diagnosis of carcinomas. Instead, local stromal invasion has been identified as the single best histologic evidence of malignancy in mammary tumors (Yager et al., 1993). When stromal invasion is present, 80% of affected dogs will be dead within 2 years, usually within the first year. In the absence of stromal invasion, 80% of affected dogs will be alive after 2 years (Yager et al., 1993). Using stromal invasion as the primary criteria for malignancy, a lifespan study of over a thousand beagles was recently reported which correlated the various histologic classifications of epithelial mammary tumors with biologic behavior (Benjamin et al., 1999). Specifically, the study showed that ductular carcinomas accounted for 65.8% of all fatalities due to mammary neoplasia, even though these tumors composed only 18.7% of all mammary carcinomas. Of the malignant tumors, squamous cell carcinomas exhibited the lowest metastatic rate (20%), with carcinosarcomas exhibiting the highest rate of metastasis (100%). Ductular carcinomas metastasized more frequently than adenocarcinomas, 45% versus 35%, respectively.

FNA of mammary masses is easy to perform in a clinical setting and, compared to surgical biopsy, is relatively inexpensive. When combined with history, signalment, and clinical findings, cytologic examination of mammary aspirates is particularly useful for differentiation between neoplastic disease, cystic lesions, or mastitis. Exfoliative cytology is also useful for evaluation of regional lymph nodes, distant metastatic sites, and neoplastic effusions associated with mammary malignancies. Unfortunately, use of cytology to evaluate mammary neoplasms can be difficult and definitive diagnoses may not always be possible. Some of these difficulties are related to sample collection and others are simply inherent in the nature of mammary neoplasia.

Proper sample collection is important for cytology to be useful in the evaluation of mammary tumors. Because of the considerable tissue heterogeneity that may be present within mammary tumors, sampling of multiple areas within a single tumor and similar samplings of additional tumors are very important. Care should also be taken to aspirate the periphery of a mammary mass as opposed to fluctuant areas within a solid lesion or the center of large tumors. These areas tend to yield fluid of low cellularity or necrosis resulting in a nondiagnostic sample.

Aside from sample collection considerations, accurate and diagnostic exfoliative cytology of mammary tumors is associated with other difficulties. Mesenchymal tumors or tumors with a fibrous or scirrhous component may not exfoliate well, leading to a poorly cellular sample inadequate for diagnosis. Tissue imprints or smears of tissue scrapings taken from biopsy samples may improve cytologic diagnosis in these cases, however, imprints generally do not yield as good a sample for evaluation as aspirates (Baker and Lumsden, 1999a). Also, mammary hyperplasia, dysplasia, benign tumors, and well-differentiated carcinomas tend to form a continuum of morphologic appearance, making cytologic differentiation of these lesions difficult (Benjamin et al., 1999). Lastly, the presence of stromal invasion, one of the most important criteria for determining the malignant potential of a mammary neoplasm, cannot be assessed by the cytologist. All of these factors can result in either false-positive or false-negative diagnosis of malignant mammary tumors using aspiration cytology. A few studies have examined the accuracy of cytology for detecting mammary malignancies as compared to histologic findings. Allen et al. (1986) reported cytologic sensitivities for detecting malignancies of 25% and 17% for the two cytopathologists involved in the study. Reported specificities for cytologic evaluation of malignant mammary tumors were 62% and 49% for the two cytopathologists (Allen et al., 1986). Positive (PPV) and negative (NPV) predictive values were generally similar between the two pathologists, with PPVs of 90% and 100% and NPVs of 75% and 59% (Allen et al., 1986). The diagnostic accuracy was reported as 79% and 66% (Allen et al., 1986). In another study, the sensitivity for cytologic detection of mammary malignancies was found to be 65% with a specificity of 94% (Hellman and Lindgren, 1989). The PPV was reported as 93% with an NPV of 67% and diagnostic accuracy of 79% (Hellman and Lindgren, 1989). These studies did not correlate cytologic diagnosis with disease-free intervals or survival times, thus the use of cytologic criteria to accurately predict the biologic behavior of MGT is uncertain.

Cytological examination of most mammary tumors reveals a background containing variable amounts of blood, basophilic proteinaceous material, lipid, and foam cells. Aspirates of benign epithelial tumors (adenomas and papillomas) typically reveal moderate to large numbers of epithelial cells arranged in sheets and clusters (Fig. 11–7). These cells are uniform in appearance with smooth nuclear chromatin and occasionally prominent, single, small, round nucleoli (Shull and Maddux, 1999). Acinar structures may be seen in samples from adenomas. Benign complex adenomas or pap-

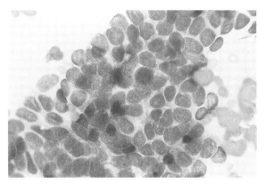

FIGURE 11–7. Sheet of epithelial cells from an aspirate of a mammary adenoma. The cells are of uniform size and shape with a high nuclear-to-cytoplasmic ratio and fine nuclear chromatin. The cytoplasm is lightly basophilic and scant in amount. Feline. (Wright-Giemsa; ×250.)

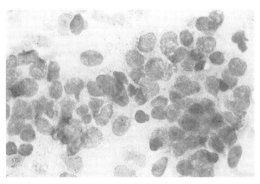

FIGURE 11–8. Epithelial cells from an aspirate of a mixed mammary tumor. The cells display slightly coarse nuclear chromatin, high nuclear-to-cytoplasmic ratios, and mild to moderate anisokaryosis and anisocytosis. Canine. (Wright-Giemsa; ×250.)

illomas, fibroadenomas, and benign mixed tumors may yield sheets and clusters of uniform-appearing epithelial cells and individualized or clumped spindle-shaped cells of myoepithelial (complex tumors) or mesenchymal (mixed tumors) origin. Myoepithelial cells may also appear as oval free nuclei (Shull and Maddux, 1999). Examination of mixed mammary tumors may reveal the presence of cartilage or bone elements

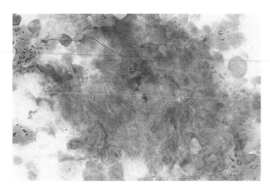

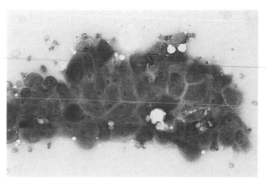

FIGURE 11–9. Clump of spindle-shaped cells associated with large amounts of extracellular pink material from the same aspirate shown in Figure 11–8. Canine. (Wright-Giemsa; ×250.)

FIGURE 11–10. Sheet of epithelial cells displaying prominent cell-to-cell junctions from an aspirate of a mammary adenocarcinoma. These cells also exhibit prominent, large nucleoli, moderate anisokaryosis, and deeply basophilic cytoplasm. Canine. (Wright-Giemsa; ×250.)

such as osteoblasts, osteoclasts, hematopoietic cells, and/or bright-pink extracellular material representative of osteoid (Shull and Maddux, 1999; Fernandes et al., 1998) (Figs. 11–8 and 11–9). Mixed mammary tumors can be difficult to diagnose using exfoliative cytology. For instance, the presence of spindle-shaped cells may not be sufficient for diagnosis of mixed or complex tumors. Allen et al. (1986) have noted that spindle cells were identified in the mammary tumors evaluated in their study, yet the presence of these cells did not correlate significantly with histologic classification of complex or mixed tumors. Aspirates of mixed tumors also may not reveal all of the cells composing the tumor. In a recent case report, aspiration of a mammary mass in a dog revealed the presence of osteoblasts displaying moderate anisokaryosis and anisocytosis, osteoclasts, hematopoietic cells, and pink extracellular material (Fernandes et al., 1998). No epithelial cells were noted in the sample. Thus, the multiple differentials included benign or malignant mixed mammary tumor, osseous metaplasia, and osteosarcoma. Histopathology confirmed that the neoplasm was a benign mixed mammary tumor.

Malignant mammary tumors may be di-

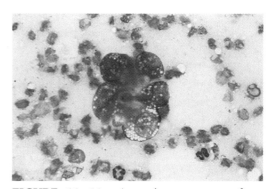

FIGURE 11–11. An acinar structure from an aspirate of a mammary adenocarcinoma. Note the presence of punctate cytoplasmic vacuoles as well as prominent nucleoli and moderate anisokaryosis. Canine. (Wright-Giemsa; ×250.)

agnosed based upon the cytologic appearance of the cell types present and the observation of more than three criteria of malignancy. Adenocarcinomas are characterized by epithelial cells arranged in sheets (Fig. 11–10) and clusters, or sometimes individualized. Acinar structures may be observed (Fig. 11–11). The epithelial cells are typically round, with round to oval, eccentrically located nuclei and moderate

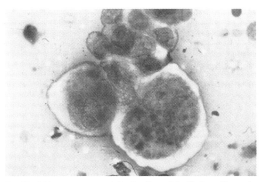

FIGURE 11–12. Marked epithelial cell anisokaryosis and anisocytosis in an aspirate from a mammary adenocarcinoma. The epithelial cells contain basophilic secretory material as well as diffuse, peripheral cytoplasmic vacuolation. Canine. (Wright-Giemsa; ×250.)

amounts of basophilic cytoplasm that may contain amorphous basophilic secretory product and/or clear vacuoles (Shull and Maddux, 1999) (Fig. 11–12). Some of these vacuoles may appear as punctate vacuoles of variable number or as a diffuse clearing of the cytoplasm that distends the cell and displaces the nucleus peripherally. Criteria of malignancy that may be seen in these cells include increased nuclear-to-cytoplasmic ratio; moderate to marked variation in nuclear and cell size; nuclear molding; large, prominent, multiple, and/or abnormally shaped nucleoli; and binucleation and multinucleation. Increased mitotic activity and abnormal mitotic figures may be present (Figs. 11–13 and 11–14). Ductular carcinomas typically present with sheets and clusters of pleomorphic epithelial cells with high nuclear-to-cytoplasmic ratios and round, basal nuclei. These cells usually display more than three malignant criteria. Acinar structures, secretory product, and cytoplasmic vacuoles are not characteristic features of ductular carcinomas.

Anaplastic carcinomas may present with very large, extremely pleomorphic epithelial cells occurring singly and in small clusters (Shull and Maddux, 1999). These cells tend to have bizarre nuclear and nucleolar forms. Multinucleation and abnormal mitotic figures are frequently seen (Shull and Maddux, 1999). Inflammatory carcinomas, which are a locally aggressive form of mammary carcinoma, also present with large, pleomorphic epithelial cells exhibiting various criteria of malignancy as well as large numbers of nondegenerate neutrophils and

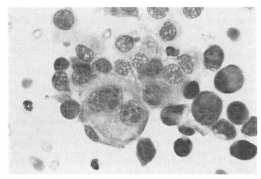

FIGURE 11–13. Marked anisokaryosis, anisocytosis, prominent nucleoli, coarse nuclear chromatin, and binucleation in cells from an aspirate of a mammary carcinoma. The cells also display poor cellular adhesion. Canine. (Wright-Giemsa; ×250.)

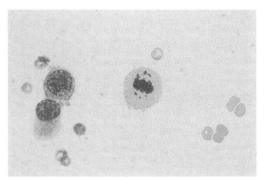

FIGURE 11–14. Abnormal mitotic figure with lag chromatin from the mammary carcinoma shown in Figure 11–13. Lag chromatin results from abnormal formation of the mitotic spindle apparatus. Abnormal mitotic figures are considered one criterion of malignancy. Canine. (Wright-Giemsa; ×250.)

macrophages (MacEwen and Withrow, 1996). The cytologic appearance of inflammatory carcinoma may resemble mastitis. However, history, signalment, and presence of very anaplastic epithelial cells should be helpful for differentiation of these two conditions.

Squamous cell carcinomas of the mammary gland appear cytologically similar to those found in other body sites. The malignant squamous cells tend to occur individually or in small sheets. The nuclei may vary from small and pyknotic to large, round and immature with prominent nucleoli. The nuclear-to-cytoplasmic ratio is variable and binucleation may be noted. The cytoplasm of the tumor cells is moderately to deeply basophilic (nonkeratinized) or may have a blue-green color characteristic of keratinization. Mammary squamous cell carcinomas may ulcerate, leading to the presence of inflammatory cells and phagocytized bacteria in the cytologic sample (Shull and Maddux, 1999).

Aspirates of malignant mixed mammary tumors may reveal epithelial cells and spindle-shaped, individualized cells of mesenchymal origin with one of these populations displaying nuclear and cellular criteria of malignancy. However, the presence of either population or predominance of one cell type over the other may depend on the area of tumor aspirated (Shull and Maddux, 1999). In carcinosarcomas, both epithelial and mesenchymal populations should display malignant features. Mammary sarcomas, such as osteosarcoma, fibrosarcoma, and liposarcoma, are of similar cytologic appearance to those found in other body sites. Sarcomas tend to exfoliate poorly, often resulting in samples of low cellularity. Depending on the type of tumor, pink extracellular material or lipid may be present in the background. In general, sarcomas are characterized by spindle-shaped to irregular cells arranged individually and in small

clumps. The cytoplasm of these cells is moderately to deeply basophilic and the cytoplasmic borders tend to be indistinct. The cells display similar cytologic features of malignancy as described for epithelial neoplasms.

Feline Mammary Gland Tumors

Mammary tumors are common in cats and follow hematopoietic, skin, and, in some studies, alimentary tumors in prevalence (Hayes and Mooney, 1985; MacVean et al., 1978; Patnaik et al., 1975; Dorn et al., 1968). The median age for MGT development in the cat is 10 years of age or older (Hayes and Mooney, 1985; MacEwen and Withrow, 1996). Almost all (99%) of feline MGT occur in intact females (Moulton, 1990). Although some researchers believe that there is no breed predisposition for mammary neoplasia in the cat, Hayes et al. (1981) reported an increased incidence and a younger age at diagnosis of MGT in the Siamese breed.

Development of feline MGT is thought to have a hormonal component. Intact females have an almost seven-fold greater risk of developing mammary neoplasms as compared to neutered females, and ovariohysterectomy has been reported to decrease the risk of MGT to 0.6% compared to intact females (Dorn et al., 1968; Hayes et al., 1981). Regular, but not irregular, administration of exogenous progesterone was associated with a significantly increased risk of benign mammary tumors and mammary carcinomas in cats (Misdorp, 1991). Hormone receptor analysis has shown that normal feline mammary tissue contains estrogen and progesterone receptors in levels similar to those found in the dog (Rutteman et al., 1991). However, unlike canine MGT, the majority of feline mammary neoplasms express very low levels of estrogen and progesterone receptors, which may be related to the high rate of malignancy found with mammary neoplasia in the cat (Rutteman et al., 1991).

In contrast to the dog, the majority of feline mammary tumors are malignant with some studies reporting a greater than 80% incidence of malignant neoplasms (Mac-Vean et al., 1978; Hayes et al., 1981; Priester Mamel, 1971). Adenocarcinomas are the most prevalent malignant mammary tumor followed by carcinomas and sarcomas (Hayes et al., 1981; MacEwen et al., 1984). Malignant MGT in cats tend to grow rapidly and metastasize to regional lymph nodes and lung (Hayes et al., 1981; Mac-Ewen et al., 1984). The single most important prognostic indicator for feline MGT is tumor size at time of diagnosis. Median survival times for cats with mammary tumors greater than 3 cm, between 2 and 3 cm, and less than 2 cm is 6 months, 2 years, and greater than 3 years, respectively (MacEwen et al., 1984). Thus, early diagnosis and treatment is very important for feline mammary malignancies.

The cytologic features of benign and malignant mammary neoplasms in the cat are similar to those described in the dog (Figs. 11–10, 11–13, 11–14). The reliability of cytologic criteria to differentiate between hyperplasia, benign tumors, and malignancies in the cat does not appear to have been reported (Baker and Lumsden, 1999a). Given the high rate of mammary malignancy in cats, cytologic findings of a benign-appearing population of epithelial cells, particularly in an older cat with no history of progesterone administration, should be treated with some caution. In these cases, samples should be submitted for histopathologic examination to rule out the presence of a malignancy.

Treatment considerations will follow clinical and cytologic and/or histologic identification of a mammary neoplasm in a dog or cat. A thorough evaluation of health status involving a complete physical examination, complete blood count, and serum biochemical profile should be performed. If a malignancy is present, staging the extent of the disease should include radiographs of the lungs and any other potential metastatic sites as well as cytologic analysis of regional lymph nodes, metastatic lesions, and/or body cavity effusions. Surgical excision is the treatment of choice for both canine and feline mammary neoplasms. The benefits of adjuvant therapy involving chemotherapeutics, radiation, or immune stimulation are uncertain in treatment of canine and feline mammary malignancies (Hahn et al., 1992). Doxorubicin in dogs (Hahn et al., 1992) and a combination of doxorubicin and cyclophosphamide in cats (MacEwen and Withrow, 1996) have been shown to have some benefit in cases of disseminated, inoperable mammary malignancies. Antihormonal therapy using the estrogen agonist/antagonist tamoxifen produced mixed results in regards to tumor response and can be associated with undesirable estrogen-related side-effects (Morris et al., 1993). To be effective, antihormonal therapy should be accompanied by determination of tumor hormone receptor status using methods validated for the species of interest. In veterinary medicine, this technology is available only for research purposes. Currently, tamoxifen is not recommended for treatment of canine MGT (MacEwen and Withrow, 1996).

Vagina

Examination of exfoliated vaginal cells for staging the estrous cycle is one of the most common uses of cytology in veterinary practice. This technique is easy to perform and, with some experience, can be successfully used by the clinician to optimize breeding of client animals. Cytologic examination of vaginal mucosal imprints and discharges is also useful for evaluation of vaginal inflammation and neoplasia of the female reproductive tract.

Special Collection Techniques

Several techniques have been described for obtaining vaginal cells for cytologic examination (Olson et al., 1984a; Thrall and Olson, 1999; Mills et al., 1979). Most commonly, a saline-moistened cotton swab or thin glass rod with a rounded tip is directed craniodorsally into the caudal vagina. The vestibule and clitoral fossa should be avoided since keratinized superficial squamous cells present in these sites may alter cytologic interpretations (Thrall and Olson, 1999). Once craniad to the urethral orifice, vaginal cells are obtained by gently passing the swab or glass rod over the epithelial lining. In an alternate method of sample collection, a small glass bulb pipette containing sterile saline is passed into the caudal vagina and cells are obtained by repeatedly flushing and aspirating the saline fluid (Olson et al., 1984a). Once collected, the exfoliated cells are gently transferred onto a clean microscope slide for staining. Although several types of stains have been used for cytologic evaluation of vaginal cells, Romanowsky-type stains or modified Romanowsky stains are most commonly used. These stains are easy to use in a clinical setting and provide good morphologic detail for determining the degree of maturation of the epithelial cells. Papanicolau or trichrome stains have also been used for estrous cycle staging. These stains impart a distinctive orange staining to the keratin precursors abundant in superficial cells. The ratio of orange or eosinophilic cells to no-neosinophilic cells, termed the *eosinophilic index,* can be used to assess the degree of

maturation of the epithelial cells and subsequently stage the estrous cycle. However, these stains may yield variable staining results and the need for multiple solutions limits their practical use (Mills et al., 1979; Olson et al., 1984a).

Normal Anatomy and Histology

The vagina is a musculomembranous canal extending from the uterus to the vulva. The vaginal wall is composed of an inner mucosal layer, a middle smooth muscle layer, and an external coat of connective tissue and peritoneum (cranially) (Banks, 1986b). The mucosal layer consists of stratified squamous epithelium, which undergoes characteristic morphologic changes in association with the estrous cycle. Although the mucosa is typically nonglandular, intraepithelial glands have been observed during estrus in the dog (Banks, 1986b). The vulva is anatomically similar to the caudal vagina. The vulva is composed of the vestibule containing the urethral orifice, the clitoral fossa, and the labia. The mucosa is lined by stratified squamous epithelium; some keratinized epithelial cells may be found in the vestibule and clitoral fossa (Thrall and Olson, 1999). Vestibular glands within the submucosal layer of the vestibule are responsible for mucus production, which is most notable during estrus and at parturition (Banks, 1986b).

Normal Cytology

Four types of vaginal epithelial cells may be identified by exfoliative cytology. In order from the deepest and most immature cells to the most superficial and mature, these cells are basal, parabasal, intermediate, and superficial.

Basal cells are located along the basement membrane and give rise to the other epithelial cell types seen in a vaginal smear

(Thrall and Olson, 1999). Round nuclei and scant amounts of basophilic cytoplasm characterize these small cells. Because of their deep location, basal cells are rarely seen in vaginal preparations.

Parabasal cells are the smallest of the epithelial cells seen in routine vaginal cytologic samples. These cells have a high nuclear-to-cytoplasmic ratio, round nuclei of uniform size and shape, and basophilic cytoplasm. Parabasal cells containing cytoplasmic vacuoles are called *foam cells;* the significance of the vacuoles is unknown (Olson et al., 1984a). Large numbers of parabasal cells may be seen in vaginal smears of prepubertal animals and should not be confused with neoplastic cells (Olson et al., 1984a).

Intermediate cells may vary in size, but are generally twice the size of parabasal cells (Thrall and Olson, 1999). The nuclear-to-cytoplasmic ratio is decreased with abundant amounts of blue to blue-green (keratinized) cytoplasm. The cytoplasmic borders are round to irregular and folded (Baker and Lumsden, 1999b). Intermediate cells may also be called *superficial intermediate* or *transitional intermediate cells* (Thrall and Olson, 1999).

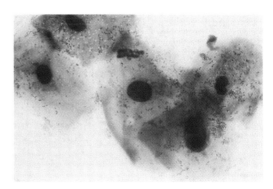

FIGURE 11–16.   **Late proestrus.** Intermediate and superficial cells with round to pyknotic nuclei and moderately basophilic cytoplasm with angular to folded borders. The cells are associated with large numbers of bacteria. Canine. (Wright-Giemsa; ×250.) (Sample provided by Rolf Larsen, University of Florida.)

Superficial cells are characterized by small round to pyknotic nuclei, abundant amounts of light blue to blue-green (keratinized) cytoplasm, and angular to folded cell borders. Some superficial cells contain dark-staining bodies of unknown significance (Olson et al., 1984a). As superficial cells age and become degenerate, the nuclei are lost and the cells become anucleated. Superficial cells with pyknotic nuclei and anucleated superficial cells have the same physiologic significance (Thrall and Olson, 1999). The maturation of squamous epithelial cells into folded, angular cells with pyknotic or absent nuclei is called *cornification,* therefore superficial cells are sometimes referred to as *cornified cells* (Thrall and Olson, 1999).

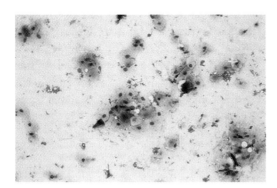

FIGURE 11–15.   **Proestrus.** Intermediate epithelial cells with lower numbers of superficial cells from a vaginal smear. Red blood cells are present. The background has a basophilic appearance due to the presence of mucus. Canine. (Wright-Giemsa; ×125.) (Sample provided by Rolf Larsen, University of Florida.)

Staging the Canine Estrous Cycle

Proestrus

In the dog, the average length of proestrus (Figs. 11–15 and 11–16), which is the preovulatory follicular phase of the estrous cycle, is 9 days with a range of 3 to 17 days (Freshman, 1991). Proestrus is characterized by rising concentrations of estradiol and low progesterone concentrations (Freshman, 1991). As the estradiol concentrations increase, the vaginal epithelium proliferates and red blood cells move via diapedesis through uterine capillaries (Baker and Lumsden, 1999b). In early to mid proestrus, neutrophils and a mixture of parabasal, intermediate, and superficial epithelial cells (Olson et al., 1984a) characterize the vaginal smear. Red blood cells may be abundant or absent (Olson et al., 1984a). The background of the smear may have a "dirty" appearance due to the presence of mucus (Baker and Lumsden, 1999b). Variable numbers of bacteria may also be seen in the background. As proestrus progresses, the neutrophils decrease in number and superficial epithelial cells begin to predominate (Olson et al., 1984a).

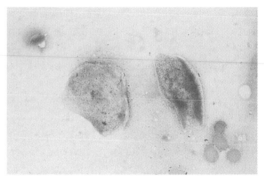

FIGURE 11–17. Estrus. Anucleated (cornified) superficial epithelial cells from a vaginal smear. Note the presence of red blood cells in the background. Canine. (Wright-Giemsa; ×250.) (Sample provided by Rolf Larsen, University of Florida.)

Estrus

The onset of estrus (Fig. 11–17) is characterized by declining estradiol concentrations and rising progesterone concentrations (Freshman, 1991). The average duration of estrus is 9 days with a range of 3 to 21 days (Freshman, 1991). The primary cytologic characteristic of estrus is the presence of 90% or greater superficial cells. Parabasal or intermediate cells comprise 5% or less of the epithelial population (Olson et al., 1984a). Neutrophils are absent and red blood cells may or may not be seen (Olson et al., 1984a). Clearing of the background may be noted (Baker and Lumsden, 1999b). Bacteria associated with the superficial cells are usually present (Olson et al., 1984a).

For optimal breeding efficiency, sperm should be present in the female reproductive tract as near to ovulation as possible. Although vaginal cytology has been shown to be a more accurate indicator of estrus and, subsequently, ovulation than behav-

ioral signs, evidence of vaginal maturation or cornification is not closely associated with ovulation. Maximum cornification of vaginal superficial cells ranges from 6 days before the luteinizing hormone (LH) peak to 3 days after the LH peak (Olson, 1984a). Since ovulation usually occurs 1 to 2 days after the LH peak, vaginal cytology is not an accurate predictor of ovulation. Ova are viable for up to 2 days postovulation and sperm may remain viable for up to 4 days within the canine reproductive tract during estrus (Freshman, 1991). Therefore, bitches should be bred every 2 to 3 days during cytologic estrus (greater than 90% superficial cells) for optimal breeding (Freshman, 1991). Use of plasma progesterone concentrations in combination with vaginal cytology may indicate more accurately the time of ovulation, allowing for even greater breeding efficiency and more accurate estimation of the time of expected parturition (Wright, 1990).

Diestrus

Diestrus (Figs. 11–18 and 11–19) is the luteal phase of the estrous cycle character-

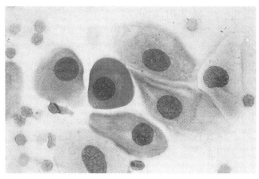

FIGURE 11–18. Diestrus. Parabasal and intermediate epithelial cells are present in this vaginal smear. The parabasal cells have round nuclei, moderate nuclear-to-cytoplasmic ratios, moderately to deeply basophilic cytoplasm, and round cell borders. The intermediate cells are larger with increased amounts of cytoplasm and angular borders. Red blood cells are present in the background. Canine. (Wright-Giemsa, ×250.) (Sample provided by Rolf Larsen, University of Florida.)

ized by high concentrations of progesterone (Freshman, 1991). The length of diestrus is usually 2 months, whether or not the bitch is pregnant (Freshman, 1991). Cytologically, an abrupt 20% decrease in superficial cells and a 15% to 20% increase in small intermediate cells characterize diestrus (Olson et al., 1984a; Holst and Phemister, 1974). The decrease of superficial cells at the beginning of diestrus is usually more rapid than the increase of superficial cells occurring at estrus (Holst and Phemister, 1974). Neutrophils frequently reappear during diestrus. Some neutrophils from normal bitches in diestrus contain ingested bacteria (Olson et al., 1984b). Red blood cells may also be present in diestrus vaginal smears (Olson et al., 1984a). The cytologic appearance of early proestrus and diestrus can be very similar, thus one vaginal smear is not adequate for differentiation of these two stages (Olson et al., 1984a). Once cytologic evidence of diestrus is apparent, breeding is unlikely to be successful (Olson et al., 1984a).

Anestrus

Anestrus, the period between the end of diestrus and the beginning of the next proestrus, is a time of uterine involution and endometrial repair (Freshman, 1991). Parabasal and intermediate cells characterize anestrus. Superficial cells are absent. Neutrophils and bacteria are either absent or present in low numbers (Olson et al., 1984a).

Staging the Feline Estrous Cycle

Cats are seasonally polyestrous. Coitus is necessary for ovulation, with successive estrous cycles occurring until ovulation takes place (Thrall and Olson, 1999). The average duration of estrus is 8 days (range 3 to 16 days) with an intermediate period of 9 days (range 4 to 22 days) if ovulation does not occur (Thrall and Olson, 1999). In the presence of ovulation without pregnancy, the

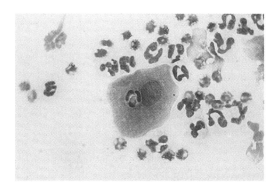

FIGURE 11–19. Diestrus. Note the large number of neutrophils and red blood cells in the background. An intermediate epithelial cell containing a neutrophil (metestrum cell) is located in the center. These cells are not specific for diestrus and may be found whenever increased numbers of neutrophils are present. Canine. (Wright-Giemsa; ×250.) (Sample provided by Rolf Larsen, University of Florida.)

return to estrus may be delayed for about 45 days (Olson et al., 1984a). Vaginal cytology has been shown to accurately predict the various stages of the estrous cycle in the cat (Shille et al., 1979; Mills et al., 1979). Collection of smears for cytologic evaluation is similar to those described for the dog; collection of feline vaginal samples may rarely result in ovulation (Thrall and Olson, 1999).

Changes in feline vaginal cytology during the estrous cycle are similar to those seen in the dog, however, some differences should be noted. Red blood cells are rarely seen in smears made at any stage of the cycle (Mills et al., 1979). Neutrophils are rare in smears from proestrus and are an inconsistent feature of diestrus (Mills et al., 1979; Thrall, 1999). Superficial cells are the predominant cell type seen during estrus (Mills et al., 1979). In contrast to dogs, superficial cells comprise only 40% to 88% of the epithelial cells seen during feline estrus (Shille et al., 1979; Mills, 1979). Anucleated cells increase to about 10% of the epithelial population on the first day of estrus, with a maximum average of 40% anucleated cells by the fourth day of estrus (Shille et al., 1979). A prominent clearing of the vaginal smear background in association with estrus has been observed. This clearing occurred in 90% of feline estrus smears and was suggested to be a sensitive indicator of estrus in the cat (Shille et al., 1979).

Inflammation

Vaginitis

Inflammatory disease of the vaginal mucosa is often related to noninfectious factors such as vaginal anomalies, clitoral hypertrophy, foreign bodies, neoplasia, or vaginal immaturity ("puppy vaginitis") (Olson et al., 1984b). Smears for cytologic evaluation of inflammation may be obtained from the vaginal mucosa, vaginal discharges, or FNA of vaginal/vulvar masses. Moderate to large numbers of neutrophils characterize acute vaginitis. In addition to neutrophils, lymphocytes and macrophages may be seen in more chronic inflammatory conditions (Thrall and Olson, 1999). If an infectious component is involved in the inflammatory process, degenerate neutrophils and phagocytized bacteria may be seen (Figs. 11–20 and 11–21). Less commonly, hyphal elements related to fungal infection or pythiosis may be observed. Cytologic specimens may be submitted for silver stains to identify hyphae if fungal infection or pythiosis is suspected (Figs. 11–22 and 11–23).

Treatment of vaginitis should involve identification and correction of any underlying conditions responsible for the inflammation. If sepsis is present, appropriate antibiotic therapy based upon culture and sensitivity results should be instituted. Vaginitis can be associated with the presence of

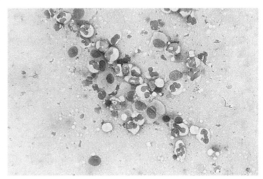

FIGURE 11–20. Increased numbers of neutrophils from an imprint of a tissue scraping of vaginal papules. The neutrophils display degenerative nuclear changes of moderate to marked karyolysis. Degenerative changes are typically associated with bacterial infections. A few parabasal and intermediate epithelial cells are also present. Canine. (Wright-Giemsa; ×125.)

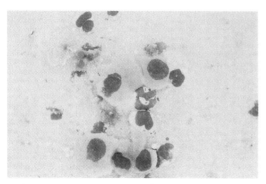

FIGURE 11–21. Two degenerative neutrophils containing phagocytized bacteria from the vaginal scraping shown in Figure 11–20. Cytologic diagnosis was septic vaginitis. Canine. (Wright-Giemsa; ×250.)

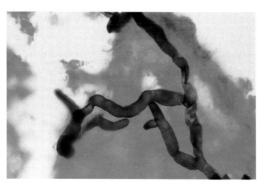

FIGURE 11–23. Fungal stain of sample shown in Figure 11–22. Positive-staining, poorly septated, linear structures approximately 6 to 8 μm in width are present. Culture confirmed the presence of *Pythium* sp. (Gomori's methenamine silver; ×250.)

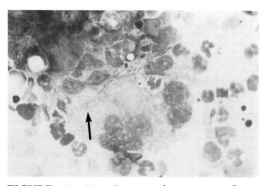

FIGURE 11–22. Pyogranulomatous inflammation in an aspirate from a vulvar mass. Large numbers of neutrophils, lower numbers of eosinophils, and a multinucleated macrophage are present. Pale-staining linear structures suspicious for hyphae are seen associated with the macrophage (*arrow*). Canine. (Wright-Giemsa; ×250.)

epithelial cells displaying atypical cellular features in response to the inflammatory process. In the absence of a tumor, therapy to alleviate the inflammation should eliminate the atypical cells. However, if an observable mass is present and/or atypical cells remain after appropriate treatment, further tests to rule out the presence of neoplasia should be considered.

Pyometra/Metritis

Cytologic examination of vaginal discharges may be useful for diagnosis of inflammatory disease of the uterus. Pyometra is the accumulation of pus within the uterus associated with diestrus. The common presentation involves older, unbred bitches presenting several weeks following estrus with mild to severe evidence of systemic illness (Gilbert, 1992). Clinical signs may include anorexia, depression, polyuria, and/or polydipsia. A vaginal discharge may be present in open-cervix pyometra. Closed-cervix pyometra is usually not associated with a discharge (Gilbert, 1992). An inflammatory leukogram may be present in some, but not all, cases of pyometra (Gilbert, 1992). Pyometra is considered to be less common in cats, probably because cats are induced ovulators, which limits uterine exposure to progesterone (Gilbert, 1992). Metritis usually follows parturition and is characterized by a systemically ill animal with a malodorous uterine/vaginal discharge (Olson et al., 1984b). Treatment of choice for pyometra is ovariohysterectomy with supportive therapy including appropriate antibiotic administration (Gilbert, 1992). The treatment of metritis is also ovariohysterectomy if the owner is not interested in further breeding or if severe systemic illness is present. Nursing puppies or kittens should be weaned and hand raised. If future breeding is desired, medical treatment of metritis includes antibiotic therapy, intravenous fluids, and uterine drainage (Stone, 1985).

Large numbers of neutrophils, many of which are degenerate (Olson et al., 1984b), characterize smears prepared from vaginal discharges resulting from open-cervix pyometra or metritis. Bacteria may be seen extracellularly and within the neutrophils (Olson et al., 1984b). Muscle fibers from decomposing fetuses may rarely be visible in samples from metritis (Thrall and Olson, 1999).

Vaginal Neoplasia

Vaginal and vulvar tumors are uncommon and tend to occur in older animals (Olson et al., 1984b). Leiomyomas and fibromas are the most common vaginal neoplasm in dogs and cats (Baker and Lumsden, 1999b). These benign mesenchymal tumors are characterized by variable numbers of spindle-shaped cells of uniform size and shape arranged individually and in small clumps (Fig. 11–24). The nuclei are typically oval and scant to moderate amounts of wispy cytoplasm are present. Vaginal epithelial tumors that may be seen include fibropapillomas (polyps), squamous cell carcinomas, and urethral transitional cell carcinomas invading the vagina (Olson et al., 1984b). The cytologic appearance of these tumors is similar to those found in other body sites. Treatment of vaginal tumors usually involves surgical excision. In cases of malignant tumors, further evaluation to determine extent of local invasion or metastasis should be performed.

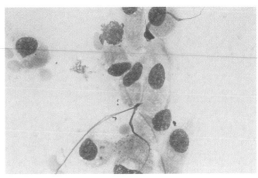

FIGURE 11–24. Imprint of a vaginal leiomyoma. The cells are arranged individually or in small clumps and display round to oval nuclei with coarse nuclear chromatin, moderate nuclear-to-cytoplasmic ratios, and inconspicuous nucleoli. The cytoplasm is moderately basophilic and cell borders are indistinct. Canine. (Wright-Giemsa; ×250.)

Transmissible venereal tumors (TVT) may also be diagnosed using cytologic examination of vaginal smears or fine-needle aspirates. TVT are contagious, sexually transmitted tumors occurring in both genders. The tumors may be located in genital areas and extragenital sites such as the rectum, skin, and oral and nasal cavities. They appear as firm, friable, tan, ulcerated, nodular or polypoid masses (Fig. 11–25). In bitches, TVT may spread directly to the cervix, uterus, and oviducts (Rogers, 1997). Although metastasis is uncommon, TVT can spread to regional lymph nodes, skin, and subcutaneous tissue. Other reported metastatic sites include lips, oral mucous membranes, eye, musculature, abdominal viscera, lungs, and the central nervous system (Rogers, 1997).

Aspirates of TVT generally yield large numbers of individualized, round cells (Figs. 11–26 and 11–27). The nuclei are round with clumped nuclear chromatin and one or two prominent nucleoli (Rogers, 1997). Moderate amounts of pale-blue cytoplasm frequently contain multiple punctate

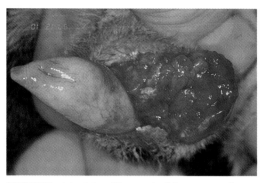

FIGURE 11–25. Transmissible venereal tumor (TVT) appears as a soft, friable, hemorrhagic mass on the external genitalia of a dog.

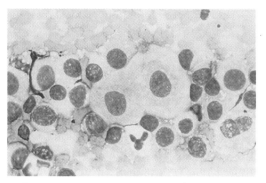

FIGURE 11–27. Two intermediate epithelial cells (center) and individualized tumor cells from the TVT shown in Figure 11–26. Note the larger size and increased amounts of cytoplasm in the epithelial cells compared to the tumor cells. Canine. (Wright-Giemsa; ×250.)

vacuoles. Mitotic activity is often high. Inflammation, as indicated by increased numbers of plasma cells, lymphocytes, macrophages, and neutrophils, may be present (Rogers, 1997).

Marginal surgical resection is not considered effective treatment for TVT. Although surgery may be effective with small, localized TVT, the recurrence rate may approach 68% (Rogers, 1997). The most effective treatments for TVT are chemotherapy and radiation. Single-agent therapy with vincristine has been shown to be very effective for TVT even in cases of metastatic disease. Doxorubicin is the drug of choice for TVT resistant to vincristine (Rogers, 1997).

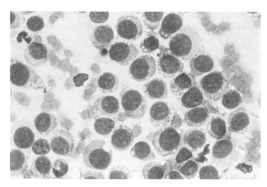

FIGURE 11–26. Large numbers of round cells from an imprint of a vaginal transmissible venereal tumor. The cells have round nuclei, coarse nuclear chromatin, variably prominent nucleoli, and scant to moderate amounts of lightly basophilic cytoplasm. Many of the cells contain punctate cytoplasmic vacuoles, which is a characteristic feature of this tumor. Canine. (Wright-Giemsa; ×250.)

MALE REPRODUCTIVE SYSTEM: PROSTATE AND TESTES

Prostate Gland

Although the prostate gland is present in cats, the vast majority of prostatic disease is reported in the dog. Therefore, the following discussion of normal and abnormal findings associated with the prostate gland will be limited to the dog. Prostatic disease is common in middle-aged and older male dogs. Canine prostatic illness may be separated into infectious and noninfectious categories. Infectious prostatic diseases include acute and chronic prostatitis and prostatic abscesses. Noninfectious prostatic diseases include benign hyperplasia, prostatic cysts, and neoplasia. Infectious and noninfectious prostatic disease may occur simultaneously (Baker and Lumsden, 1999b).

The primary presenting clinical findings associated with prostatic disease are signs of systemic febrile illness, lower urinary tract symptoms (hemorrhagic urethral discharge), abnormalities of defecation, and locomotion problems (Dorfman and Barsanti, 1995). Some cases of canine prostatic disease may be present without obvious clinical signs, therefore palpation of the prostate per rectum should be a part of all physical examination in mature intact and neutered male dogs. Normally, the prostate should be smooth, symmetrical, and nonpainful (Dorfman and Barsanti, 1995). Abdominal palpation can be used to evaluate an enlarged prostate that has moved into the abdominal cavity. Ancillary diagnostic tests that may be used to evaluate suspected cases of prostatic disease include urinalysis, bacterial culture, radiography, and ultrasonography. Complete blood counts and serum biochemical profiles are usually normal in cases of prostatic illness, however, the presence of hemogram and biochemical abnormalities may help in diagnosis (Dorfman and Barsanti, 1995). Cytology, microbiology, and/or histopathology may be necessary for classification of the type of prostatic disease (Baker and Lumsden, 1999b).

Special Collection Techniques

Urethral Discharge

Sampling of urethral discharge is a simple method for evaluation of prostatic abnormalities, but is the least effective technique (Baker and Lumsden, 1999b). If present, urethral discharge is collected by retracting the prepuce, cleaning the glans, and collecting the discharge into a vial or onto a microscope slide for microscopic evaluation. Some samples may also be collected into sterile containers for bacterial culture and colony counts. Concurrent analysis of urine collected by catheterization should be performed to differentiate between normal urethral flora and cystitis (Baker and Lumsden, 1999b).

Semen Evaluation

Ejaculate material for evaluation of prostatic disease can be obtained from intact dogs via manual stimulation; however, collection of semen may not be possible if the dog is inexperienced or in pain (Dorfman and Barsanti, 1995). A collection funnel may be used to separate the clear prostatic third fraction of the ejaculate from the sperm-rich first and second fractions (Olson et al., 1987). An aliquot for microbiologic analysis should be placed into a sterile culture tube with the remaining fluid retained for cytologic evaluation. If inflammation is suspected, the cytologic aliquot should be placed into a vial containing EDTA (Baker and Lumsden, 1999b). Because of the presence of normal bacterial flora in the lower urethra, a quantitative culture should be performed on the ejaculate fluid. In the presence of inflammatory cells, high numbers (>100,000/ml) of gram-negative or gram-positive bacteria indicate an infectious process (Dorfman and Barsanti, 1995). If cytologic and microbiologic results are equivocal in regards to prostatic infection versus urethral contamination, a quantitative lower urethral culture to compare to the semen culture results may be useful (Dorfman and Barsanti, 1995).

Prostatic Massage

Prostatic massage is used primarily to collect prostatic fluid in dogs unable to ejaculate (Dorfman and Barsanti, 1995; Olson et al., 1987). The simplest method for prostatic massage involves passing a urinary catheter, guided by rectal palpation, to the caudal pole of the prostate. A syringe is attached to the catheter and fluid is aspirated as the prostate is gently massaged per rectum (Olson et al., 1987). A few milliliters of sterile saline may be flushed into the catheter and aspirated to facilitate collection of fluid for analysis (Olson et al., 1987). Urinary tract infection often accompanies infectious prostatitis, which may confound the results of prostatic massage. For these cases, an alternative massage procedure may be used to determine the source of the infection (Olson et al., 1987). The urinary bladder is catheterized, emptied of urine, and flushed with 5 ml of sterile physiologic saline. The fluid from this first flush is collected as the preprostatic massage fraction. The catheter is then retracted to the caudal pole of the prostate. Another 5 ml of sterile physiologic saline is injected through the catheter while the prostate is massaged per rectum. The catheter is then advanced back into the bladder and all the fluid in the bladder is collected. This fluid is the postprostatic massage fraction, which should be relatively free of urinary contamination. Bacterial colony counts and presence or absence of inflammatory cells from the pre- and postprostatic massage fractions can be compared to isolate the source of the infection. Ampicillin, which concentrates in urine but reaches lower concentrations in the prostate owing to its inability to cross the prostatic–lipid barrier, may be administered one day prior to prostatic massage to aid in isolation of the source of infection (Barsanti et al., 1983). In general, prostatic massage should be reserved for evaluation of prostatitis in dogs without urinary tract infection or in which the urinary tract infection is controlled (Barsanti et al., 1983).

Fine-Needle Aspiration

Fine-needle aspiration (FNA) of the prostate gland has been shown to produce more reliable results and more prostatic cells than prostatic massage (Thrall and Olson, 1985). If the gland is enlarged, a transabdominal approach may be used. Transperineal and perirectal approaches have also been described (Olson et al., 1987; Thrall and Olson, 1985). Ultrasound is particularly useful for guiding the aspiration needle, particularly if focal prostatic disease is present (Zinkl, 1999). The method of aspiration of the prostate gland is similar to that used for other tissues. A 22-gauge needle attached to a 12-cc syringe is directed into the gland and cells and/or fluid are aspirated. A drop of aspirate material or fluid is placed onto a slide. If necessary, any remaining material may then be submitted for culture.

Use of FNA in cases of acute prostatitis or abscessation may be associated with a risk of peritonitis or seeding the infection along the needle tract (Dorfman and Barsanti, 1995). Dogs with suspected prostatic disease presenting with an inflammatory leukogram and fever should not undergo FNA (Dorfman and Barsanti, 1995). If purulent fluid is obtained during aspiration of the prostate, aspiration should continue until all pressure is reduced to prevent leakage of the material (Baker and Lumsden, 1999b). FNA of the prostate gland has several advantages compared to other collection methods. Identification of squamous epithelial cells from a prostatic aspirate allows diagnosis of squamous metaplasia, whereas the presence of these cells in prostatic massage fluid could be misinterpreted as normal lower urinary tract squamous epithelial cells (Thrall and Olson, 1985). Also, the greater cellular detail obtained via FNA increases the confidence of a diagnosis of neoplasia (Thrall and Olson, 1985). The primary disadvantage of prostatic FNA is that focal lesions, such as neoplasia, may be missed (Thrall and Olson, 1985). However, use of ultrasound to guide the aspirate can lessen this possibility.

Normal Anatomy and Histology

The prostate gland secretes a fluid that promotes sperm survival and motility (Dorfman and Barsanti, 1995). Normal prostatic fluid is clear and represents the third fraction of the canine ejaculate, although some have suggested that the first fraction also originates from the prostate (Dorfman and Barsanti, 1995). The prostate gland is a glandular, muscular structure completely surrounding the proximal portion of the male urethra (Lowseth et al., 1990). Prior to 2 months of age, the prostate is located within the abdominal cavity. After breakdown of the urachal ligament until sexual maturity, the prostate lies in the pelvic canal. With increasing age, the prostate enlarges and moves over the pelvic brim into the abdomen. Bladder distension can also pull the prostate cranially into the abdomen (Dorfman and Barsanti, 1995).

The prostate gland is composed of compound tubuloalveolar glands radiating from the urethral opening (Dorfman and Barsanti, 1995) (Figs. 11–28 and 11–29). The secretory alveoli contain primary and secondary enfoldings of epithelium that project

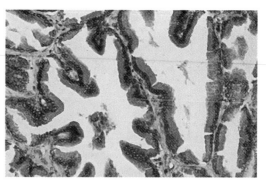

FIGURE 11–29. Higher magnification of normal prostate gland. Cuboidal and columnar epithelium line the prostatic lumens and ducts. Canine. (H & E; ×50.) (Case material supplied by Roger Reep and Don Samuelson, University of Florida.)

into the alveolar lumen. A fibromuscular stroma surrounds the prostatic ducts, which are lined by cuboidal to columnar epithelium. Transitional epithelium lines the excretory ducts that open onto the urethra (Dorfman and Barsanti, 1995).

Normal Cytology

The number and type of prostatic cells in cytologic samples from the prostate vary depending on the collection technique. Prostatic epithelial cells obtained via aspiration from normal dogs occur in frequent clusters and are cuboidal to columnar. These cells are uniform in size and shape and contain round to oval nuclei, which may be basilar in columnar cells. Nucleoli are usually small and inconspicuous. The cytoplasm is finely granular and basophilic (Thrall and Olson, 1985). Other cell types that may be seen, particularly from semen samples or prostatic massages, include spermatozoa, squamous epithelial cells, and transitional epithelial cells (urothelial cells) (Zinkl, 1999). Spermatozoa stain blue-green with Romanowsky and modified Romanowsky stains and may adhere to other cells. Squamous cells are large with abun-

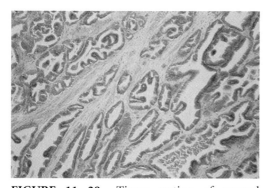

FIGURE 11–28. Tissue section of normal prostate gland. The tubuloalveolar glands are surrounded by a fibromuscular stroma. Primary and secondary enfoldings of epithelium project into the alveolar lumen. Canine. (H & E; ×25.) (Case material supplied by Roger Reep and Don Samuelson, University of Florida.)

dant amounts of blue to blue-green (keratinized) cytoplasm. The nuclei of these cells may be round to pyknotic or absent. Cell borders are typically angular to folded. Transitional cells (urothelial cells) are larger than prostatic epithelial cells and have lighter-staining cytoplasm with a lower nuclear-to-cytoplasmic ratio (Thrall and Olson, 1985; Zinkl, 1999). Normal ejaculate fluid may contain low numbers of neutrophils and red blood cells (Barsanti et al., 1980). Use of excessive amounts of ultrasound gel during ultrasound-guided FNA can result in large amounts of purple, variably sized granular background debris that may obscure cellular detail (Zinkl, 1999). To prevent this artifact, excess gel should be removed prior to inserting the aspiration needle.

Prostatic Cysts

Prostatic cysts may occur as multiple, small cysts associated with benign hyperplasia, large prostatic retention and paraprostatic cysts, and cysts associated squamous metaplasia. Except for hyperplasia-associated cysts, prostatic cysts account for only 2% to 5% of prostatic abnormalities (Dorfman and Barsanti, 1995). Small cysts may be palpated per rectum as small, fluctuant areas in an asymmetrically enlarged prostate (Dorfman and Barsanti, 1995). Large, discrete cysts may be palpated in the caudal abdomen or in the perineal area. Unless the cyst(s) become secondarily infected, clinical signs are uncommon (Olson et al., 1987). A bloody urethral discharge, dysuria, and tenesmus may be present owing to increased prostatic size (Olson et al., 1987).

Aspiration of prostatic cysts typically yields variable amounts of serosanguinous to brown fluid (Baker and Lumsden, 1999b). Cytologic examination of the fluid usually reveals low numbers of normal-appearing epithelial cells with rare neutrophils and erythrocytes on a red to brown background (Thrall and Olson, 1985; Baker and Lumsden, 1999b).

Benign Prostatic Hyperplasia

Benign prostatic hyperplasia (BPH) is a common finding in older intact male dogs. In one study of 15 beagles, all dogs 6 years of age or older had evidence of prostatic hyperplasia (Lowseth et al., 1990). BPH is associated with increases in gland size and weight related to increases in interstitial tissue and gland lumens (Lowseth et al., 1990). Symmetrical cystic dilation of the glands results from increases in the interstitium and gland lumens (Lowseth et al., 1990). Development of BPH is hormonally dependent and requires the presence of functioning testes (Dorfman and Barsanti, 1995). Circulating levels of testosterone are often decreased in older male dogs; however, dihydrotestosterone concentrations are often increased in the hyperplastic tissue (Olson et al., 1987). Nuclear androgen receptor expression is increased in hyperplastic tissue of older beagles, suggesting an increased tissue sensitivity to circulating androgens (Olson et al., 1987). Additionally, estrogens appear to act synergistically with androgens in potentiating BPH and may also act directly on the prostate, resulting in stromal hypertrophy and squamous epithelial metaplasia (Olson et al., 1987). The treatment of choice for canine BPH is castration.

In men, the prostate is fixed anatomically such that enlargement causes urinary obstruction resulting in the most common presenting sign of dysuria (Lowseth et al., 1990). In dogs, the prostate gland is not fixed so that enlargement occurs in an outward direction resulting in constipation and tenesmus. Mild hemorrhagic urethral discharge can also be noted (Dorfman and Barsanti, 1995). However, clinical signs are

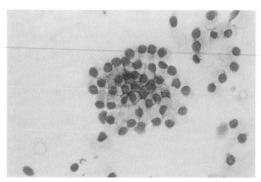

FIGURE 11–30. Normal-appearing prostatic epithelial cells from an aspirate of an enlarged prostate. The cells are uniform in size and shape and are arranged in clusters and individually. The cluster of cells in the center display a characteristic "honeycomb" appearance. These findings are consistent with benign prostatic hyperplasia. Canine. (Wright-Giemsa; ×125.)

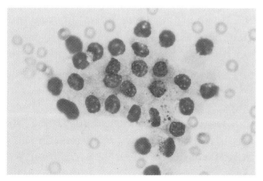

FIGURE 11–31. Aspirate from a dog with benign prostatic hyperplasia. The prostatic epithelial cells display round nuclei, slightly coarse nuclear chromatin, and moderate amounts of lightly basophilic cytoplasm. A few cells contain small amounts of basophilic secretory product. Canine. (Wright-Giemsa; ×250.)

often absent in canine BPH. Palpation of the prostate usually reveals a symmetrically enlarged, nonpainful gland; however, an irregular surface is occasionally felt (Dorfman and Barsanti, 1995).

Epithelial cells obtained from a hyperplastic prostate gland are generally arranged in variably sized sheets and clusters (Figs.

11–30 and 11–31). The cells are uniform in appearance with round nuclei and small round nucleoli. The nuclear-to-cytoplasmic ratio is low to moderate and the cytoplasm is basophilic. Mild increases in cell size and anisokaryosis may be noted (Baker and Lumsden, 1999). Cytologic samples yielding a normal-appearing population of prostatic epithelial cells from an enlarged prostate, particularly if the enlargement is symmetrical, is consistent with a diagnosis of benign hyperplasia.

Squamous Metaplasia

Increased circulating concentrations of estrogen can result in squamous metaplasia of the prostatic epithelium. During this process, the epithelial cells develop staining and morphologic characteristics of squamous epithelial cells. Estrogen receptors, which are present on ductal, stromal, and 10% of the prostatic epithelial cells, may mediate this responsiveness (Baker and Lumsden, 1999b). Although chronic irritation and inflammation can result in squamous metaplasia, the most common endogenous source of estrogen is Sertoli cell tumors (Baker and Lumsden, 1999b). The prostate may be small as a result of decreased concentrations of testosterone or enlarged if cysts or abscessation is present (Baker and Lumsden, 1999b). Clinical signs usually relate to hyperestrogenism. Treatment for squamous metaplasia is removal of the estrogen source.

Prostatic Inflammation

Inflammation may be seen in histopathologic samples from experimental animals with uncomplicated BPH without evidence of infectious organisms (Olson et al., 1987). However, infectious causes of prostatitis are more common and are implicated in 20% to 70% of dogs with prostatic disease

(Cowan and Barsanti, 1991). Ascending infection through the urethra is the usual route of infection, although hematogenous and local spread from other urogenital organs is possible (Dorfman and Barsanti, 1995). *Escherichia coli* is the most commonly isolated organism from both acute and chronic cases of prostatitis. Other organisms that may be cultured are *Proteus* sp., *Staphylococcus* sp., and *Streptococcus* sp. (Dorfman and Barsanti, 1995). Alteration of normal architecture by diseases such as BPH, squamous metaplasia, and neoplasia can interfere with normal defense mechanisms or provide a medium (i.e., blood in cysts) for bacterial growth (Olson et al., 1987). Coalescing of focal areas of septic prostatitis or infection of prostatic cysts may result in prostatic abscessation (Baker and Lumsden, 1999b).

Acute prostatitis is usually associated with systemic signs of illness (fever, anorexia, and lethargy) as well as urethral discharge and an enlarged, painful gland (Dorfman and Barsanti, 1995). The dog may also experience locomotor problems due to caudal lumbar or abdominal pain (Dorfman and Barsanti, 1995). An inflammatory leukogram with or without a left-shift is often present (Dorfman and Barsanti, 1995). In dogs with chronic prostatitis, the primary presenting problem is recurrent urinary tract infection (Dorfman and Barsanti, 1995). Intermittent or constant urethral discharge may also be noted. Prostatic abscesses may present with signs related to enlargement of the prostate (tenesmus, dysuria), constant or intermittent urethral discharge, and evidence of systemic illness related to endotoxemia or peritonitis (Dorfman and Barsanti, 1995). Treatment of prostatitis involves appropriate antibiotic therapy as determined by culture and sensitivity. In acute prostatitis, most antibiotics will reach the site of infection since the prostate–lipid barrier is disrupted (Olson

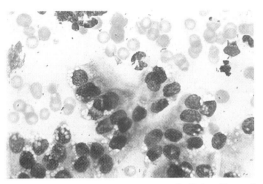

FIGURE 11–32. Prostatic epithelial cells and neutrophils are present in this aspirate from a dog with acute septic prostatitis. The neutrophils are degenerate as indicated by moderate karyolysis. Bacteria are present in the background and within the neutrophils. Canine. (Wright-Giemsa; ×250.)

et al., 1987). Antibiotics for treatment of chronic prostatitis should be selected for the ability to cross the lipid barrier, which is usually intact, and for the ability to concentrate in the prostate (Olson et al., 1987). In addition to appropriate antibiotic therapy, prostatic abscesses can be treated surgically with marsupialization of the gland, placement of a drain, or prostatectomy. All of these surgical procedures are associated with significant complications (Dorfman and Barsanti, 1995). Castration should also be performed in dogs with prostatitis (Dorfman and Barsanti, 1995).

Cytologic evaluation of samples from bacterial prostatitis contain large numbers of neutrophils, many of which exhibit degenerative changes of karyolysis and karyorrhexis (Fig. 11–32). Macrophages may also be present, especially in chronic prostatitis (Fig. 11–33). In the absence of previous antibiotic therapy, intracellular and extracellular organisms may be seen. Epithelial cells that are present may appear normal or hyperplastic as evidenced by increased cytoplasmic basophilia, increased nuclear-to-cytoplasmic ratios, and mild anisokaryosis.

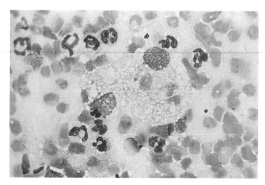

FIGURE 11–33. Prostatic aspirate from a dog with chronic prostatitis. Increased numbers of neutrophils, the majority of which are nondegenerate, and two reactive macrophages are present. Infectious organisms were not seen in this sample. Canine. (Wright-Giemsa; ×250.)

Cellular atypia associated with prostatic epithelial cells in the presence of inflammation should be interpreted cautiously to avoid a false-positive diagnosis of neoplasia (Thrall and Olson, 1984).

Prostatic Neoplasia

Prostatic carcinoma in the dog is rare, with reported prevalences of 0.2% and 0.6% (Bell et al., 1991). The disease most frequently occurs in dogs 8 to 10 years of age, and both intact and neutered dogs are at risk for developing prostatic carcinoma (Dorfman and Barsanti, 1995; Bell et al., 1991). The disease carries a poor prognosis in dogs; survival time in treated and untreated dogs is usually less than 2 months (Bell et al., 1991). In one study, metastases were present at necropsy in 89% of dogs with prostatic carcinoma (Bell et al., 1991). The primary site for metastasis of prostatic carcinoma is the iliac lymph nodes followed by lungs, urinary bladder, mesentery, and bone (Dorfman and Barsanti, 1995). Bone metastases are most often located in the pelvis, lumbar vertebrae, and femur and can be lytic or proliferative (Dorfman and Bar-

santi, 1995). Canine prostatic carcinoma is an insidious disease, with many dogs showing no evidence of clinical abnormalities until late in the course of the malignancy. In one study, owners most commonly reported the presence of tenesmus, dyschezia, anorexia, and weight loss (Bell et al., 1991). The most frequently detected abnormality during physical examination was prostatomegaly, which was identified in 52% of the dogs with carcinoma (Bell et al., 1991). The enlargement was primarily asymmetrical (32%), however, some symmetrical enlargement (6%) was noted. Other physical abnormalities included depression, painful abdominal palpation, cachexia, pyrexia, dyspnea, and presence of an abdominal mass (Bell et al., 1991). Therapy for prostatic carcinoma is usually palliative and may include prostatectomy or intraoperative radiation (Dorfman and Barsanti, 1995).

Adenocarcinoma is the most commonly reported neoplasm of the prostate followed by transitional cell carcinoma arising from the prostatic urethra (Dorfman and Barsanti, 1995). These two neoplasms can be difficult to distinguish cytologically, and histopathology may be required for definitive diagnosis (Baker and Lumsden, 1999b). FNA is most useful for diagnosis of prostatic neoplasia. Cytologic evaluation of FNA samples from prostatic adenocarcinoma usually reveals large numbers of deeply basophilic epithelial cells arranged in variably sized clusters and sheets (Figs. 11–34 and 11–35). The nuclear-to-cytoplasmic ratio is often high and anisokaryosis and anisocytosis can be moderate to marked. Nuclei are round to pleomorphic and nucleoli are large, prominent, and often multiple. Binucleation may be noted. Some acinar structures may be noted which can help to differentiate the neoplasm from transitional cell carcinoma (Zinkl, 1999). Bell et al. (1991) reported that a diagnosis of neoplasia was established in 15 of 19 (79%) of

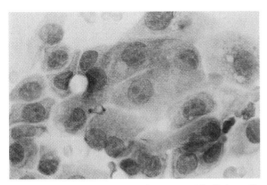

FIGURE 11–34. Neoplastic epithelial cells from a prostatic carcinoma. The cells display prominent, large, multiple nucleoli, coarse nuclear chromatin, moderate anisokaryosis and anisocytosis, variable nuclear-to-cytoplasmic ratios, and binucleation. Canine. (Wright-Giemsa; ×250.)

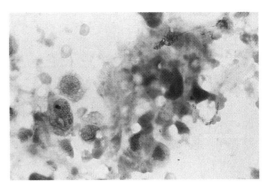

FIGURE 11–35. Amorphous basophilic material from the carcinoma shown in Figure 11–34. This material is compatible with necrosis, which can be found in aspirates of malignant tumors. Canine. (Wright-Giemsa; ×250.)

samples submitted for cytologic analysis from dogs with histologically confirmed prostatic carcinoma. False-negative cytology results could have been related to small sample size, focal distribution of neoplastic lesions, or concurrent prostatitis and/or BPH (Bell et al., 1991).

Testes

Unilateral or bilateral testicular enlargement is the primary indication for fine-needle aspiration (FNA) and cytologic evaluation of the testes (Zinkl, 1999). Cytology is useful for differentiation between inflammatory or neoplastic conditions that cause testicular enlargement (DeNicola et al., 1980). Testicular FNA has also been shown to be useful for evaluation of male infertility (Dahlbom et al., 1997). Testicular FNA is usually not associated with immediate or long-term adverse effects (Dahlbom et al., 1997).

Special Collection Techniques

Routine FNA with a 22-gauge needle and 12-cc syringe is used for cytologic sampling of the testes. Because of the increased fragility of testicular cells, great care should be taken when preparing the slide of aspirated material. The material should be very lightly smeared when preparing the cell monolayer. Alternatively, gentle touch imprints from available tissue may decrease cellular disruption (Baker and Lumsden, 1999b). Imprints of testicular biopsies should be made rapidly after removal of the tissue to prevent degeneration of the cells (Baker and Lumsden, 1999b).

Normal Anatomy and Histology

The testes are the site of spermatogenesis in the adult animal and exhibit both exocrine and endocrine function (Banks, 1986c). The exocrine portion of the testes is a compound, coiled tubular gland that produces spermatozoa as its secretory product. The germinal epithelium is actively involved in spermatogenesis. The endocrine portions of the testes are composed of the interstitial (Leydig) cells, which secrete testosterone, and Sertoli (sustentacular) cells, which provide support for the developing sperm (Banks, 1986c) (Figs. 11–36 and 11–37).

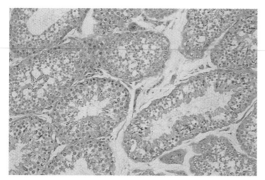

FIGURE 11–36. Multiple seminiferous tubules are present in this tissue section of a normal testis. The tubules are surrounded by connective tissue containing low numbers of interstitial cells. Canine. (H & E; ×50.)

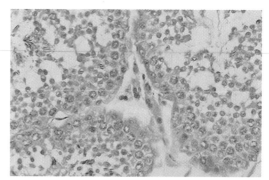

FIGURE 11–37. Higher magnification of the seminiferous tubules in normal canine testis. Interstitial cells are seen in the center of the photomicrograph. Spermatocytes as well as early and late spermatids are seen within the tubules. Spermatocytes are characterized by round nuclei and coarse nuclear chromatin. During the maturation process, developing sperm move from the periphery of the tubule to the central lumen. Low numbers of Sertoli cells with smooth nuclear chromatin and single, prominent nucleoli are seen at the periphery of the tubules. (H & E; ×125.)

Normal Cytology

Normal testicular imprints are highly cellular with a predominance of ruptured cells and streaming nuclear material (Baker and Lumsden, 1999b). When cells rupture, the nuclear chromatin becomes coarse and nucleoli are prominent. Testicular cells are generally round, with coarse nuclear chromatin, a single large, prominent nucleoli, and moderate amounts of basophilic cytoplasm. Mitotic activity is often high (Baker and Lumsden, 1999b). More mature stages of developing sperm are characterized by oval, eosinophilic to pale-staining nuclei, and tails may be noted.

Testicular Inflammation

Inflammatory disease of the testes (orchitis) or epididymis can be due to infection with *Brucella canis, Pseudomonas* sp., *E. coli,* or *Proteus* sp. (Ladds, 1993). Intranuclear or intracytoplasmic inclusions may be seen in cases of distemper-associated orchitis (Ladds, 1993). Orchitis may also be associated with infection by the dimorphic yeast, *Blastomyces dermatitidis* (DeNicola et al., 1980).

Acute orchitis is characterized by a predominance of neutrophils, some of which may exhibit nuclear degenerative changes. Macrophages, including multinucleated giant cells, and lymphocytes may be seen in chronic inflammatory disease or fungal (blastomycosis) infections. Since the infectious organisms are usually not observed cytologically, culture should be performed to identify the pathogens (Baker and Lumsden, 1999b).

Testicular Neoplasia

Seminoma

Seminomas arise from neoplastic transformation of the testicular germ cells. These tumors are fairly common in dogs, but are extremely rare in cats (Nielson and Kennedy, 1990). Seminomas may appear in association with other testicular tumors. For example, in one study, 31% of testes with a seminoma had either an interstitial cell tumor or a Sertoli cell tumor also present (Nielson and Kennedy, 1990). The mean age for development of seminoma is 10 years (Nielson and Kennedy, 1990). Cryptorchidism is a predisposing factor for development of seminomas (Nielson and Kennedy, 1990). Other than testicular enlargement, which may not be readily apparent if the tumor is involving a cryptorchid testicle, clinical symptoms related to seminomas are rare. The presence of a concurrent estrogen-secreting Sertoli cell tumor may be responsible for feminization and hemogram abnormalities (Nielson and Kennedy, 1990). Six to 11% of canine seminomas metastasize, with primary metastatic sites including the inguinal, iliac, and sublumbar lymph nodes and the lungs or abdominal organs (Nielson and Kennedy, 1990).

Cytologic differentiation of seminomas from other testicular tumors may be difficult. Cytologic preparations from seminoma

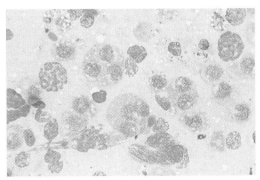

FIGURE 11–39. Several multinucleated cells are seen in this aspirate of a seminoma. Note the large number of lysed cells and free nuclei in the background. The tendency of testicular cells to rupture can make cytological evaluation difficult. Canine. (Wright-Giemsa; ×250.)

mas often contain large numbers of lysed cells and free nuclei. In general, tumor cells from a seminoma occur individually or in small clusters. These cells are large, round with one, two, or occasionally multiple nuclei and large prominent nucleoli (Fig. 11–38). Moderate anisokaryosis, anisocytosis, and binucleation and multinucleation may be present (Fig. 11–39). The cytoplasm is lightly to moderately basophilic with a moderate to high nuclear-to-cytoplasmic ratio. Mitotic activity is often high.

Sertoli Cell Tumor

Sertoli cell tumors are fairly common in the dog, particularly in retained testicles (Nielson, 1990). As with the other testicular neoplasms, Sertoli cell tumors are extremely rare in cats (Nielson and Kennedy, 1990). Most dogs with Sertoli cell tumors are greater than 6 years of age, although tumors in dogs as young as 3 years of age have been reported (Nielson and Kennedy, 1990). About one third of canine Sertoli cell tumors are associated with excess produc-

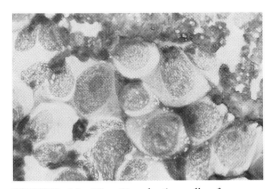

FIGURE 11–38. Neoplastic cells from an aspirate of a seminoma. The cells are large and have round nuclei, coarse nuclear chromatin, and prominent, large nucleoli. The cytoplasm is lightly basophilic and some cells contain small numbers of punctate cytoplasmic vacuoles. Canine. (Wright-Giemsa; ×250.)

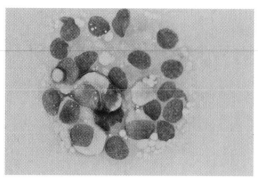

FIGURE 11–40. Aspirate of a Sertoli cell tumor from a dog presenting with infertility, dermatitis with hyperpigmentation, and a testicular mass. The tumor cells have round to oval nuclei, slightly coarse nuclear chromatin, and moderate nuclear-to-cytoplasmic ratios. The nucleoli are small and variably prominent. The cytoplasm is lightly basophilic and cell borders are often indistinct. Canine. (Wright-Giemsa; ×250.)

tion of estrogen. High levels of estrogens produced by the tumor cells can be associated with clinical signs of feminization and/or bone marrow suppression (Baker and Lumsden, 1999b). Metastasis occurs in 10% to 14% of Sertoli cell tumors. Sites of metastasis are similar to those for seminomas (Nielson and Kennedy, 1990).

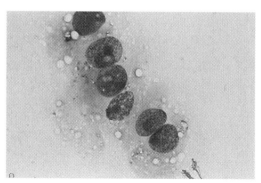

FIGURE 11–41. A row of tumor cells from the Sertoli cell tumor shown in Figure 11–40. Variably sized cytoplasmic vacuoles are seen in several of the cells. Canine. (Wright–Giemsa; ×250.)

Cytologically, variable numbers of round to elongated, pleomorphic cells characterize Sertoli cell tumors. These cells may occur individually or in small clusters. Nuclei are generally round with fine nuclear chromatin and one to three prominent, large nucleoli (DeNicola et al., 1980) (Fig. 11–40). The lightly basophilic cytoplasm may vary from scant to abundant in amount and some cytoplasmic granulation may be present (DeNicola et al., 1980). The presence of small to moderately sized cytoplasmic vacuoles is typical (Fig. 11–41).

Interstitial Cell Tumors

Interstitial cell tumors are very common in the dog and extremely rare in the cat (Nielson and Kennedy, 1990). However, only 16% of these tumors are associated with testicular enlargement, therefore they are infrequently aspirated for cytologic analysis (Nielson and Kennedy, 1990; Baker and Lumsden, 1999). Clinical signs associated with interstitial cell tumors are uncommon. Cytologic samples from interstitial cell tu-

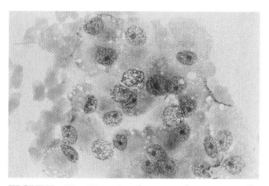

FIGURE 11–42. A cluster of tumor cells from an interstitial cell tumor. The cells display coarse nuclear chromatin, prominent, single nucleoli, and large amounts of moderately basophilic cytoplasm. The nuclei are often located at the periphery of the cell. Punctate cytoplasmic vacuoles are present in the majority of the cells. Canine. (Wright-Giemsa; ×250.)

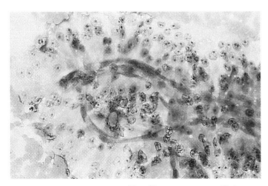

FIGURE 11–43. Palisading arrays of interstitial cells surrounding a central capillary are seen in this aspirate of an interstitial cell tumor. Canine. (Wright-Giemsa; ×125.)

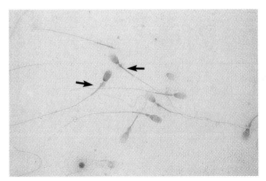

FIGURE 11–44. Noninflammatory semen sample from a dog with infertility. Sperm have prominent proximal protoplasmic droplets (*arrows*). Canine. (Wright; ×250.)

mors are of variable cellularity. The cells vary in size, but usually contain abundant amounts of lightly to moderately basophilic cytoplasm. The nuclei are round and exhibit criteria of malignancy including moderate to marked anisokaryosis, one to multiple prominent nucleoli, fine to clumped chromatin patterns, and variable nuclear-to-cytoplasmic ratios. The cytoplasmic margins are often indistinct and variable numbers of small, uniform cytoplasmic vacuoles are common (DeNicola et al., 1980) (Fig. 11–42). Clusters of cells may be arranged in a palisading array around a central, endothelial-lined capillary space (DeNicola et al., 1980) (Fig. 11–43). Dark, irregularly shaped cytoplasmic granules may be present in some cells (DeNicola et al., 1980; Zinkl, 1999).

Semen Abnormalities

A detailed discussion of semen analysis is not covered in this text and may be found elsewhere (Johnson, 1999). However, the cytologist is occasionally presented with seminal material from dogs with infertility or suspected testicular disease, thus the ability to recognize certain abnormalities is useful. Romanowsky-type or modified Roma-

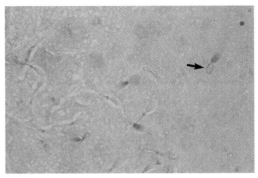

FIGURE 11–45. Noninflammatory semen sample from a dog with infertility. Against a heavy proteinaceous background, several sperm display coiled tails (*arrow*) and proximal protoplasmic droplets. Canine. (Wright; ×250.)

nowsky stains are often used but sperm morphology may be better viewed using India ink or new methylene blue stains. In high-quality semen, nearly all of the sperm should be of similar morphology. Dogs with good fertility usually do not have more than 20% to 25% abnormal sperm (Johnson, 1999). Abnormalities may relate primarily to defective spermatogenesis or secondarily to defective maturation in the epididymis or during sample handling. Severe abnormalities include abnormal size or shape of the sperm head or acrosomal cap, proximal or midpiece protoplasmic droplets, and coiled tails (Figs. 11–44 to

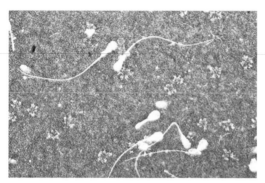

FIGURE 11–46. Noninflammatory semen sample from a dog with infertility. Sperm abnormalities include proximal protoplasmic droplets, coiled tails, and bent tails. Canine. (India ink; ×250.) (Photo courtesy of Rose Raskin, Gainesville, FL.)

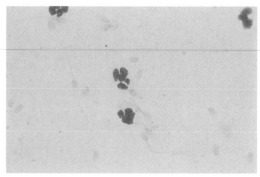

FIGURE 11–47. An ejaculate sample from a dog with intermittent preputial bleeding. Mildly degenerate neutrophils are present. Several morphological abnormalities of the sperm (detached heads, bent tails, and coiled tails) are present. Canine. (Wright-Giemsa; ×250.)

11–46). Less severe abnormalities include detached normal-appearing heads and bent tails (Figs. 11–46 and 11–47). Semen should also be evaluated for evidence of inflammation as indicated by the presence of neutrophils and/or macrophages (Figs. 11–47 and 11–48). If neutrophils exhibit degenerative changes, a search for infectious organisms should be performed. However, culture of the fluid may be necessary for identification of pathogens. Lower urinary tract inflammation and/or prostatitis should also be considered when inflammatory cells are present in semen. Abnormalities in sperm morphology may be observed in conjunction with the inflammatory cells. The presence of abnormal prostatic epithelium in the semen sample warrants further evaluation of the prostate gland (Zinkl, 1999).

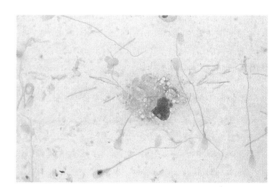

FIGURE 11–48. A reactive macrophage and several relatively normal appearing sperm from the same ejaculate demonstrated in Figure 11–47. Canine. (Wright-Giemsa; ×250.)

References

Allen SW, Prasse KW, Mahaffey EA: Cytologic differentiation of benign from malignant canine mammary tumors. Vet Pathol 1986; 23:649–655.

Baker R, Lumsden JH: The mammary gland. *In* Baker RH, Lumsden JH (eds): *Color Atlas of Cytology of the Dog and Cat.* CV Mosby, St. Louis, 1999a, pp 253–262.

Baker R, Lumsden JH: Reproductive tract. *In* Baker RH, Lumsden JH (eds): *Color Atlas of Cytology of the Dog and Cat.* CV Mosby, St. Louis, 1999b, pp 235–251.

Banks WJ: Integumentary system. *In* Banks, WJ (ed): *Applied Veterinary Histology.* Williams & Wilkins, Baltimore, 1986a, pp 348–378.

Banks WJ: Female reproductive system. *In* Banks,

WJ (ed): *Applied Veterinary Histology.* Williams & Wilkins, Baltimore, 1986b, pp 506–523.

Banks WJ: Male reproductive system. *In* Banks, WJ (ed): *Applied Veterinary Histology.* Williams & Wilkins, Baltimore, 1986c, pp 489–504.

Barsanti JA, Prasse KW, Crowell WA, et al: Evaluation of various techniques for diagnosis of chronic bacterial prostatitis in the dog. J Am Vet Med Assoc 1983; 183:219–224.

Barsanti JA, Shotts EB, Prasse KW, et al: Evaluation of diagnostic techniques for canine prostatic diseases. J Am Vet Med Assoc 1980; 177: 160–163.

Bell FW, Klausner JS, Hayden DW, et al: Clinical and pathologic features of prostatic adenocarcinoma in sexually intact and castrated dogs: 31 cases (1970–1987). J Am Vet Med Assoc 1991; 199:1623–1630.

Benjamin SA, Lee AC, Saunders WJ: Classification and behavior of canine mammary epithelial neoplasms based on life-span observations in beagles. Vet Pathol 1999; 36:423–436.

Brodey RS, Goldschmidt MH, Roszel JR: Canine mammary gland neoplasms. J Am Anim Hosp Assoc 1983; 19:61–90.

Cowan LA, Barsanti JA: Prostatic disease. *In Small Animal Medicine.* JB Lippincott, Philadelphia, 1991, pp 780–791.

Dahlbom M, Makinen A, Suominen J: Testicular fine needle aspiration cytology as a diagnostic tool on dog infertility. J Small Anim Pract 1997; 38:506–512.

DeNicola DB, Rebar AH, Boon GD: Cytology of the canine male urogenital tract. Ralston Purina, St. Louis, 1980.

Donnay I, Rauis J, Devleeschouwer N, et al: Comparison of estrogen and progesterone receptor expression in normal and tumor mammary tissues from dogs. Am J Vet Res 1995; 9:1188–1193.

Dorfman M, Barsanti J: Diseases of the canine prostate gland. Comp Cont Ed Pract 1995; 17: 791–810.

Dorn CR, Taylor DON, Schneider R, et al: Survey of animal neoplasms in Alameda and Contra Costa counties, California. II. Cancer morbidity in dogs and cats from Alameda county. J Ntl Cancer Inst 1968; 40:307–318.

Fernandes PJ, Guyer C, Modiano JF: What is your diagnosis? Mammary mass aspirate from a Yorkshire terrier. Vet Clin Pathol 1998; 27: 79, 91.

Freshman JL: Clinical approach to infertility in the cycling bitch. Vet Clin North Am Small Anim Pract 1991; 21:427–435.

Gilbert RO: Diagnosis and treatment of pyometra in bitches and queens. Compend Contin Educ Pract 1992; 14:779–784.

Gruffydd-Jones TJ: Acute mastitis in a cat. Feline Pract 1980; 10:41–42.

Hahn KA, Richardson RC, Knapp DW: Canine malignant mammary neoplasia: biological behavior, diagnosis, and treatment alternatives. J Am Anim Hosp Assoc 1992; 28:251–256.

Hayden DW, Barnes DM, Johnson KH: Morphologic changes in the mammary gland of megestrol acetate-treated and untreated cats: a retrospective study. Vet Pathol 1989; 26:104–113.

Hayden DW, Johnston SD, Kiang DT, et al: Feline mammary hypertrophy/fibroadenoma complex: clinical and hormonal aspects. Am J Vet Res 1981; 42:1699–1703.

Hayes AA, Mooney S: Feline mammary tumors. Vet Clin North Am Small Anim Pract 1985; 15: 513–520.

Hayes HM, Milne KL, Mandell CP: Epidemiological features of feline mammary carcinoma. Vet Rec 1981; 108:476–479.

Hellman E, Lindgren A: The accuracy of cytology in diagnosis and DNA analysis of canine mammary tumors. J Comp Pathol 1989; 101:443–450.

Holst PA, Phemister RD: Temporal sequence of events in the estrous cycle of the bitch. Am J Vet Res 1974; 36:705–706.

Inaba T, Takahashi N, Matsuda H, et al: Estrogen and progesterone receptors and progesterone metabolism in canine mammary tumours. Jpn J Vet Sci 1984; 46:797–803.

Johnson CA: Reproductive disorders. *In* Willard MD, Tvedten H, Turnwald GH (eds): *Small Animal Clinical Diagnosis by Laboratory Methods,* 3rd ed. WB Saunders, Philadelphia, 1999, pp 270–278.

Ladds PW: The male genital system: the testes. *In* Jubb KVF, Kennedy PC, Palmer N (eds): *Pathology of Domestic Animals,* 4th ed. Academic Press, San Diego, 1993, pp 485–512.

Lowseth LA, Gerlach RF, Gillett NA, et al: Age-related changes in the prostate and testes of the beagle dog. Vet Pathol 1990; 27:347–353.

MacEwen EG, Hayes AA, Harvey J, et al: Prognostic factors for feline mammary tumors. J Am Vet Med Assoc 1984; 185:201–204.

MacEwen EG, Withrow SJ: Tumors of the mammary gland. *In* Withrow SJ, MacEwen EG (eds): *Small Animal Clinical Oncology,* 2nd ed. WB Saunders, Philadelphia, 1996, pp 356–372.

MacVean DW, Monlux AW, Anderson PS, et al: Frequency of canine and feline tumors in a defined population. Vet Pathol 1978; 15:700–715.

Mesher CI: What is your diagnosis? A 14-month old domestic cat. Vet Clin Pathol 1997; 26:4, 13

Mills JM, Valli VE, Lumsden JH: Cyclical changes of vaginal cytology in the cat. Can Vet J 1979; 20:95–101.

Misdorp W: Progestagens and mammary tumours in dogs and cats. Acta Endocrinol (Copenh) 1991; 125:27–31.

Morris JS, Dobson JM, Bostock DE: Use of tamoxifen in the control of canine mammary neoplasia. Vet Rec 1993; 27:539–542.

Moulton JE: Tumors of the mammary gland. *In* Moulton JE (ed): *Tumors in Domestic Animals,* 3rd ed. University of California Press, Berkeley, 1990, pp 518–522.

Nielsen SW, Kennedy PC: Tumors of the genital systems. *In* Moulton JE (ed): *Tumors in Domestic Animals,* 3rd ed. University of California Press, Berkeley, 1990, pp 479–513.

Olson PN, Thrall MA, Wykes PM, et al: Vaginal cytology: Part I. A useful tool for staging the canine estrous cycle. Compend Contin Educ Pract 1984a; 6:288–297.

Olson PN, Thrall MA, Wykes PM, et al: Vaginal cytology. Part II. Its use in diagnosing canine reproductive disorders. Compend Contin Educ Pract 1984b; 6:385–390.

Olson PN, Wrigley RH, Thrall MA, et al: Disorders of the canine prostate gland: pathogenesis, diagnosis, and medical therapy. Compend Contin Educ Pract 1987; 9:613–623.

Patnaik AK, Liu SK, Hurvitz AI, et al: Nonhematopoietic neoplasms in cats. J Natl Cancer Inst 1975; 54:855–860.

Priester WA, Mamel N: Occurrence of tumors of domestic animals. Data from 12 United States and Canadian colleges of veterinary medicine. J Natl Cancer Inst 1971; 47:1333–1344.

Rogers KA: Transmissible venereal tumor. Compend Contin Educ Pract 1997; 19:1036–1044.

Roudebush P, Wheeler KG: Peracute gangrenous mastitis in a cat. Feline Pract 1979; 9:35–38.

Rutteman GR, Blakenstein MA, Minke J, et al: Steroid receptors in mammary tumours of the cat. Acta Endocrinol (Copenh) 1991; 125:32–37.

Rutteman GR, Misdorp W, Blakenstein MA, et al: Oestrogen (ER) and progestin receptors (PR) in mammary tissue of the female dog: different receptor profile in non-malignant and malignant states. Br J Cancer 1988; 58:594–599.

Shille VM, Lundstrom KE, Stabenfeldt GH: Follicular function in the domestic cat as determined by estradiol-17β concentrations in plasma: relation to estrous behavior and cornification of exfoliated vaginal epithelium. Biol Reprod 1979; 21:953–963.

Shull RM, Maddux JM: Subcutaneous glandular tissue: mammary, salivary, thyroid, and parathyroid. *In* Cowell RL, Tyler RD, Meinkoth JM (eds): *Diagnostic Cytology and Hematology of the Dog and Cat.* CV Mosby, St. Louis, 1999, pp 90–92.

Stone EA: The uterus. *In* Slatter DH (ed): *Textbook of Small Animal Surgery.* WB Saunders, Philadelphia, 1985, pp 1661–1665.

Thrall MA, Olson PN: The vagina. *In* Cowell RL, Tyler RD, Meinkoth JM (eds): *Diagnostic Cytology and Hematology of the Dog and Cat.* CV Mosby, St. Louis, 1999, pp 240–248.

Thrall MA, Olson PN, Freemyer EG: Cytologic diagnosis of canine prostatic disease. J Am Anim Hosp Assoc 1985; 21:95–102.

Van Garderen E, de Wit M, Voorhout WF, et al: Expression of growth hormone in canine mammary tissue and mammary tumors; evidence for a potential autocrine/paracrine stimulatory loop. Am J Pathol 1997; 150:1037–1047.

Wright PJ: Application of vaginal cytology and plasma progesterone determinations to the management of reproduction in the bitch. J Small Anim Pract 1990; 31:335–340.

Yager JA, Scott DW, Wilcock BP: The skin and appendages: neoplastic disease of skin and mammary gland. *In* Jubb KVF, Kennedy PC, Palmer N (eds): *Pathology of Domestic Animals,* 4th ed. Academic Press, San Diego, 1993, pp 706–737.

Zinkl JG: Cytology of the male reproductive tract. *In* Cowell RL, Tyler RD, Meinkoth JM (eds): *Diagnostic Cytology and Hematology of the Dog and Cat.* CV Mosby, St. Louis, 1999, pp 230–239.

CHAPTER 12

Musculoskeletal System

David J. Fisher

Lameness is the cardinal clinical sign associated with disease of the musculoskeletal system. Other signs include stiffness, weakness, pain, fever, limb and joint swelling, and deformity. Depending on the type of disorder, other organ systems may also be involved, including neurologic, endocrine, urologic, hemolymphatic, digestive, respiratory, and cardiovascular systems. Because of this, an animal with musculoskeletal disease may present with a variety of problems and signs.

Cytology may be a component of the work-up in an animal with a suspected musculoskeletal disorder. Material that may be sampled include synovial fluid as well as fine-needle aspirates of soft tissue masses involving muscle or proliferative/lytic lesions of the bone. Cytologic evaluation alone is rarely the sole diagnostic test necessary to completely define a musculoskeletal problem. Other important information includes signalment, history, physical examination, radiographs, complete blood count, and biochemistry. In addition, many lesions will require histopathology for definitive

characterization. Some types of muscle, bone, and joint disease cause changes that cannot be detected by cytologic methods.

JOINT DISEASE

Synovial fluid analysis is part of the minimum database when assessing an animal for joint disease. It is important to recognize that evaluation of the synovial fluid is only a component of the work-up of an animal with suspected joint disease. The data obtained from joint fluid analysis must be integrated with other clinical and laboratory findings, including appropriate ancillary diagnostic tests (culture, serology, antinuclear antibody (ANA) titer, rheumatoid factor (RF) titer). Nevertheless, when an animal has suspected joint disease, fluid evaluation is a critical component in determining the cause of disease.

As with other body cavity effusions, a complete fluid analysis is helpful when evaluating a synovial effusion. Routine synovial

TABLE 12–1.   Classification of Synovial Fluid

	Normal	Hemarthrosis	Degenerative Arthropathy	Inflammatory Arthropathy
Appearance	Clear to straw-colored	Red, cloudy, or xanthochromic	Clear	Cloudy
Protein	<2.5 g/dl	Increased	Normal to decreased	Normal to increased
Viscosity	High	Decreased	Normal to decreased	Normal to decreased
Mucin clot	Good	Normal to poor	Normal to poor	Fair to poor
Cell count (/μl)	<3000	Increased RBCs	1000 to 10,000	5000 to >100,000
PMN	<5%	Relative to blood	<10%	>10 to 100%
Mononuclear	>95%	Relative to blood	>90%	10 to <90%
Comments	Only a small amount should be present (<0.5 ml in most joints).	Erythrophagia helps confirm previous hemorrhage.	Cells are typically macrophages or found in thick sheets (synoviocytes).	Septic and nonseptic etiologies. Bacteria are rarely observed in infected joints.

fluid analysis should include evaluation of color, transparency, protein concentration, viscosity, mucin clot test, nucleated cell count, differential, and cytologic evaluation. These tests are discussed in further detail below. If the sample is limited, the most important component of analysis is the cytology. Typical results for different kinds of joint disease are shown in Table 12–1.

Sample Collection and Handling

Collection of synovial fluid varies to some degree depending on the joint sampled. Descriptions of approaches to various joints have been described. In general, collection of synovial fluid requires the following materials: 3- to 6-ml syringe, 20- to 22-gauge 1-inch needles (25-gauge in very small joints), and red-top and/or lavender-top tubes. The amount of restraint and necessary levels of sedation and anesthesia will vary from animal to animal. Enough restraint should be used to minimize struggling during collection. In general, many animals will require at least some degree of sedation or anesthesia. The site should be prepared using routine aseptic technique. Palpation and slight flexion of the joint will help to identify insertion points of the needle. The needle should be advanced slowly through the joint capsule into the joint cavity. The amount of fluid withdrawn is dependent on the size of animal and joint as well as the amount of effusion present. Synovial fluid will be aspirated easily if there is a significant effusion but a few drops may be obtained from joints without an increase in synovial fluid volume. Care should be taken to note the color of the fluid as aspirated. If at some point blood is seen to enter in a trailing wisp, contamination rather than true hemorrhage is implied. Prior to removing the needle from the synovial cavity, the plunger of the syringe should be released to remove any negative pressure effect. Normal synovial fluid has a gel-like consistency that should not be mistaken for a clot. The gel-like consistency will become less viscous when shaken and return to the original viscosity upon standing; this property is referred to as *thixotropy*. Clotting is likely to occur if there is significant blood contamination and inflamed joints may form fibrin precipitates or clots. For these reasons, some joint fluid should be put into an EDTA tube (lavender-top tube). The EDTA will interfere with tests such as the mucin clot test and culturing. The synovial fluid should be refrigerated if not immediately evaluated. For samples that may be cultured dependent on the cytologic findings, the fluid should be put into a red-top tube, left in the sterile syringe, and/or placed in an aerobic culturette. There are advocates of putting fluid in blood culture media to improve the chances for bacterial growth. The laboratory should be contacted for their recommendations. In many smaller-sized animals, only one or two drops of joint fluid can be obtained. In these cases, immediate preparation of direct smears is the critical component of sample management (refer to Chapter 1). Regardless of the amount of fluid collected, it usually is advantageous to make direct smears immediately to best preserve cell morphology. These slides should not be refrigerated prior to staining.

Appearance and Viscosity

Normal joint fluid is typically present in small amounts (<0.5 ml) and is clear to straw-colored (Fig. 12–1). The fluid should be viscous as evident by a stringiness when suspended between fingertips or expelled from the syringe. The fluid viscosity is related to the concentration and quality of

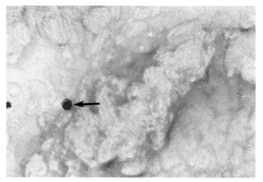

FIGURE 12–1. Normal synovial fluid has low nucleated cell numbers with a thick granular to ropy background material separating the cells. The granular background is related to the mucin content of the fluid. The low cellularity generally means that fewer than 1 to 3 small to medium-sized mononuclear cells are cells seen on high-power examination (*arrow*). (Wright; ×125.)

hyaluronic acid. Normal synovial fluid has good viscosity and demonstrates thixotropy (see above).

Cell Counts and Differential

Cell counts and the differential are done by routine methods. If enough fluid is present, cell counts can be made using a hemocytometer. Some reference laboratories utilize automated cell counters for cell enumeration. The cells may occur in clumps and accurate assessment of cell numbers may be difficult. In an effort to minimize cell clumping, hyaluronidase can be added to the synovial fluid. Various methods have been described. The easiest procedure is to add a small amount of hyaluronidase powder (amount adherent to an applicator stick) directly into the sample tube, which may result in more accurate cell counts. If only slides are prepared, cell numbers can be roughly estimated by counting the number of cells per high-power field. Normal joints will have low nucleated cell numbers, typically less than $3000/\mu l$, although this may vary slightly based on breed, age, and joint sampled. Consequently, only 1 to 3 cells per high-power field will be observed depending on the thickness of the direct smear. Of these few nucleated cells, the majority are mononuclear. Neutrophils typically account for less than 5% to 10% of nucleated cells in normal joints.

Mucin Clot Test

The mucin clot test is done to semiquantitatively assess the amount and/or degree of polymerization of hyaluronic acid in the joint fluid. Since EDTA interferes with this test, heparin can be used if an anticoagulant is required prior to performing this test. One to two drops of undiluted joint fluid are added to four to eight drops of 2%

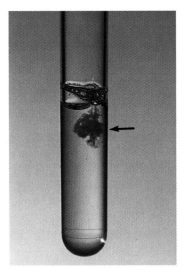

FIGURE 12–2. Mucin clot test. This sample is from a normal joint. The mucin clot is thick and ropy indicative of good mucin content and quality (*arrow*). (Courtesy of Dr. Sonjia Shelly.)

acetic acid. In a sample with normal hyaluronic acid concentration and quality, a thick ropy clot will form (Fig. 12–2). As the amount and/or quality of hyaluronic acid decreases in various forms of joint disease, the mucin clot is less well formed. This test is typically interpreted as good, fair, or poor. Normal joints have good mucin clot results.

Protein Concentration

Protein concentration is often measured by refractometry, which usually provides a value that is useful for routine clinical classification and interpretation of the synovial fluid. The most accurate measurement of protein requires chemical methods. Normal synovial fluid generally has a low protein concentration (<2.5 g/dl). Protein concentration will increase with inflammatory disease.

Classification of Joint Disease

The primary goal in synovial fluid evaluation is to distinguish inflammatory joint disease from degenerative joint disease. Other types of joint disease that may be distinguished include hemarthrosis and neoplastic disease. Further defining the disease process, as noted above, requires integrating the synovial fluid findings with other historical, physical, and laboratory findings. It is important to note that synovial fluid analysis alone rarely differentiates or identifies the specific cause from among the multiple etiologic factors involved in inflammatory and noninflammatory joint diseases.

Inflammatory Joint Disease

Inflammatory joint disease is characterized by finding increased numbers of neutrophils (Fig. 12–3) in the joint fluid. Absolute

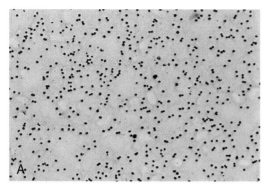

FIGURE 12–3. A, Inflamed joints have an absolute increase in the numbers of neutrophils and often exceed 50,000/μl, as in this specimen. The total cell number occasionally may be within normal limits (i.e., <3000/μl) in a septic joint but the neutrophil number will represent greater than 70% of the total cell number emphasizing the need for microscopic examination. (Wright; ×50.)

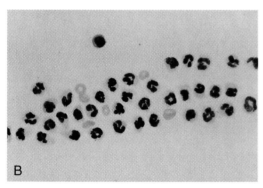

FIGURE 12–3. B, The cells in this figure are found in rows. This is referred to as "windrowing" and is commonly seen in fluids with increased viscosity or increased protein concentration. Inflamed joints may have decreased viscosity by gross visual examination, but prominent windrowing of cells microscopically. (Wright; ×250.)

numbers of segmented neutrophils are typically moderately to markedly increased. However, the inflammatory process appears to cytologically wax and wane with time and, if polyarticular, involve other joints with varying intensity. Consequently, repeating joint sampling and, more importantly, sampling multiple joints, even if not clinically affected, has diagnostic value. A key point is that inflammatory joint disease has both infectious and noninfectious causes.

Infectious Arthritis

Some cases of joint disease are caused by bacterial (Fig. 12–4) or fungal infection (Fig. 12–5). In general, septic joints have very high cell counts. In most cases, the cells are primarily segmented neutrophils. When neutrophil degeneration is observed (lack the nuclear integrity of clumped chromatin), the presence of bacteria is highly suspect. Most of the time, all or the great

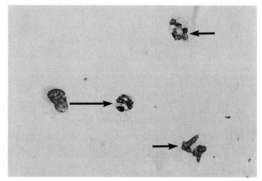

FIGURE 12–4. Bacterial arthritis may be caused by direct inoculation or hematogenous spread. Infected joints typically have high neutrophil counts (>50,000/μl). In this example, the neutrophils display degenerative changes, including nuclear swelling (*short arrows*), and cytoplasmic vacuolization. The presence of degenerative changes strongly supports infection, however, the lack of degenerative changes or observable microorganisms does not rule out the possibility of infection. The bacteria may be located in the joint tissue and not present in the synovial fluid. Rare bacteria were observed after prolonged searching (*long arrow*). (Wright; ×250.)

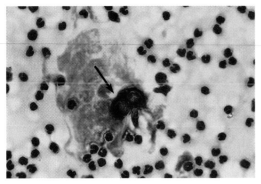

FIGURE 12–5. In addition to bacteria, other types of infectious agents may also involve the joint. This photomicrograph contains numerous neutrophils that are "rounded up" and almost appear like mononuclear cells owing to the thickness of the smear. In the center of the photo, broad-based budding yeast are found that are consistent with *Blastomyces dermatitidis* (*arrow*). Fungal organisms may be present infrequently and are best found on low-power examination. As with bacteria, the lack of observable organisms does not rule out infection. Fungal culture and serology is advisable in suspected cases. (Wright; ×250.)

tissue. Other types of organisms that have been implicated as causative agents of joint disease include mycoplasma, bacterial L-forms, spirochetes (*Borrelia burgdorferi*), protozoa (*Leishmania donovani*), viruses (calicivirus, coronavirus), and rickettsia (*Ehrlichia canis, Ehrlichia equi, Ehrlichia ewingii, Rickettsia rickettsii*).

Noninfectious Arthritis

Many animals with inflamed joints have nonerosive disease. Causes of nonerosive polyarthritis include borreliosis (Lyme disease), ehrlichiosis (Fig. 12–6), polyarthritis secondary to infection or neoplasia elsewhere, breed-specific polyarthritis, drug-induced disease, immune-mediated polyarthritis, and systemic lupus erythematosus. Although crystal-induced arthritis (e.g., gout) has been described in animals, it is extremely uncommon in dogs and cats. As the name implies, polyarthritis typically af-

majority of the neutrophils will not show a degenerate appearance in septic arthritis. Organisms may gain access to joints either hematogenously or via direct inoculation. In addition, there may be infection elsewhere in the body (e.g., endocarditis) with immune complex deposition in the synovial tissue and resultant nonseptic inflammation in the fluid. Bacterial and fungal arthritis most commonly present with solitary joint involvement but on occasion may have multiple joint involvement. Because infectious and noninfectious arthritis can have a similar presentation, it may be advisable to always culture inflamed joints, keeping in mind that a negative culture does not rule out infection as the microorganisms are sometimes limited to the synovial lining

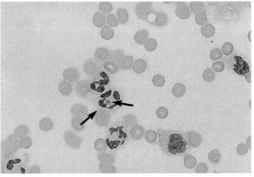

FIGURE 12–6. The neutrophil in the center (*arrows*) contains an ehrlichia morula in the cytoplasm. Granulocytic ehrlichiosis may be caused by *E. equi* or *E. ewingii*. These organisms may cause polyarthritis as well as a variety of other clinical signs and laboratory problems. It is unusual to find the organisms in clinical samples except for acute infections. Diagnosis is usually based on recognition of clinical signs with appropriate serologic testing. (Wright; ×250.)

fects multiple joints, but on occasion may present with only a solitary affected joint.

Joints affected by immune-mediated disease have increased numbers of nondegenerate neutrophils. In rare cases, increased numbers of lymphocytes and plasma cells may be found. Smaller distal joints are most commonly affected. Diagnosis of immune-mediated disease is dependent not only on demonstrating joint inflammation, but also on ruling out infection via culture, serology, and/or empiric therapy. Some cases of immune-mediated disease will have ragocytes (Fig. 12–7) or LE cells (Fig. 12–8). These are rare findings and should not be relied upon to make a diagnosis of immune-mediated disease.

Erosive arthritis is suggested when there are lucent cyst-like areas in the subchondral

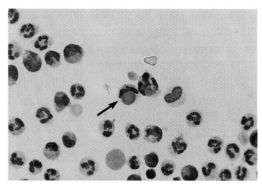

FIGURE 12–8. Synovial fluid from a dog with shifting leg lameness. The total cell number is moderately increased and composed of predominantly nondegenerate neutrophils with lesser numbers of lymphocytes and monocytes. The neutrophil in the center contains a large round homogeneous eosinophilic inclusion in the cytoplasm that displaces the nucleus to the periphery of the cell membrane (*arrow*). This is an LE cell. The phagocytozed material is thought to be nuclear material that has been structurally altered by antinuclear antibody. The homogeneous light staining appearance of the material distinguishes it from normal nuclear material. LE cells are rare, but when found, support the diagnosis of systemic lupus erythematosus. (Wright; ×250.) (Courtesy of Dr. Linda L. Werner.)

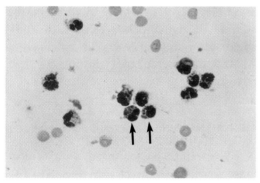

FIGURE 12–7. Ragocytes are neutrophils with multiple small, variably sized, purple cytoplasmic inclusions (*arrows*). They are thought to represent nuclear remnants or phagocytosed immune complexes. They should be distinguished from bacteria. Observations suggest that these cells are seen more commonly in association with immune-mediated polyarthropathies but are not considered diagnostic. Serologic evaluation for immune-mediated disease and extra-articular nonbacterial infections such as ehrlichiosis and borreliosis is recommended when polyarthritis is identified. (Wright; ×250.)

bone with narrowing or widening of the joint spaces found on joint radiographs. Types of erosive arthritis described in animals include rheumatoid arthritis, polyarthritis of greyhounds, and feline chronic progressive polyarthritis. The classic finding is progressive loss of subchondral bone with deformation and destruction of affected joints. Infection or neoplasia may also cause erosive joint disease. Erosive arthritis, as with other types of inflammatory joint disease, is characterized by increased numbers of neutrophils in the synovial fluid. Synovial fluid analysis alone cannot distinguish erosive disease from nonerosive disease and, for this reason, radiographs should be done on animals with inflammatory joint disease. Other clinical features of noninfectious erosive arthritis include morning stiffness, swelling of same or multiple joints within a 3-month period, symmetric swelling of joints, mononuclear infiltrates observed microscopically in a synovial membrane biopsy, and positive RF titer.

Degenerative Joint Disease

Degenerative joint disease (osteoarthritis, osteroarthropathy) is characterized by degeneration of articular cartilage with secondary changes in associated joint structures. The disorder usually occurs secondary to conditions such as osteochondrosis, hip dysplasia, joint instability, and trauma. Changes in the synovial fluid are not as

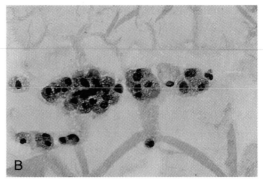

FIGURE 12–9. **B,** Joints with degenerative disease typically have increased numbers of macrophages or synoviocytes. The cells are usually large and vacuolated, and contain numerous pink-staining cytoplasmic granules. Mucin content may remain good as is evident in this figure by the thick pink background. (Wright; ×125.)

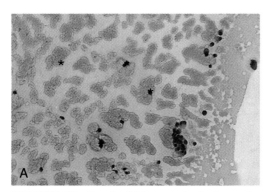

FIGURE 12–9. **A,** This sample is from the stifle joint of a large dog with chronic hind limb lameness. Cell numbers appear to be slightly increased although difficult to estimate because of clumping and thickness of the smear (see Chapter 1 for sample management). The granular background that includes clumps of mucin (asterisks), is suggestive of good mucin content. The majority of the cells are mononuclear with some having a macrophage appearance consistent with a cytologic interpretation of degenerative joint disease. Further evaluation for underlying disease such as osteochondrosis or meniscal disease is warranted. (Wright; ×50.)

remarkable as seen with inflammatory disease (Fig. 12–9). A mild increase in the number of mononuclear cells is the predominant finding. These cells are likely a mixture of macrophages (histiocytes) and synovial cells.

Hemarthrosis

If recent trauma has occurred, joint hemorrhage may be appreciated (Fig. 12–10). True hemorrhage must be distinguished from the much more common artifact of blood contamination. This is best done at the time of sample collection. If previous hemorrhage has occurred, the withdrawn fluid will appear xanthochromic (yellowish color due to old hemorrhage) to homogeneously red and cloudy. Besides trauma, other causes of hemorrhagic joint fluid include coagulation defects and neoplasia. A congenital coagulation factor deficiency should be considered in a puppy or kitten that presents with repeated episodes of he-

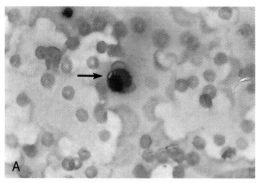 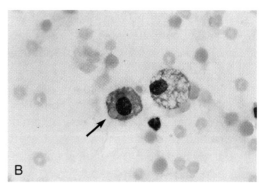

FIGURE 12–10. Because of the small size of canine and feline joints, it is common to get some degree of blood contamination in most joint aspirates. To help distinguish true hemorrhage from blood contamination, the smears should be routinely examined for erythrophagia, hematoidin crystals, hemosiderin, and platelet clumps. In (A), the macrophage contains a small golden hematoidin crystal (arrow), while the smaller of two macrophages in (B) contains a phagocytosed erythrocyte in the lower left area of its cytoplasm (arrow). These findings indicate that there has been previous hemorrhage in the joint. Potential causes of hemarthrosis include trauma, coagulopathy, and neoplasia. Coagulopathies may have evidence of multiple joint involvement and bleeding elsewhere. Abnormal hemostasis is documented by coagulation testing. (Wright; ×250.)

marthrosis or with hemarthrosis and a history of minimal trauma.

MUSCULOSKELETAL DISORDERS

The amount of information garnered by cytologic evaluation of other tissues in suspected musculoskeletal disorders is limited. Although inflammation may be appreciated in aspirates from muscle tissue, it cannot be architecturally related to the muscle and for this reason is a poor diagnostic aid for myositis. On the other hand, neoplastic lesions such as rhabdomyosarcoma and synovial sarcoma (Fig. 12–11) may exfoliate enough cells to make a diagnosis. Aspiration of muscle, connective tissue, or bone lesions is much the same as aspiration of other lesions. In aspiration of a bony lesion, use of a needle with a stylet (such as bone marrow needle) may be advisable when en-

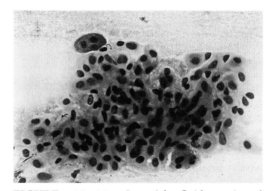

FIGURE 12–11. Synovial fluid aspirated from a dog with lameness localized to a solitary joint. The sample is predominated by large sheets of pleomorphic spindle cells that are sometimes separated by a fine pink streaming stroma. The cells display moderate pleomorphism. This joint had an associated soft tissue mass that was ultimately diagnosed as synovial sarcoma. The cells in this photograph display some cytologic features of malignancy and may be neoplastic, but could potentially be reactive synovial cells. As with many mesenchymal tumors, it is difficult to definitively diagnose malignancy based solely on cytologic detail. (Wright; ×125.)

tering the lesion to prevent plugging of the needle with cortical bone. In many instances, however, core biopsy specimens and histopathology will be necessary for diagnosis. In addition, it is important to note that in most animals with a bone or muscle disorder, diagnosis is reliant on integrating information from the signalment, history, physical examination and radiographic examination, and/or histopathology.

Diagnosis of myositis typically requires consideration of history, signalment, chemistry findings (increased creatine kinase and aspartate transaminase) as well as electromyographic (EMG), immunologic, and se-

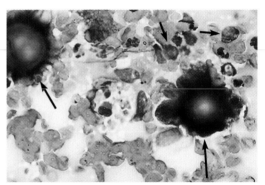

FIGURE 12–13. Aspirate from a lytic lesion in the scapula of a middle-aged dog with pain and lameness of the foreleg. This aspirate contains blood with a mixture of inflammatory cells and smudged nuclei (*short arrows*). There are two large blue spherical structures in this field (*long arrows*) that are *Coccidioides immitis* spherules. The size of the spherules prevents sharp focusing on both the spherules and the background cells. When focusing up and down on these spherules, variable numbers of endospores may be seen within. Aspiration of fungal myelitis lesions does not always yield observable organisms (particularly *Coccidiodes*) and if infection is suspected, culture and appropriate serology is indicated. Because of the zoonotic potential of some fungal organisms, extreme care should be taken when culturing these lesions. (Wright; ×250.)

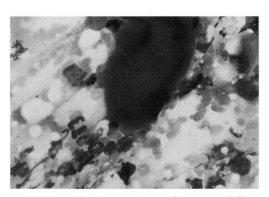

FIGURE 12–12. Aspirate from a diffuse swollen lesion in the thigh region. This photomicrograph contains a background of blood with increased numbers of degenerating neutrophils and some macrophages. The large blue structure at the top center of the picture is a fragment of skeletal muscle tissue. These typically stain a dark blue color with Wright stain. Aspiration of muscle typically yields fragments of tissue instead of individualized cells. When focusing up and down on the fragments, striations can be seen. This animal had suppurative myositis and cellulitis due to a bite wound. Because aspiration of this type of lesion frequently is bloody, it is difficult to be certain whether the leukocytes are due to inflammation or blood contamination. (Wright; ×250.) (Courtesy of Dr. Sonjia Shelly.)

rologic tests. Aspirates of swollen muscle tissue may be taken (Fig. 12–12), but interpretation is typically limited because of blood contamination as well as lack of architectural relationship of the cells. Muscle biopsy is typically necessary for definitive characterization of inflammatory as well as degenerative lesions.

Osteomyelitis is a difficult cytologic diagnosis as aspiration of bony lesions may be contaminated with marrow and blood. Nevertheless, on occasion, clearly increased numbers of inflammatory cells may be found as well as specific etiologic agents such as *Nocardia, Actinomyces,* other bacte-

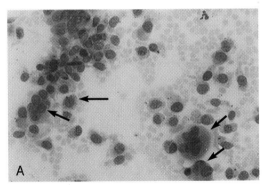

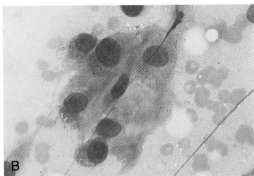

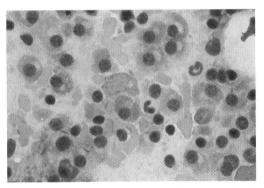

FIGURE 12–15. Aspirate from a lytic "punched out" lesion in a vertebral spinous process of an 8-year-old dog. The aspirate is predominated by mildly pleomorphic plasma cells. This finding in combination with the presence of lytic bony lesions is diagnostic for multiple myeloma. (Wright; ×200.)

FIGURE 12–14. Aspirate from a lytic and proliferative lesion of the proximal tibia. Figure **(A)** is bloody and cellular with a mixture of ellipsoid and multinucleated cells (*arrows*). In some areas, the cells are found in thick accumulations, occasionally contain cytoplasmic granules (*long arrow*), and a fine pink extracellular material swirls around them. (Wright; ×500.) Figure **(B)** shows a high-power view of individualized cells that are presumptively osteoblasts. Note cell size by contrasting to the greenish-stained erythrocytes. This pattern is most consistent with a sarcoma. It is difficult to cytologically distinguish different types of sarcoma and additional tests such as radiography and biopsy are necessary for definitive morphologic diagnosis. Biopsy of this lesion indicated osteosarcoma. (Wright; ×250.)

ria and fungi (Fig. 12–13). If osteomyelitis is suspected, a specimen should also be collected for culture.

Primary bone tumors such as osteosarcoma (Fig. 12–14) and chondrosarcoma may be recognized on cytologic samples,

however, the cytologic interpretation may be limited to a general classification of sarcoma with histopathologic examination of tissue architecture required defining the specific cell type. Lytic, "punched-out" lesions may be aspirated to investigate the possibility of multiple myeloma (Fig. 12–15). Because the plasma cells in this tumor typically are well differentiated and large numbers of plasma cells may be found in some infectious conditions (e.g., ehrlichiosis), it is important to also demonstrate other findings of myeloma such as monoclonal gammopathy, Bence–Jones proteinuria, and lytic bone lesions. Not all of these will be found in every case of multiple myeloma.

Finally, metastatic tumors (e.g., carcinoma) may present with lameness and lytic bone lesions or pathologic fractures. Rarely, metastatic tumors may also affect the joint cavity (Fig. 12–16). Aspiration of these lesions may demonstrate metastatic tumor cells, although defining the primary tumor will require complete physical examination and histopathology of the primary tumor.

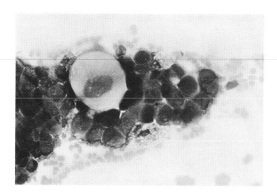

FIGURE 12–16. This sample is from the stifle joint of a 12-year-old golden retriever. The joint was swollen and painful with evidence of bony lysis. Numerous clusters of pleomorphic cells are present. These cells display marked anisocytosis and anisokaryosis with prominent irregularly shaped nucleoli. The atypia of the cells is consistent with the diagnosis of metastatic carcinoma. (Wright; ×125.)

Recommended Literature

Boon GD: Synovial fluid analysis: A guide for small-animal practitioners. Vet Med 1997; May: 443.

Carr AP: Infectious arthritis in dogs and cats. Vet Med 1997; Sept: 786.

Carr AP, Michels G: Identifying noninfectious erosive arthritis in dogs and cats. Vet Med 1997; Sept: 804.

Ellison RS: The cytologic examination of synovial fluid. Semin Vet Med Surg (Sm Anim) 1988; 3(2):133.

Fernandez FR, Grindem CB, Lipowitz AJ, et al: Synovial fluid analysis: Preparation of smears for cytologic examination of canine synovial fluid. J Am Anim Hosp Assoc 1983; 19:727.

Harari J: Clinical evaluation of the osteoarthritic patient. Vet Clin North Am (Small Anim Pract) 1997; 27(4):725.

Johnson AJ, Watson ADJ: Skeletal diseases. In Ettinger SJ, Feldman EC (eds): Textbook of Veterinary Internal Medicine, 5th ed. WB Saunders, Philadelphia, 2000, p 1887.

Lewis RM: Rheumatoid arthritis. Vet Clin North Am (Small Anim Pract) 1994; 24(4):697.

Marchevsky AM, Read RA: Bacterial septic arthritis in 19 dogs. Aust Vet J 1999; 77:233.

Michels GM, Carr AP: Noninfectious nonerosive arthritis in dogs. Vet Med 1997; Sept: 798.

Pedersen NC, Morgan JP, Vasseur PB: Joint diseases of dogs and cats. In Ettinger SJ, Feldman EC (eds): Textbook of Veterinary Internal Medicine, 5th ed. WB Saunders, Philadelphia, 2000, p 1862.

Schrader SC: The use of the laboratory in the diagnosis of joint disorders of dogs and cats. In Bonagura JD (ed): Kirk's Current Veterinary Therapy XII: Small Animal Practice. WB Saunders, Philadelphia, 1995, p 1166.

Schrader SC: Differential diagnosis of nontraumatic causes of lameness in young growing dogs. In Bonagura JD (ed): Kirk's Current Veterinary Therapy XII: Small Animal Practice. WB Saunders, Philadelphia, 1995, p. 1171.

CHAPTER 13

Cytology of the Central Nervous System

Kathy P. Freeman

Rose E. Raskin

CEREBROSPINAL FLUID

Cerebrospinal fluid (CSF) evaluation is a mainstay in the diagnosis of central nervous system (CNS) disease because it is relatively simple to collect and has the potential to provide valuable information (Fenner, 1995). Lesions of the CNS do not consistently cause CSF abnormalities related to the location and extent of the lesion. Although CSF evaluation infrequently provides a definitive diagnosis, it may be of benefit in documenting normal or abnormal features and, in combination with other tests, determining a diagnosis or differential diagnoses (Chrisman, 1992; Cook and DeNicola, 1988; Fenner, 1995; Evans, 1988; Oliver et al., 1997; Parent and Rand, 1994; Rand, 1995). CSF collection is recommended as a part of virtually any diagnostic investigation of CNS disease of unknown cause when contraindications to its collection are not present (Cook and DeNicola, 1988; Coles, 1986; Fenner, 1995).

The submission of a properly collected specimen is necessary to obtain reliable and accurate information. Proper interpretation of the sample requires knowledge of the clinical presentation, collection site, and specimen-handling considerations. The presence of artifacts or contaminants may interfere with an appropriate interpretation unless the conditions surrounding the collection are known. Experience in interpretation of cytologic specimens from the species of interest and knowledge of the limitations of cytology or types of pathologic processes likely to be reflected in CSF are also important and can only be gained by diligent study of the literature and specimens over time.

Cerebrospinal fluid is formed primarily by the ultrafiltration and secretion through the choroid plexuses of the lateral, third, and fourth ventricles. Other sites that secrete CSF include the ependymal linings of the ventricles and blood vessels of the subarachnoid spaces and pia mater. Fluid then escapes from the fourth ventricle into the subarachnoid spaces and central canal of the spinal cord. It is then absorbed predominantly from the subarachnoid spaces via veins in the arachnoid and subarachnoid villi that project into subdural venous sinuses (Hoerlein, 1971).

Collection of Cerebrospinal Fluid

Contraindications to CSF Collection

Cerebrospinal fluid collection is not indicated in cases in which a cause is obvious, such as known trauma or intoxication (Parent and Rand, 1994). Because anesthesia is required for collection of CSF in small animals, CSF collection is contraindicated in cases in which anesthesia is contraindicated (Carmichael, 1998; Cook and DeNicola, 1988; Evans, 1988).

Cerebrospinal fluid collection is contraindicated in cases with increased intracranial pressure. Increased intracranial pressure should be suspected with acute head trauma, active or decompensated hydrocephalus, anisocoria, papilledema, or cerebral edema. Expansile mass lesions and unstable CNS or systemic conditions may result in increased intracranial pressure or decreased pressure in the spinal compartment relative to the intracranial compartment. In these situations herniation of the brain may result in severe compromise of brain function, tetraplegia, stupor/coma, and/or death (Evans, 1988; Oliver et al., 1997; Parent and Rand, 1994). Physical and neurologic examination, history, presentation, and results of imaging studies are of benefit in determining if these conditions are likely prior to the decision to collect CSF.

Even in cases with potential for brain herniation, the risks associated with CSF collection may be acceptable if the cause of patient deterioration is not apparent (Parent and Rand, 1994). Risk of herniation may be reduced by administration of dexamethasone (0.25 mg/kg IV) just prior to induction of anesthesia and by hyperventilation of the patient with oxygen during the procedure (Fenner, 1995; Parent and Rand, 1994). Except in cases in which dexamethasone is administered prophylactically because of suspected increased intracranial pressure, CSF collection should predate corticosteroid administration because of potential alteration of CSF composition (Rand, 1995).

Complications of CSF Collection

As with any medical procedure, the risks and benefits of CSF collection should be considered for individual cases. The potential exists for iatrogenic trauma to the spinal cord and/or brainstem from the collection needle, but is minimized by attention to anatomic landmarks and careful collection procedures (Carmichael, 1998; Parent and Rand, 1994). Risk of introduction of infectious agents into the CNS is minimized by adherence to the basic principles of aseptic technique and correct preparation of the site of collection (Cook and DeNicola, 1988).

Slight to moderate blood contamination is a common complication of collection associated with penetration of the dorsal vertebral sinuses or small vessels within the meninges; this may complicate interpretation of the fluid analyses and cytology, but has not been found to be harmful to the patient (Carmichael, 1998; Fenner, 1995).

Ketamine should not be used to anesthetize cats for CSF collection because it increases intracranial pressure and may induce seizures; gas anesthesia should be used (Parent and Rand, 1994).

If three unsuccessful attempts at CSF collection occur, abandonment of the procedure is recommended to decrease the probability of repeated penetration of the spinal cord, which may result in serious complications or death (Rand, 1995). Practice on cadavers prior to performing collection in live clinical cases has been recommended (Carmichael, 1998; Parent and Rand; 1994; Rand, 1995).

Equipment for CSF Collection

Clippers, scrub, and alcohol to surgically prepare the site of collection are needed. Sterile gloves should be worn during the procedure. A sterile disposable or resterilizable spinal needle with stylet is used. A 20- to 22-gauge, 1.5-inch needle is recommended for most cases, although smaller needles may be needed in very small dogs and cats and longer needles may be needed in large dogs (Carmichael, 1998; Cook and DeNicola, 1988; Evans, 1988; Parent and Rand, 1994; Rand, 1995). Several needles should be available since replacement may be needed if the needle is inserted off the midline and enters a venous sinus (Cook and DeNicola, 1989).

Sterile plain tubes for collection of CSF are recommended. Some authors indicate that EDTA is not used because clotting is rare and EDTA may falsely elevate the protein concentration of CSF (Parent and Rand, 1994). However, others recommend addition of samples to EDTA if blood contamination is present or if elevated nucleated cell count, bacteria, elevated protein concentration, and/or the presence of fibrinogen are suspected because these may lead to clotting (Carmichael, 1998; Evans, 1988). Evans (1988) recommends collection into fluoride/oxalate if glucose determination is desired; this may not be necessary if CSF contains few erythrocytes and is analyzed rapidly.

Plastic containers are recommended because leukocytes may adhere to glass (Fenner, 1995). In the authors' experience, use of only a few plain, sterile containers makes collection easier and simpler and increases the probability of maximum yield of CSF.

Collection Volume

Carmichael (1998) indicates that approximately 1 ml of CSF per 5 kg of body weight can be collected safely. Coles (1986) indicates that it may be dangerous to remove more than 1 ml of CSF per 30 seconds, more than 4 to 5 ml of CSF from the dog, more than 0.5 to 1 ml of CSF from the adult cat or more than 10 to 20 drops of CSF from the kitten. Rand (1995) indicates that 1.0 to 1.5 ml of CSF can usually be collected from the cat. The cat may be susceptible to meningeal hemorrhage if too much fluid is withdrawn (Coles, 1986).

Cerebellomedullary Cistern Collection

Collection at this site is indicated to classify lesions affecting the meninges of the head and neck when the clinical signs involve seizures, generalized incoordination, head tilt, or circling.

Preparation of the site should include clipping of the hair from the head and neck, from the anterior margin of the pinna to the level of the third cervical vertebra and laterally to the level of the lateral margins of the pinnae. This area should be scrubbed for a sterile procedure (Carmichael, 1998; Fenner, 1995; Rand, 1995).

The animal is positioned in lateral recumbency with the head and vertebral column positioned at an angle of approximately 90 degrees. Excessive flexion of the neck may result in elevation of intracranial pressure and increase the potential for brain herniation (Fenner, 1995) or may result in occlusion of the endotracheal tube (Carmichael, 1998; Rand, 1995). The nose should be held or propped so that its long axis is parallel to the table and it should not be allowed to rotate in either direction. The point of insertion is located on the midline approximately half way between the external occipital protuberance and the craniodorsal tip of the dorsal spine of C2 (axis) and just rostral to the anterior margins of the wings of C1 (atlas). The needle is inserted at the intersection of a line connecting the anterior borders of the wings of the atlas and a line drawn from the occipital crest to the dorsal border of the axis along the midline (Carmichael, 1998; Coles, 1986; Cook and DeNicola, 1989; Evans, 1988; Fenner, 1995). Puncture of the skin first with an 18-gauge needle or a scalpel blade is helpful in overcoming skin resistance in thick-skinned animals (Rand, 1995). Alternatively, the skin can be pinched and lifted so that the needle can be safely pushed through the skin with a twisting motion (Parent and Rand, 1994).

The needle should be inserted with the bevel oriented cranially. It should be held perpendicular to the skin surface and gradually advanced with the stylet in place. Periodically the needle should be stabilized and the stylet withdrawn to determine if CSF is present (Cook and DeNicola, 1989; Evans, 1988; Parent and Rand, 1994; Rand, 1995). Occasionally, a sudden loss of resistance may be felt as the subarachnoid space is entered, but this may not be recognized in all cases (Cook and DeNicola, 1989; Evans, 1988; Rand, 1995). If the collector suspects that the needle has been inserted too deeply, the stylet may be removed and the needle slowly withdrawn a few millimeters at a time, watching for the appearance of fluid in the hub (Cook and DeNicola, 1989; Rand, 1995). If the needle hits bone during insertion, slight redirection of the needle cranially or caudally should be attempted to enter the atlanto-occipital space.

If pressure readings are taken, CSF fluid sample is taken by directing the flow of CSF through the manometer by way of a three-way stopcock (Cook and DeNicola, 1989). If pressure readings are not obtained, CSF may be collected directly from the spinal needle hub by dripping into a test tube or gentle aspiration of drops as they collect at the hub using a syringe (Rand, 1995). Attachment of a syringe to the needle with aspiration of CSF is not recommended because suction may result in contamination with blood, meningeal cells or obstruction of CSF flow by aspirated meningeal trabeculae (Cook and DeNicola, 1989; Rand, 1995). Careful aspiration is acknowledged to be necessary for collections in some cases (Fenner, 1995). Passage of the needle through the spinal cord to underlying bone should be avoided at the cerebellomedullary cistern because it may cause damage to the cord and/or cause blood contamination of the CSF sample (Rand, 1995). Upon completion of collection of CSF, the needle is smoothly withdrawn. Replacement of the stylet is not necessary (Cook and DeNicola, 1988).

If the fluid appears bloody at the onset of collection, replacement of the stylet for 30 to 60 seconds may result in clearing of the blood (Fenner, 1995). If the first few drops of CSF are still slightly bloody, they can be collected separately from the following drops that are often clear (Carmichael, 1998; Fenner, 1995). If rate of flow of CSF is slow, the needle should be rotated slightly to make sure that it is clear at the luminal tip (Fenner, 1995). If this not effective, rate of flow may be increased by compression of the jugular veins, resulting in expansion of the venous sinuses and increased CSF pressure (Coles, 1986; Cook and DeNicola, 1988; Fenner, 1995).

Appearance of abundant fresh blood from the collection needle indicates that the point of the needle is most likely off the midline and in a lateral venous sinus. A new approach with a fresh, clean needle is recommended if the first attempt results in frank blood consistent with puncture of the venous sinus (Cook and DeNicola, 1988).

Lumbar Cistern

Both cerebellomedullary and lumbar cistern specimens may be collected. Cook and DeNicola (1988) recommend collection of a cerebellomedullary specimen prior to thoracolumbar myelography to ensure that a diagnostic CSF sample will be obtained because lumbar puncture alone may not be sufficient. The collection of CSF from the lumbar cistern is more difficult and more likely to be contaminated with blood than that from the cerebellomedullary cistern (Cook and DeNicola, 1988; Chrisman, 1992). Sometimes no fluid or only a very small amount of fluid can be obtained owing to the small size of the lumbar subarachnoid space (Cook and DeNicola, 1988; Chrisman, 1992). Lumbar puncture may be preferred in cases with localized spinal disease because it may be more likely to confirm abnormality than cerebellomedullary cistern collections (Thomson et al., 1990).

The dorsal midline is clipped and prepared between the midsacrum and L3, extending laterally to the wings of the ilium. The animal is placed in lateral recumbency and the back is flexed slightly to open the spaces between the dorsal laminae of the vertebrae. The L5-6 or L6-7 spaces are most commonly used in dogs because the subarachnoid space rarely extends to the lumbosacral junction. In cats collection can frequently be made from the lumbosacral space (Cook and DeNicola, 1988; Evans, 1988).

The dorsal spinous process of L7 lies between the wings of the ilia and is usually smaller than that of L6. To collect from the L5-6 interspace, the needle is inserted just off the midline at the caudal aspect of the L6 dorsal spinous process and advanced at an angle cranioventrally and slightly medially to enter the spinal canal between the dorsal laminae of L5 and L6 (Cook and DeNicola, 1988). Misdirection laterally into the paralumbar muscles or underestimation of the length of needle required might result in advancement of the needle to the hub without encountering bone (Cook and DeNicola, 1988).

Cerebrospinal fluid may be collected from the dorsal subarachnoid space, or the needle may be passed through the nervous structures to the floor of the spinal canal and CSF collected from the ventral subarachnoid space (Evans, 1988). The stylet is removed and the needle may be carefully withdrawn a few millimeters to allow for fluid flow. The rate of flow is usually slower than from the cerebellomedullary cistern. Rate of flow may be increased by jugular compression (Coles, 1986; Cook and DeNicola, 1988).

Handling of Cerebrospinal Fluid Specimens

Cells lyse rapidly in the low-protein milieu of CSF, so cell counts and cytologic preparations of unfixed fluid should be done within 30 to 60 minutes of collection (Carmichael, 1998; Oliver et al., 1997; Parent and Rand, 1994). Addition of an equal volume of 4% to 10% neutral buffered formalin or 50% to 90% alcohol is recommended for fixation of specimens that cannot be immediately delivered to a laboratory and processed immediately (Carmichael, 1998; Duncan et al., 1996; Evans, 1988; Roszel, 1972). Alternatively, the addition of one drop of 10% formalin to 1 to 2 ml of CSF may be used to preserve cells for cell counts and morphologic examination when submitted to a referral laboratory, keeping in mind that cell counts will be affected but may not be clinically significant. Refrigeration will help retard cellular degeneration (Fenner, 1995). Cellular stability can be increased by addition of fresh, frozen, or thawed serum or plasma (Cook and De-Nicola, 1988) or by addition of 20% albumin (Fenner, 1995). Protein and enzyme concentrations in CSF are relatively stable and submission to the laboratory by routine delivery, postal delivery, or courier is usually sufficient for accurate determinations (Carmichael, 1998; Evans, 1988).

Laboratory Analysis of CSF

Usually at least 1 to 2 ml of CSF is available from dogs or cats. The analysis for cell counts requires approximately 0.5 ml (500 μl total or 250 μl for duplicate erythrocyte

count and nucleated cell count, respectively). The volume required for chemical protein determination will vary, depending on the equipment and method used, but can be expected to be on the order of 200 to 250 μl for large, automated pieces of equipment. Taking these figures into account, approximately 0.25 to 1.25 ml of CSF should be available for cytologic evaluation and/or other tests.

Routine analysis of CSF is recommended in all cases in which it is collected; specialized analyses may be needed in selected cases. Routine analyses of CSF includes the following: macroscopic evaluation, quantitative analysis (erythrocyte count, nucleated cell count, and total protein), and microscopic evaluation as summarized in Table 13–1 (Carmichael, 1998; Chrisman, 1992;

TABLE 13–1	Routine Evaluation of CSF		
Component of CSF Evaluation	Normal CSF	Abnormal CSF	Comments/Notes
Macroscopic Evaluation			Compare with tube containing water
Color	Colorless	Pink, red xanthochromic (yellow to yellow-orange). Occasional gray to green color may be seen.	Red or pink suggests blood; if due to intact erythrocytes, it will clear with centrifugation. Xanthochromia is an indication of previous hemorrhage with accumulation of oxyhemoglobin or methemoglobin from erythrocyte degradation; may occur with hyperbilirubinemia. May be graded as slight, moderate, or marked.
Turbidity	Clear Turbidity absent	Turbid or cloudy—slight, moderate, or marked	Evaluate ability to read printed words through the tube. Detectable turbidity corresponds to nucleated cell count > 500 cells/μl

Component of CSF Evaluation	Normal CSF		Abnormal CSF		Comments/Notes
Quantitative Analysis					
Erythrocyte (RBC) count	Zero RBC considered normal, but frequently present in small numbers		Variable		Standard hemocytometer
Nucleated cell count	Most commonly cited reference intervals: 0–5 cells/μl (dog) 0–8 cells/μl (cat)		Variable		Standard hemocytometer
Specific gravity	1.004–1.006		Most within reference interval for normal CSF		Of questionable value because only relatively marked increases in total protein result in changes that are detectable by specific gravity measurement
Total protein (microprotein)					
Quantitation	Most commonly cited reference intervals indicate usually <30 mg/dl (cerebellomedullary) or <45 mg/dl (lumbar cistern)		Increased total protein seen in a variety of conditions		Microprotein method and reference values may vary with laboratory; use laboratory-established reference values.
Estimation Ames Multistix* (urine dipstick) (Jacobs et al, 1990)	Ames Multistix Trace 1+ Trace to 1+ protein on urine dipstick is within normal limits	Microprotein Concentration <30 mg/dl 30 mg/dl	Ames Multistix 2+ 3+ 4+	Microprotein Concentration 100 mg/dl 300 mg/dl >2000 mg/dl	Most sensitive to albumin; detects ranges of protein that are useful for evaluation of most canine and feline CSF specimens; good correlation with standard dye-binding microprotein determinations.
Microscopic Evaluation					
Cell population	Lymphocytes and monocytoid cells predominate; very few mature, nondegenerated neutrophils may be present. A few erythrocytes may be seen.		Variable		See other sections for more details of cytologic features and specific conditions. Preparatory techniques for concentrating cells: Cytospin preparation Membrane filter Sedimentation chamber

* N-Multistix SG, Bayer, Miles, Diagnostic Division, Elkhart, IN.

Coles, 1986; Cook and DeNicola, 1988; Evans, 1988; Parent and Rand, 1994; Rand, 1995). If the volume of CSF is small and all tests are not likely to be obtainable, the clinician should rank the tests in order of preference when the specimen is submitted to the laboratory. Rand (1995) indicates that the most useful diagnostic tests, in decreasing order, are nucleated and erythrocyte counts, sedimentation cytology, protein concentration, and cytocentrifuge cytology.

Effect of Blood Contamination

Various formulas have been used to predict the effect of blood contamination on protein concentration and nucleated cell count in CSF (Coles, 1986; Parent and Rand, 1994; Rand, et al., 1990; Wilson and Stevens, 1977). Rand (1995) indicates that red blood cell (RBC) counts greater than 30 cells/μl in CSF will have a profound effect on the total and differential cell counts. However, in a recent study of iatrogenic blood contamination effects of total protein and nucleated cell counts in CSF, Hurtt and Smith (1997) found that the RBC count was not significantly correlated with nucleated cell count or protein concentration in CSF from clinically normal dogs or those with neurologic disease. They concluded that high CSF nucleated cell counts and protein concentrations are indicative of neurologic disease, even if samples contain up to 13,200 RBC/μl. Although blood contamination may make interpretation of CSF more difficult, red or pink CSF or CSF with a high RBC count should not be discarded as a useless specimen because cytologic evaluation may detect abnormalities (Chrisman, 1992).

Macroscopic Evaluation

Normal CSF is clear, colorless, and transparent and does not coagulate. Deviations

from normal should be recorded as part of the macroscopic evaluation and are often graded 1 to 4 + or as slight, moderate, or marked (Coles, 1986; Evans, 1988). Turbidity is reported to be detectable if greater than 500 cells/μl are present (Coles, 1986; Duncan et al., 1996; Fenner, 1995) or if at least 200 leukocytes/μl or 700 leukocytes/μl are present (Parent and Rand, 1994).

Red to pink discoloration may be associated with iatrogenic contamination with blood or pathologic hemorrhage (Coles, 1986; Evans, 1988). Erythrophages or siderophages in a rapidly processed CSF specimen with fixative added immediately following collection support pathologic hemorrhage as an underlying cause (Evans, 1989). Xanthochromia is the yellow to yellow-orange discoloration associated with pathologic hemorrhage due to trauma, vasculitis, severe inflammation, disc extrusion, or necrotic or erosive neoplasia (Coles, 1986; Evans, 1989). Occasionally xanthochromia will be seen with leptospirosis, cryptococcosis, toxoplasmosis, ischemic myelopathy, coagulopathy, or hyperbilirubinemia (Evans, 1989).

Cell Counts

Erythrocyte and nucleated cell counts are done using standard hemocytometer techniques (Carmichael, 1998; Parent and Rand, 1994). In general, collections from normal animals from the cerebellomedullary cistern have slightly higher numbers of cells and slightly lower protein levels than those from the lumbar cistern.

To count nucleated cells, charge both chambers of the hemocytometer with undiluted CSF and place the unit in a humidified petri dish for 15 minutes to allow cells to adhere to the glass. All nucleated cells are counted in the 10 large squares (four corner squares and one center square on each side) for a total nucleated cell count per microliter. Cell counts for erythrocytes are performed similarly.

Reference intervals for feline CSF erythrocyte counts are reported to range from 0 to 30 red blood cells per microliter (Parent and Rand, 1994). Reference intervals for feline CSF nucleated cell counts are reported to be less than 5 cells/μl (Coles, 1986; Evans, 1989; Oliver et al., 1997) 0 to 2 cells/μl (Parent and Rand, 1994), less than 3 cells/μl (Chrisman, 1992), and less than 8 cells/μl (Cook and DeNicola, 1988; Duncan et al., 1996).

Reference intervals for canine CSF erythrocyte counts are reported to be zero (Chrisman, 1992). Reference intervals for canine CSF nucleated cell counts are reported to be less than 5 cells/μl (Cook and DeNicola, 1988; Oliver et al., 1997), less than 8 cells/μl (Duncan et al., 1996), and less than 6 cells/μl for cerebellomedullary cistern collections or less than 5 cells/μl for lumbar cistern collections (Chrisman, 1992).

Absence of elevation of nucleated cell counts in CSF does not preclude the need for cytomorphologic evaluation with a differential cell count or estimate because abnormalities in cell type or morphology may be present even when CSF nucleated cell counts are within normal limits (Christopher et al., 1988).

Protein

Reference intervals for CSF total protein values may vary slightly with the laboratory and testing method used (Chrisman, 1992), but cerebellomedullary CSF protein is usually less than 25 to 30 mg/dl and lumbar cistern collections less than 45 mg/dl in dogs and cats (Chrisman, 1992; Fenner, 1995). Refractometer total protein evaluation is not accurate for assessment of CSF since the concentration of protein is quite low compared to serum or plasma and clin-

ically significant changes may not be easily detectable on the refractometer scale. Special analytic techniques most often available at commercial or reference laboratories and not available in practice are needed owing to the minute protein concentration in CSF (Chrisman, 1992; Parent and Rand, 1994); therefore, CSF protein analysis may be referred to as "microprotein." An estimate of CSF protein content can be obtained using urine dipsticks (Jacobs et al., 1990). Increased CSF protein concentration may be caused by an alteration in the blood–brain barrier and leakage from plasma or increased local synthesis (Duncan et al., 1996). Quantitative tests for detection of the components of CSF protein are covered under the heading of Other Tests. Differential diagnoses and examples of processes causing elevated CSF protein are covered under the heading of Protein Abnormalities in CSF.

Albumin accounts for 80% to 95% of the total protein in normal CSF (Evans, 1988). Qualitative tests to detect increased globulins in CSF are the Pandy and Nonne–Apelt tests (Coles, 1986; Evans, 1988). Use of these tests is limited because of the qualitative nature and absence of specificity regarding underlying cause. Normal CSF contains little if any globulin that can be detected by these methods (Coles, 1986).

Other Tests

Other tests that have been recommended by various authors or used in specific situations include electrophoretic determination of albumin and determination of total immunoglobulin levels. In combination with the serum albumin level and serum immunoglobulin, these can be used to calculate the albumin quotient (AQ) and immunoglobulin G (IgG) index (Chrisman, 1992; Duncan et al., 1996). The AQ is equal to the CSF albumin divided by serum albumin times 100. AQ greater than 2.35 suggests an altered blood–brain barrier with increased protein in CSF associated with leakage from plasma. The IgG index is equal to the (CSF IgG/serum IgG) divided by (CSF albumin/serum albumin). An IgG index greater than 0.272 with a normal AQ suggests intrathecal production of IgG. An increased IgG index and increased AQ are suggestive of an altered blood–brain barrier as the source of IgG (Chrisman, 1992).

Alterations in electrophoretic protein fractions have been reported to be useful in identifying inflammatory, degenerative, and neoplastic disease in combination with clinical signs (Sorjonen, 1987; Sorjonen et al., 1989). In general, dogs with canine distemper often have elevated CSF gamma globulins most likely related to intrathecal production, while dogs with granulomatous meningoencephalitis (GME) may have elevated CSF beta and gamma globulins (Chrisman, 1992). Detection of specific antibodies within the CSF and comparison with serum levels may be useful in diagnosis of infectious meningoencephalitides, including infectious canine hepatitis, canine herpesvirus, canine parvovirus, canine parainfluenza virus, canine distemper virus, ehrlichiosis, Rocky Mountain spotted fever, Lyme disease (borreliosis), *Toxoplasma gondii, Neospora caninum,* and *Encephalitozoon cuniculi* infection, *Babesia* spp. infection, cryptococcosis, and blastomycosis (Berthelin et al., 1994; Bichsel et al., 1984; Chrisman, 1992; Fenner, 1995; Mandel et al., 1993; Tyler and Cullor, 1989). Serial titers for serum IgG to show rising titer are helpful to demonstrate active disease. The presence of IgM in serum or CSF is considered more specific than IgG or total immunoglobulin levels for detection of active disease (Chrisman, 1992).

Glucose measurement in CSF and its comparison with serum or plasma glucose levels are frequently cited (Coles, 1986; Duncan et al., 1996). Normal CSF glucose is approximately 60% to 80% of the serum or plasma concentration (Fenner, 1995; Duncan et al., 1996). However, changes in CSF glucose concentration in serum or plasma are not immediately reflected in CSF and may take 1 to 3 hours before they are apparent in CSF (Cook and DeNicola, 1988; Duncan et al., 1996). The ratio between blood glucose and CSF glucose is frequently reduced in bacterial infections of the CNS in humans and has been reported to occur in some cases of pyogenic infections of the CNS, CSF hemorrhage, or blood contamination that may result in increased utilization of glucose by cells (Duncan et al., 1996). However, the relationship between bacterial encephalitis and decreased CSF glucose compared with serum or plasma glucose may depend on multiple factors, including the blood glucose level, degree of permeability of the blood–brain barrier, and presence or absence of glycolytic cells or microorganisms (Coles, 1986; Duncan et al., 1996). Fenner (1995) states that this reduction does not occur in dogs.

Measurement of various electrolytes and enzymes in CSF has been reported (Chrisman, 1992; Cook and DeNicola, 1988; Evans, 1988). Their interpretation may be limited because of increases associated with altered blood–brain barrier permeability, concurrent evaluation of serum values, low benefit for cost, and poor correlation or specificity for particular pathologic processes or conditions (Chrisman, 1992; Cook and DeNicola, 1988; Evans, 1988; Parent and Rand, 1994).

Aerobic and anaerobic bacterial cultures are recommended for all CSF samples with degenerated neutrophils or when bacteria are identified cytologically (Chrisman, 1992). *Staphylococcus, Streptococcus,* and *Pasteurella* are aerobic bacteria that may cause CNS infection; *Fusobacterium, Bacteroides, Peptostreptococcus,* and *Eubacterium* are anaerobic species that have been reported.

Cytologic Evaluation of CSF

Cytologic evaluation of CSF is recommended for all collections as a valuable part of CSF evaluation (Carmichael, 1998; Cook and DeNicola, 1988). In our experience, clinicians are asked to rank tests in order of preference if less than 1-ml total volume is submitted. Usually, cell counts and total protein concentration are requested, followed by cytology. If additional CSF is available, other tests may be requested, depending on the differential diagnoses suggested by clinical signs, presentation, history, imaging studies and results of cell counts, protein, and cytologic evaluation. Rand (1995) indicates that the most useful diagnostic tests, in decreasing order, are nucleated cell and erythrocyte counts, sedimentation cytology, protein concentration, and cytocentrifuge cytology.

Methods of Cytologic Preparation

Standardization of the volume used for cytologic evaluation may be of benefit in minimizing analytic variation and aid in interpretation, although evaluation of multiple preparations or preparations from larger volumes of CSF may increase the likelihood of detection of minor abnormalities. Because CSF is normally of low cellularity and increases in cellularity may not result in large numbers of cells, concentration of the cells is required (Carmichael, 1998; Chrisman, 1992; Coles, 1986; Cook and De-

Nicola, 1988; Fenner, 1995; Parent and Rand, 1994; Roszel, 1972). Cytocentrifugation, sedimentation, or membrane filtration techniques may be used for concentration of cells (Chrisman, 1992; Cook and DeNicola, 1988; Fenner, 1995; Parent and Rand, 1994; Roszel, 1972).

Cytocentrifugation is most commonly available in reference or commercial laboratories in which the volume of submissions justifies purchase of specialized equipment (Chrisman, 1992; Cook and DeNicola, 1988; Fenner, 1995; Parent and Rand, 1994). The membrane filtration technique requires special staining that is not commonly available in practice, but which may be available at some reference or commercial laboratories (Roszel, 1972). Several sedimentation techniques have been described and are suitable for use in practice or commercial or reference laboratories to which rapid submission of CSF specimens is possible (Cook and DeNicola, 1988; Parent and Rand, 1994). Readers are referred to these sources for more detail on construction of a sedimentation apparatus and preparation of sedimentation specimens. A sample device is demonstrated in Figure 13–1.

Sedimentation preparations should be made if a specimen cannot be delivered immediately to the laboratory for cytologic processing. Prepared slides can then be sent to a commercial or reference laboratory for interpretation or stained and evaluated by clinicians at the practice (Cook and DeNicola, 1988; Parent and Rand, 1994).

Cytocentrifuge or sedimentation preparations are most commonly air-dried and stained with Romanowsky stains that are commonly available in commercial or reference laboratories and clinical practice laboratories (Cook and DeNicola, 1988; Parent and Rand, 1994). Membrane-filtration specimens require wet-fixation and stains ap-

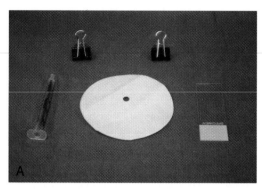

FIGURE 13–1. A, Unassembled in-house CSF sedimentation device. Materials needed include 1-ml tuberculin syringe, filter paper with hole punch, glass slide, and two binder clips.

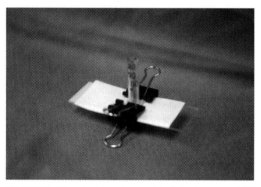

FIGURE 13–1. B, Assembled in-house CSF sedimentation device. The syringe barrel is cut in half and the flanged portions are attached to the filter paper and glass slide with the binder clips. As little as 100 μl CSF is added and allowed to sit undisturbed for 1 hour.

propriate for this method, commonly Papanicolaou, Trichrome, or H & E (Cook and DeNicola, 1988; Roszel, 1972). Wet-fixation and these staining methods may also be used on cytocentrifuge or sedimentation preparations and are appropriate for formalin- or alcohol-fixed specimens (Carmichael, 1998). Cytocentrifuge or membrane-filtration preparatory and staining techniques may vary with laboratory, technical training,

and pathologist preference. Summaries of cytopreparatory and staining techniques for cytospin and membrane filtration specimens and specimens fixed in formalin or alcohol are available from a variety of sources. Interested readers are referred to Keebler (1997) as a recent comprehensive review.

Special stains may be indicated in some cases. Gram stain may be useful for confirmation and identification of categories of bacteria (Evans, 1988; Cook and DeNicola, 1988). India ink or new methylene blue preparations have been reported to be helpful in identification of fungal infections, especially cryptococcosis (Cook and DeNicola, 1988). Periodic acid–Schiff stain may be used to demonstrate positive intracellular material in dogs with globoid cell leukodystrophy (Roszel, 1972). Luxol fast blue can be used to demonstrate myelin in CSF specimens (Mesher et al., 1996).

Cytologic Features of CSF

Several reviews of differential diagnoses and features of normal and abnormal cytologic features in canine and feline CSF with photomicrographs of selected features are available (Baker and Lumsden, 2000; Chrisman, 1992; Cook and DeNicola, 1988; Duncan et al., 1996; Jamison and Lumsden, 1988; Meinkoth and Crystal, 1999; Parent, 1995; Parent and Rand, 1994). Cytologic features that may be found in canine and feline CSF are summarized in Table 13–2. Differential diagnoses associated with abnormal CSF findings are summarized in Table 13–3.

Cytologic Features of Normal CSF

Normal CSF from healthy dogs and cats contains primarily mononuclear cells (Fig. 13–2), and is indicated to be a mixture of

Text continued on page 340

Cell or Feature	Description	Significance
Lymphocytes	Morphologically similar to those in peripheral blood; 9–15 μm in diameter, scant to moderate, pale basophilic cytoplasm with round to ovoid, slightly indented nucleus	Predominant cell type in normal CSF from healthy dogs; present in normal CSF from healthy cats
Reactive lymphocytes	Morphologically similar to those in peripheral blood; greater amount of cytoplasm and more deeply basophilic cytoplasm than normal lymphocytes; may see prominent perinuclear clear zones and coarse chromatin patterns	Not present in normal CSF from healthy animals, but not specific for underlying condition
Monocytoid cells	Large mononuclear cell; 12–15 μm diameter; moderate amount, pale basophilic, often finely foamy cytoplasm nuclear shape variable to amoeboid; chromatin pattern open to lacy	Present in CSF from healthy animals in low numbers
Activated monocytoid cells	Morphologically resemble macrophages in many sites; larger than "normal" monocytoid cells (>12–15 μm diameter); increased amount of cytoplasm that is often paler than normal and possibly vacuolated; nuclei become round to oval and eccentric; chromatin with increased coarseness	Activation associated with irritation, inflammation or degenerative processes; often phagocytic Reported in cats to be commonly associated with extensive necrosis
Neutrophils	Morphologically similar to those in peripheral blood; polymorphonuclear leukocytes	May be present in low numbers (up to 25% of total nucleated cells) in normal CSF from healthy animals
Ependymal lining cells	Uniform round to cuboidal mononuclear cells; individual cells or in cohesive clusters; eccentric, round nuclei; uniformly granular to coarse chromatin; moderate amount of finely granular cytoplasm	May be present in normal CSF from healthy animals in low numbers; not consistently present in normal or abnormal conditions
Choroid plexus cells	Indistinguishable from ependymal lining cells (see above description)	May be present in normal CSF from healthy animals in low numbers; not consistently present in normal or abnormal conditions
Subarachnoid lining cells/ leptomeningeal cells	Mononuclear cells with moderate to abundant pale basophilic cytoplasm; round to oval eccentric nuclei; uniform, delicate chromatin pattern; indistinct cytoplasm margins; single or in small clusters	May be present in CSF from healthy animals in low numbers; not consistently present in normal or abnormal conditions
Hematopoietic cells	Morphologically similar to those in bone marrow or other locations	Myeloid and erythroid precursors and erythroblastic island reported as contaminants of canine CSF with lumbar collections

Cell or Feature	Description	Significance
Eosinophils	Morphologically similar to those in peripheral blood	Occasionally cells seen in normal CSF from healthy dogs or cats
	Polymorphonuclear leukocytes with eosinophilic granules with shape characteristic for species	May be seen as a nonspecific part of an active inflammatory response Also consider parasitic, hypersensitivity or neoplastic processes (primary or metastatic)
Plasma cells	Morphologically similar to those in other locations; eccentric nuclei with prominent chromatin ("clockface" pattern); moderately abundant cytoplasm, moderately to deeply basophilic with perinuclear clear zone (Golgi apparatus)	Not present in normal CSF from healthy dogs or cats; may be part of nonspecific reactive or inflammatory process with response to antigenic stimulation
Bacteria	Morphology varies with type, may include cocci, rods of various sizes, coccobacilli or filamentous forms	Not present in normal CSF from healthy dogs or cats; may be contaminants if collection process or tube are not sterile or if CSF collected close to death; pathologic role likely if suppurative meningitis is present, and supported by intracellular location
Neural tissue	Nerve cells morphologically similar to those in nervous tissue; very large cell with prominent nucleolus, abundant cytoplasm and three to four tentacle-like cytoplasmic processes Neuropil/myelin represented by amorphous, acellular background material	Reported as contaminant in canine CSF associated with accidental puncture of spinal cord; myelin fragments may be associated with demyelination
Paracellular coiled "ribbons"	Coiled, homogeneous, basophilic material within phagocytic vacuoles	Reported in CSF obtained at postmortem; hypothesized to represent denatured myelin, myelin figures, or myelin fragments
Neoplastic cells	Abnormal cell type or number for location (benign tumors) or atypical features fulfilling criteria for malignancy (malignant tumors); morphology may vary with cell type of origin and degree of differentiation	May be primary or metastatic; presence requires communication with subarachnoid space or ventricles; absence of tumor does not rule out its presence without contribution of cells to the CSF
Fungi/Yeast/Protozoa	Appearance varies with type; may be primary or opportunistic infections	Characteristic morphology associated with various common pathologic organisms; demonstration of organisms in conjunction with clinical signs and results of other testing increases confidence in diagnosis of fungal or protozoal disease
Mitotic Figures	Recognized by characteristic nuclear configurations of cells undergoing mitosis; cell type of origin not identifiable during the mitotic cycle	Rare mitotic figures reported in normal CSF from healthy animals; presence indicates proliferative process, often neoplasia

TABLE 13–3	Differential Diagnoses Associated with Cytologic Features of Inflammation in the CSF	
Cytologic Features	**Special Considerations or Differential Diagnoses**	**Comments**
Slight to Moderate Neutrophilic Inflammation 25% to 50% neutrophils, with or without elevated CSF protein, with or without pleocytosis	Bacterial, fungal, protozoal, parasitic, rickettsial, or viral infection	Depends on species, type of infection, focal or diffuse involvement, presence of concurrent necrosis; presence of protozoa or fungi/yeast organisms or intracellular bacteria confirms diagnosis
	Neoplasia	Depends on type of neoplasm, location, presence of concurrent necrosis Neoplastic cells rarely seen in CSF
	Other noninfectious conditions	Consider traumatic, degenerative, immune-mediated, associated with metabolic conditions, ischemia
Marked Neutrophilic Inflammation (Suppurative Meningitis) Predominance of neutrophils (>50%), often with increased CSF protein	Bacterial infection	May be focal (abscess) or diffuse (meningoencephalomyelitis) Intracellular bacterial confirms diagnosis
	Severe viral encephalitis	Especially feline infectious peritonitis (FIP) in cats
	Necrotizing vasculitis	May have immune-mediated or infectious basis; Bernese mountain dogs and beagles
	Steroid responsive meningitis-arteritis	Responsive to glucocorticoids but must rule out infectious causes
	Post myelography reaction (usually within 24–48 hrs)	History of recent, previous myelography
	Neoplasms	Especially meningiomas, but may occur with any neoplasm, especially if associated with necrosis
	Trauma	History may be supportive, if trauma was observed
	Hemorrhage	History may be supportive; may have traumatic, degenerative, metabolic infectious, neoplastic or other underlying cause
	Acquired hydrocephalus	May depend on underlying cause of acquired condition

TABLE 13–3 Differential Diagnoses Associated with Cytologic Features of Inflammation in the CSF *Continued*

Cytologic Features	Special Considerations or Differential Diagnoses	Comments
Mixed Cell Inflammation with a Variety of Cell Types (No Single Cell Type Predominant) Mixture of macrophages, lymphocytes, neutrophils and sometimes plasma cells, with or without elevated CSF protein, with or without pleocytosis	Often interpreted to represent granulomatous inflammation—consider fungal, protozoal, parasitic or rickettsial infection	Presence of fungal or protozoal organisms is confirmatory
	Some idiopathic inflammatory or degenerative diseases	Especially granulomatous meningoencephalomyelitis (GME)
	Inadequately treated chronic bacterial infections or early response to antibacterial treatment	History and previous diagnosis helpful
Nonsuppurative Inflammation (Mononuclear Pleocytosis) Pleocytosis with predominance of mononuclear cells, especially lymphocytes	Viral, bacterial, fungal, protozoal, parasitic, or rickettsial infection	Especially non-FIP viral meningoencephalomyelitis in cats and canine distemper infection in dogs
	Necrotizing encephalitis of small-breed dogs	Signalment and lymphocytic predominance helpful in diagnosis but definitive diagnosis requires histopathology; not responsive to glucocorticoids
	Neoplasia	Neoplastic cells may rarely be seen in CSF
	Noninfectious or degenerative conditions	Consider GME. May require elimination of other possible causes and consideration of multiple factors in order to arrive at a clinical diagnosis
Eosinophilic Inflammation Pleocytosis with predominance of eosinophils	Parasitic, protozoal, bacterial, viral, or rickettsial infections	Uncommon manifestation reported with a variety of types of disease
	Neoplasia	Occasionally seen with neoplasia
	Hypersensitivity reaction	Consider vaccine reactions or other hypersensitivity components associated with infectious or noninfectious origin
	Inflammatory process	May be seen as part of a nonspecific inflammatory process

lymphocytes and large mononuclear (monocytoid) cells (Chrisman, 1992; Coles, 1986; Cook and DeNicola, 1988; Duncan et al., 1996; Meinkoth and Crystal, 1999; Parent and Rand, 1994; Rand, 1995). The percentages of lymphocytes and monocytoid cells may vary with the method used for cytologic preparations, but lymphocytes are re-

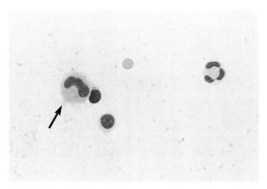

FIGURE 13–2. Cell types found in CSF. Dog. Two small mononuclear cells (lymphocytes), one large mononuclear (monocytoid) at (*arrow*), one nondegenerate neutrophil, and one erythrocyte are present. (Wright-Giemsa; ×250.)

ported to be the predominant nucleated cell type in normal canine and feline CSF by Cook and DeNicola (1988). However, Parent and Rand (1994) and Rand (1995) report monocytoid cells as the predominant type in normal CSF from healthy cats. They indicate monocytoid cells compose 69% to 100% of the nucleated cells, lymphocytes 0 to 27%, neutrophils 0 to 9%, macrophages 0 to 3%, and eosinophils 0 to less than 1% of nucleated cells (Parent and Rand, 1994; Rand, 1995). Parent and Rand (1994) describe occasional neutrophils or eosinophils as within normal limits, as long as these cell types do not represent over 10% or 1% of the nucleated cells, respectively. Chrisman (1992), Christopher et al. (1988), and Cook and DeNicola (1988) indicate that low numbers of mature, nondegenerate neutrophils are occasionally seen in normal CSF from healthy dogs and cats and that rare eosinophils may be present. Occasional choroid plexus cells, ependymal cells, meningeal lining cells, or mitotic figures may be seen in normal CSF from dogs or cats (Chrisman, 1992; Cook and DeNicola, 1988; Parent and Rand, 1994; Rand, 1995).

Accidental Puncture Contaminants

Christopher (1992) described bone marrow elements as contaminants in canine CSF associated with bone marrow aspiration during lumbar cistern collections of CSF. Neurons (Fig. 13–3A) and neurophils (Fig. 13–3B) have been reported as contaminants of canine CSF associated with accidental punc-

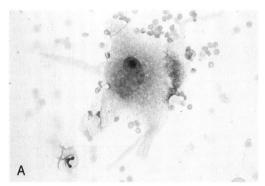

FIGURE 13–3. A, Neuron. CSF. Dog. Accidental puncture of nervous tissue during collection at the cerebellomedullary cistern demonstrating the large size of the neuron compared with a neutrophil and erythrocytes. Basophilic granular material within the neuronal cell cytoplasm is presumed to be Nissl bodies. (Wright-Giemsa; ×125.) (From Fallin CW et al: Vet Clin Pathol 25:127–129, 1996. Reprinted with permission.)

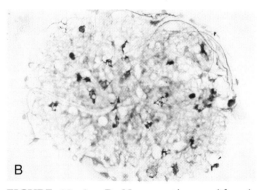

FIGURE 13–3. B, Nervous tissue with microglial cells. CSF from the same case of a dog with cervical pain as in Figure 13–3A. (Wright-Giemsa; ×125.)

ture of the spinal cord during cerebello-medullary cistern collection (Fallin et al., 1996).

Normal CSF Findings in the Presence of Disease

No abnormalities may be detected in CSF in many cases of neurologic disease, although some animals with the same conditions may have abnormalities detected in CSF (Evans, 1988). CSF abnormality is not detected in the majority of cases of idiopathic epilepsy, congenital hydrocephalus, intoxication, metabolic or functional disorders, vertebral disease, or myelomalacia (Evans, 1988). A significant proportion of cases with neurologic disease due to feline infectious peritonitis, distemper encephalitis, neoplasia or GME may have CSF that is within normal limits (Evans, 1988). Absence of cytologic abnormality does not rule out the possibility of neurologic disease that is not reflected in the CSF.

Protein Abnormalities in CSF

Elevated total protein may occur in the absence of cytologic abnormalities and may be referred to as "albuminocytologic dissociation" (Carmichael, 1998; Evans, 1988). Elevated total protein as the sole abnormality or in combination with increases in nucleated cell count and/or cytologic abnormality in CSF may occur with inflammatory, degenerative, compressive, or neoplastic disease (Carmichael, 1998). Elevated protein may occur in association with increased permeability of the blood–brain barrier, local necrosis, interruption of normal CSF flow and absorption, or intrathecal globulin production (Chrisman, 1992; Evans, 1988). Elevated CSF protein without increases in CSF nucleated cell count has been reported with viral nonsuppurative encephalomyelitis (Bichsel et al., 1984; Sorjonen, 1987; Sorjonen et al., 1989), or with neoplasia, acute spinal cord injury, and compressive spinal cord lesions (Chrisman, 1992). Evans (1988) also indicates that elevated total protein without pleocytosis may occur with neoplasia, ischemic myelopathy, seizures, fever, disc extrusion, degenerative myelopathy, myelomalacia, or GME.

Increased Cell Type Percentages without Increased Total Nucleated Cell Counts

Increased percentages of either neutrophils or eosinophils may occur without an increase in the total white cell count in a variety of neurologic disorders. If blood contamination is ruled out, increased neutrophil percentages greater than 10% to 20% (Chrisman, 1992; Meinkoth and Crystal, 1999) and eosinophil percentages greater than 1% should be considered unusual. Increased neutrophils may indicate mild or early inflammation, a lesion that does not contact the meninges or ependymal cells, or previous use of drugs such as glucocorticoids and antibiotics, which reduce the inflammatory response. Conditions to consider include degenerative intervertebral disc disease, spinal fractures, or cerebrovascular disorders such as infarcts. Increased eosinophils without increased total white blood cell (WBC) count may occur with parasite migration or protozoal disease (Meinkoth and Crystal, 1999).

Pleocytosis

Increases in the total nucleated cell count of the CSF is termed *pleocytosis*, which is further defined by the predominant cell type, that is, neutrophilic, eosinophilic, mononuclear, or mixed cell pleocytosis.

Neutrophilic Pleocytosis

Neutrophilic pleocytosis has been associated with a wide variety of active inflammatory disorders, including trauma, postmyelographic aseptic meningitis, hemorrhage, neoplasia and bacterial meningitis (Chrisman, 1992; Coles, 1986; Cook and De-Nicola, 1988; Evans, 1988). It may be seen with abscesses communicating with the ventricles or subarachnoid space, early viral infections, feline infectious peritonitis, Rocky Mountain spotted fever, discospondylitis, acquired hydrocephalus, necrosis, or GME (Evans, 1988; Chrisman, 1992). Marked neutrophilic pleocytosis is most often found with bacterial or fungal meningoencephalitis, neoplasia (Fig. 13–4), steroid-responsive meningitis, or necrotizing vasculitis (Chrisman, 1992; Evans, 1988). Demonstration of bacteria, fungi, yeast, or protozoa in CSF can confirm the presence of these infections. A variety of bacterial types, *Cryptococcus, Blastomyces, Histoplasma,* and ehrlichial organisms have been demonstrated in CSF (Berthelin et al., 1994; Chrisman, 1992; Cook and DeNicola, 1988; Meadows et al.,

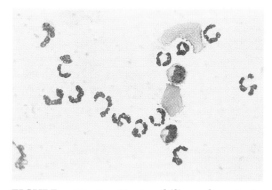

FIGURE 13–4. Neutrophilic pleocytosis. CSF. Dog. Nucleated cell count was 1018/μl and 240 mg/dl protein with a history of head tilt and hemiplegia related to a cranial meningioma. Nondegenerate neutrophils composed 83% of the cell population. (Wright-Giemsa; ×250.)

1992; Meinkoth et al., 1998). Parasites such as *Toxocara canis, Dirofilaria immitis, Cuterebra* larva, or *Cysticercus* that may cause neurologic disease have not been reported to be seen in CSF cytology preparations (Chrisman, 1992). The presence of marked neutrophilic pleocytosis or increasing numbers of neutrophils in sequential CSF collections has been reported to be an unfavorable prognostic finding (Evans, 1988). Neoplasia should be considered as the most likely diagnosis in a cat more than 7 years of age with progressive clinical neurologic signs of greater than 4 weeks' duration (Rand et al., 1994).

Feline infectious peritonitis (FIP), a coronavirus infection, is a common cause of neutrophilic pleocytosis in the cat (Fig. 13–5). The main neurologic signs are depression, tetraparesis, head tilt, nystagmus, and intention tremor (Baroni and Heinold, 1995). It accounted for 44% of 61 feline cases of inflammatory CNS disease (Rand et al., 1994). Parent and Rand (1994) indicate that marked neutrophilic pleocytosis with a nucleated count of more than 100 cells/μl and neutrophils greater than 50% is commonly seen with FIP, along with increased CSF protein (usually greater than 200 mg/dl). They indicate a high probability of FIP if a cat is less than 4 years of age and shows multifocal neurologic signs referable to the cerebellum and/or brainstem, protracted course of illness and CSF protein greater than 200 mg/dl. Later in the course of the disease, a mixed cellular population may be found with large mononuclear cells and lymphocytes present to a significant degree (Fig. 13–6). Only 11 of 19 cats in one study (Baroni and Heinold, 1995) demonstrated high serum antibody titers, indicating that CSF analysis was essential for a correct diagnosis. Non-FIP viral meningoencephalitis that involved 37% of the inflammatory cases reported by Rand et al.

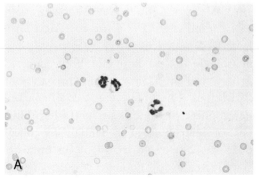

FIGURE 13–5. A, Neutrophilic pleocytosis. CSF. Cat. This direct smear is made from fluid from a kitten with a 5-day duration of ataxia. The case was diagnosed as FIP by positive titer and histologic examination. Numerous erythrocytes and several nondegenerate neutrophils characterize the cells present. Acute hemorrhage was evident but is not demonstrated in this field. (Wright; ×125.)

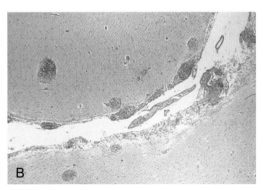

FIGURE 13–5. B, Same cat as in Figure 13–5A. Section of midbrain and third ventricle demonstrating multifocal perivascular infiltrates in a cat with FIP. The proximity of the infiltrates to the ventricle contributed to the neutrophilic pleocytosis. (H & E; ×10.)

(1994) was considered most likely with cats less than 3 years of age having progressive neurologic disease and focal neurologic signs referable to the thalamocortex. In these cases the nucleated cell count was less than 50 cells/μl and CSF protein was less than 100 mg/dl. Non-FIP viral meningoen-

cephalitis usually carries a favorable prognosis for recovery (Parent and Rand, 1994).

Steroid-responsive suppurative meningitis-arteritis (Fig. 13–7) has been recognized in young to middle-aged dogs that present with signs of fever, cervical pain, hyperesthesia, and paresis. CSF pleocytosis is often greater than 500 cells/μl with greater than 75% nondegenerate neutrophils present if glucocorticoids have not been recently administered (Chrisman, 1992). Bacteria are not observed or cultured and improvement is often seen within 72 hours following glucocorticoid administration; long-term prognosis is good. One report investigated the immunologic response in these cases finding IgG and IgA synthesis intrathecally and suggested the humoral response is primary, rather than the result of a generalized immune complex disease (Tipold et al., 1995).

Necrotizing vasculitis. Meric et al. (1985) described a syndrome of aseptic suppurative meningitis in young Bernese mountain dogs

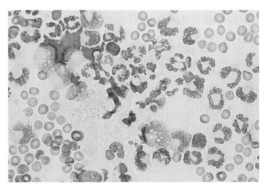

FIGURE 13–6. Mixed cell pleocytosis with neutrophilic predominance. CSF. Cat. Increased numbers of large mononuclear cells consistent with macrophages were present in a cat with fever, high titers for FIP, and histopathologic support of FIP at necropsy. Duration of disease was several months, accounting for the more mononuclear response than the case in Figure 13–5. (Wright-Giemsa; ×250.) (Courtesy of Rick Alleman, Gainesville, FL.)

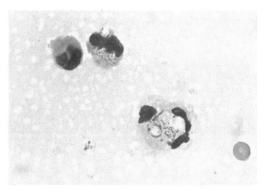

FIGURE 13–7. Neutrophilic pleocytosis. CSF. Dog. Generalized nonseptic inflammatory response in a 1-year-old dog exhibiting fever, cervical, thoracic, and lumbar pain. Nucleated cell count was 106/μl with 41 mg/dl protein and 3700 RBC/μl. Three nondegenerate neutrophils, one large mononuclear cell, and one lymphocyte are present. Multiple joints were similarly affected in this case. An immune-mediated corticosteroid-responsive meningitis was suspected. (Wright-Giemsa; $\times$125.)

FIGURE 13–8. Neutrophilic pleocytosis. CSF. Cat. Direct smear of cloudy CSF indicated increased cellularity with many degenerate neutrophils present. Associated with the karyolytic neutrophils shown are intracellular small rod-shaped bacteria that were cultured as *Enterobacter* sp. (Wright; $\times$500.)

involving the leptomeningeal arteries. Animals presented with severe cervical pain and neurologic deficits. Total WBC counts are generally greater than 1000 cells/μl. A similar condition has been reported in beagles and in both conditions, nondegenerate neutrophils predominate. Clinical improvement occurred with corticosteroid administration.

Bacterial meningoencephalitis (Fig. 13–8) is suspected if greater than 75% neutrophils are present in the CSF regardless of the total cell count. Bacteremia is usually the cause with septic emboli to the brain as a result. Untreated cases often produce marked pleocytosis with greater than 1000 cells/μl. Intracellular location of bacteria and accompanying inflammation are particularly important in eliminating the possibility of bacterial contamination associated with nonsterile collection technique or nonsterile collection tubes. Neutrophils affected may display mild to severe karyolysis.

Eosinophilic Pleocytosis

Cerebrospinal fluid pleocytosis that is predominantly eosinophilic is rare (Chrisman, 1992). Increased eosinophils in CSF may be present in association with a nonspecific acute inflammatory response, but also can be seen with parasitic, hypersensitivity, neoplastic processes, protozoal infection including toxoplasmosis (Fig. 13–9) and neosporosis, or *Cryptococcus* infection (Chrisman, 1992; Cook and DeNicola, 1988). Steroid-responsive meningoencephalitis with a predominance of eosinophils has been described in dogs and cats (Chrisman, 1992). Sometimes migrating internal parasites, *Prototheca* infection, canine distemper virus infection, or rabies may cause eosinophilic pleocytosis (Chrisman, 1992).

Steroid-responsive eosinophilic meningitis (Fig. 13–10) has been reported in dogs (Smith-Maxie et al., 1989) and a cat (Schultze et al., 1986). Finding greater than 80% eosinophils with mild to marked pleocytosis present and finding no evidence of protozoal, parasitic, or fungal infection usually supports the diagnosis. In the canine

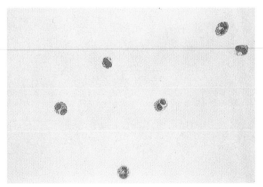

FIGURE 13–9. Eosinophilic pleocytosis. CSF. Dog. This acutely paraparetic animal with upper motor neuron dysfunction to the rear legs was diagnosed as having toxoplasmosis by serum titer. Total WBC count was 124/μl with high normal protein. Eosinophils accounted for 98% of the cell population. Peripheral eosinophilia was not evident. (Wright-Giemsa; ×125.)

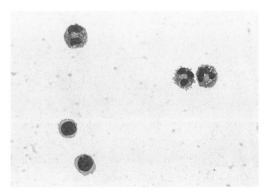

FIGURE 13–10. Eosinophilic pleocytosis. CSF. Dog. This sample is from a golden retriever whose CSF cell count was 43/μl and whose protein was 77 mg/dl. The cell differential indicated 43% eosinophils, 50% lymphocytes, and 7% large mononuclear phagocytes. Three eosinophils and two small lymphocytes are shown. An idiopathic eosinophilic meningoencephalitis associated with this breed was suspected. (Wright-Giemsa; ×250.)

study, golden retrievers were over-represented and may suggest a breed predisposition to this condition. Animals usually respond to glucocorticoid therapy with dramatic decreases in cell numbers and

changes in differential percentages. An allergic or type I hypersensitivity reaction is suspected in some cases (Schultze et al., 1986).

Mononuclear Pleocytosis

Mononuclear pleocytosis of CSF usually presents with increased lymphocytes in viral, protozoal, or fungal infection, uremia, intoxication, vaccine reaction, GME, and discospondylitis. It may be seen with necrotizing encephalitis, steroid-responsive meningoencephalomyelitis, ehrlichiosis, or treated bacterial meningoencephalitis (Chrisman, 1992; Evans, 1988). However, monocytoid/macrophage cells may also predominant in these conditions and most commonly with cryptococcosis (Figs. 13–11 and 13–12). Mononuclear pleocytosis was noted in two cats with cuterebriasis (Glass et al., 1998). A recent report of necrotizing meningoencephalitis in a young miniature poodle dog demonstrated the predominance

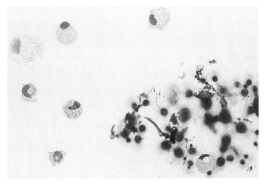

FIGURE 13–11. Cryptococcosis with mononuclear pleocytosis. CSF. Dog. Clusters of basophilic-staining extracellular yeast forms measuring approximately 10 to 20 μm in diameter are present. The fluid contained a total nucleated cell count of 60/μl of which 85% were mononuclear phagocytes. Several mononuclear cells are pictured that have abundant foamy to vacuolated pale cytoplasm indicating reactivity. (Wright-Giemsa; ×125.)

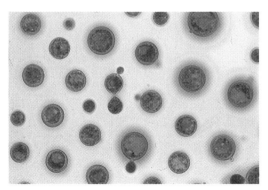

FIGURE 13–12. Cryptococcosis. CSF. Dog. These spherical organisms display frequent budding. (New methylene blue; ×250.) (Courtesy of Rick Alleman, Gainesville, FL.)

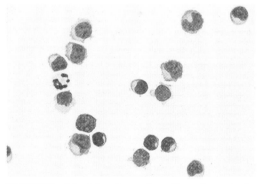

FIGURE 13–13. B, Same case as Figure 13–13A. Several vacuolated, phagocytic macrophages with engulfed erythrocytes (arrows) are shown. (Wright-Giemsa; ×250.)

and pleocytosis of large granular lymphocytes (Garma-Avina and Tyler, 1999). The most frequent noninflammatory neurologic diseases of the CNS in the cat are neoplasia and ischemic encephalopathy, which usually present with an elevated CSF protein and slight lymphocytic pleocytosis or normal nucleated cell counts (Rand et al., 1994). Hemorrhagic conditions may be accompanied by a mononuclear pleocytosis com-

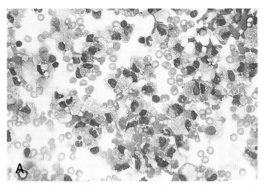

FIGURE 13–13. A, Acute hemorrhage with mononuclear pleocytosis. CSF. Dog. This animal had a history of seizures and dementia. Nucleated cell count was 190/μl and protein 72 mg/dl. Mononuclear phagocytes accounted for 91% of the cell population. (Wright-Giemsa; ×125.)

FIGURE 13–14. Lymphocytic pleocytosis. CSF. Dog. This example of pug encephalitis is characterized by pleocytosis (265 cells/μl) with lymphocytic predominance (87%). Lymphocytes shown are small to medium size with normal morphology. (Wright-Giemsa; ×250.)

posed of activated macrophages (Fig. 13–13).

Necrotizing encephalitis in small breed dogs (Figs. 13–14 and 13–15). Pug dogs, Maltese dogs, and Yorkshire terriers are reported to demonstrate multifocal to massive necrosis and nonsuppurative inflammation of the cerebrum and meninges that is fatal or leads to euthanasia (Cordy and Holliday, 1989; Uchida et al., 1999; Stalis et al., 1995; Tipold et al., 1993). These dogs are usually less than 4 years of age and present fre-

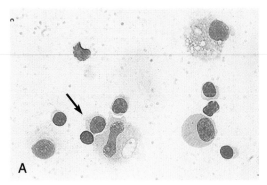

FIGURE 13–15. A, Lymphocytic pleocytosis. CSF. Dog. This 6-year-old Maltese dog presented with acute seizures that were unresponsive to glucocorticoids and anticonvulsants. Fluid indicated total nucleated cell count of 430/μl and 3+ protein on chemistry dipstick. Lymphocytes accounted for 82%, large mononuclear cells 11%, and nondegenerate neutrophils 7% of the cell population. Shown are many lymphocytes, one of which is a granular lymphocyte (*arrow*) and three large mononuclear cells demonstrating various nuclear shapes and cytoplasmic features. (Wright-Giemsa; ×250.)

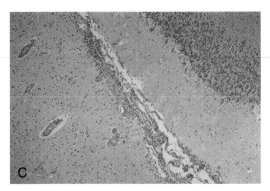

FIGURE 13–15. C, Same case as in Figure 13–15A of a Maltese dog with nonsuppurative necrotizing meningoencephalitis. Dense accumulations of mononuclear cells along the meninges that extend into the parenchyma. There is gliosis and neuronal necrosis evident in the parenchyma. (H & E; ×25.)

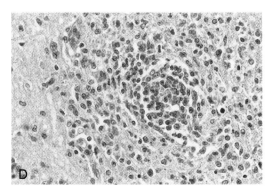

FIGURE 13–15. D, Same case as in Figure 13–15A. Severe focally extensive, perivascular meningoencephalitis. Cells present consist mostly of lymphocytes and plasma cells, with smaller numbers of large mononuclear phagocytes. (H & E; ×125.)

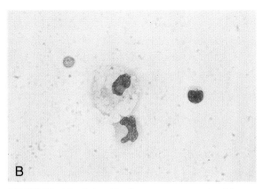

FIGURE 13–15. B, Same case as in Figure 13–15A. Mononuclear pleocytosis is evident in this field with two large mononuclear cells, one of which displays marked cytoplasmic vacuolization consistent with demyelination. One granular lymphocyte and one erythrocyte are also present. (Wright-Giemsa; ×250.)

quently with seizures, depression, and ataxia; they do not respond significantly to glucocorticoids. The CSF presents with mild to moderate pleocytosis, generally greater than 200 cells/μl, and these are predominantly lymphocytes, generally greater than 70%. CSF protein concentration is often greater than 50 mg/dl. The cause is considered unknown but some pug dogs appear to exhibit an autoantibody against astrocytes that has been detected in the CSF by indirect immunofluorescence assay, confirming an immune-mediated syndrome in those dogs (Uchida et al., 1999). A similar population of cells may be found in the CSF in GME necessitating a histologic examination of the brain to detect the necrotizing lesions.

Granulomatous meningoencephalomyelitis (GME) (Figs. 13–16 to 13–18) is an idiopathic inflammatory disease of the CNS in primarily young to middle-aged female dogs (Sorjonen, 1990). A study of 42 dogs found a high percentage of affected animals were toy or terrier breeds (Munana and Luttgen, 1998). Clinical signs of fever, ataxia, tetraparesis, cervical hyperesthesia, and seizures

have been reported (Sorjonen, 1990). Designation of the clinical signs into focal or multifocal was helpful in determining prognosis, with dogs having focal clinical signs surviving longer (Munana and Luttgen, 1998). Lesions are histologically found in both white and gray matter of the brain and predominantly the white matter of the caudal brainstem and spinal cord (Sorjonen,

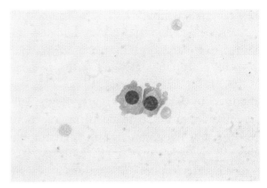

FIGURE 13–17. Flaming plasma cells. CSF. Dog. High-normal nucleated cell count and increased protein (361 mg/dl) were present in a suspected case of granulomatous meningoencephalomyelitis. The term "flaming" is used to describe the red-pink periphery of the cytoplasm. (Wright-Giemsa; ×250.)

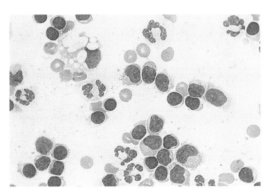

FIGURE 13–16. Lymphocytic pleocytosis. CSF. Dog. This young dog presented with neck pain. Shown are numerous small and medium-size lymphocytes (70%), several nondegenerate neutrophils (18%), and fewer numbers of large mononuclear cells (12%), one of which demonstrates large cytoplasmic vacuoles. Total WBC count was 208/µl and protein increased to 256 mg/dl. The dog died 5 days later and histopathology indicated an idiopathic condition with moderate to marked, multifocal, nonsuppurative meningoencephalitis and mild multifocal vacuolization and neuronal necrosis. (Wright-Giemsa; ×250.)

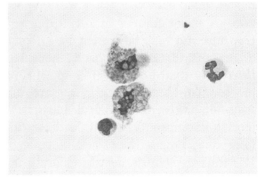

FIGURE 13–18. Granular large mononuclear phagocytes. CSF. Dog. Highly granulated and phagocytic appearing cells in a case of suspected granulomatous meningoencephalomyelitis. (Wright-Giemsa; ×250.) (Courtesy of Rick Alleman, Gainesville, FL.)

1990). The CSF may have a mild to moderate lymphocytic, mixed cell pleocytosis, or occasionally neutrophilic predominance (Chrisman, 1992). Nucleated cell counts had a median of 250 cells/μl (range 0 to 11,840), with the majority having counts greater than 100 cells/μl (Munana and Luttgen, 1998). In this same study, dogs with multifocal signs all had pleocytosis, whereas some of the dogs with focal signs had normal cell counts. The predominant cell type was lymphocytic (52%), monocytic (21%), neutrophilic (10%), and mixed cell (17%) (Munana and Luttgen, 1998). CSF protein is variably elevated, with a mean value of 256 mg/dl (range 13 to 1119) as reported by Baily and Higgins (1986). Differentiation must be made from infectious diseases and idiopathic necrotizing encephalitis, all of which may appear similar cytologically. Electrophoretic separation of CSF proteins in GME has shown increases in the alpha and beta globulin fractions (Sorjonen, 1990); however, these fractions are generally decreased in canine distemper (Chrisman, 1992). Both GME and canine distemper may have increased gamma globulins. Lesions in GME often involve parenchymal granulomas, perivascular cuffing, and meningeal infiltrates. Necrosis and demyelination are major features in necrotizing encephalitis and may be present to a minor extent in GME. GME cases with lesions that involve the caudal brainstem or spinal cord progress slowly, permitting longer survival. Radiation has been recommended as an adjunct to treatment, especially in dogs with focal clinical signs (Munana and Luttgen, 1998). The disease is poorly responsive to glucocorticoids, although an immune-mediated etiology has been suggested (Kipar et al., 1998). In this study, they determined that the GME inflammatory lesions are composed of predominantly CD3 antigen-positive T-lymphocytes and a heterogeneous population of activated macrophages with MHC class II expression suggesting a T-cell-mediated delayed-type hypersensitivity of an organ-specific autoimmune disease (Kipar et al., 1998).

Canine distemper infection (Figs. 13–19 and 13–20). The CSF in these cases exhibits a lymphocytic pleocytosis similar to that reported for steroid-responsive meningoencephalomyelitis. Cell counts may be variable, ranging from normal to greater than 50 cells/μl, and lymphocytes represent the predominant cell population, accounting for greater than 60% of the cells present. A report by Abate et al. (1998) indicated that the CSF in distemper cases had an increase in macrophages, an increase in total protein concentration, an increase of the gamma-globulin fraction by electrophoretic separation, and the presence of cellular inclusions.

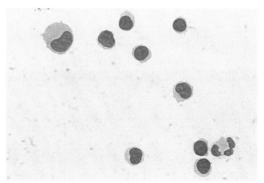

FIGURE 13–19. Lymphocytic pleocytosis. CSF. Dog. Pleocytosis (292 cells/μl), elevated CSF protein concentration (126 mg/dl), and lymphocyte predominance (72%) were detected in a cerebellomedullary cistern sample from a dog with acute ataxia and head tilt. Canine distemper titer levels were present in the CSF suggesting a viral-induced encephalopathy, which responded completely by 6 months with glucocorticoid therapy. Shown are numerous small lymphocytes, one neutrophil, and one large mononuclear cell. (Wright-Giemsa; ×250.)

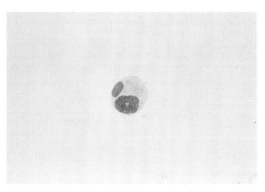

FIGURE 13–20. Distemper inclusion. CSF. Dog. Eosinophilic inclusion within a large mononuclear cell from a dog diagnosed with canine distemper. (Wright-Giemsa; ×250.) (From Alleman AR, Christopher MM, Steiner DA, et al: Identification of intracytoplasmic inclusion bodies in mononuclear cells from the cerebrospinal fluid of a dog with canine distemper. Vet Pathol 29:84-85, 1992. Reprinted with permission.)

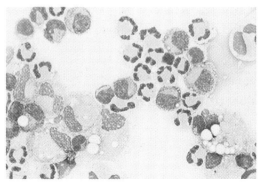

FIGURE 13–21. Mixed cell pleocytosis. CSF. Dog. This sample is from an adult female Cairn terrier with 4-month history of neck pain and muscle spasms that were responsive to glucocorticoids. Mononuclear phagocytes (52%) were mostly reactive as indicated by a foamy or vacuolated cytoplasm and evidence of phagocytized debris. Neutrophils composed 35% and lymphocytes 13% of the total cell population. (Wright-Giemsa; ×250.)

Diagnosis often involves suggestive history, clinical signs, and evidence of serum or CSF IgM in response to active infection by canine distemper virus.

Mixed Cell Pleocytosis

Pleocytosis with a mixture of cell types may be seen with a variety of underlying causes including GME, FIP, canine distemper, steroid-responsive meningoencephalomyelitis (Fig. 13–21), toxoplasmosis, neosporosis, encephalitozoonosis, cryptococcosis, blastomycosis, aspergillosis, histoplasmosis, degenerative disc disease, ischemia, and neoplasia (Chrisman, 1992; Meadows et al., 1992).

CENTRAL NERVOUS SYSTEM TISSUES

Response to Tissue Injury

In addition to blood contamination encountered during collection, the presence of erythrocytes in a cytologic preparation may result from cranial or spinal hemorrhage. Macrophages with engulfed erythrocytes (Fig. 13–22) may be seen in cases of acute

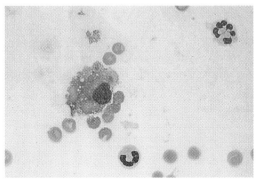

FIGURE 13–22. Erythrophagocytosis. CSF. Dog. This lumbar site collection was bloody with nucleated cells 84/μl, RBC 7000/μl, and protein 104 mg/dl. A car-related injury caused a thoracic spinal fracture that contributed to the acute hemorrhage exhibited in this example. A macrophage with engulfed red cells is present along with a hypersegmented neutrophil. (Wright-Giemsa; ×250.) (Courtesy of Rick Alleman, Gainesville, FL.)

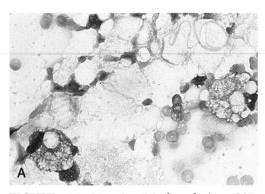

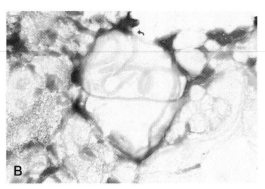

FIGURE 13–23. A, Myelomalacia. CSF. Dog. Patient presented with acute paraplegic and absent deep pain related to a disc protrusion at L1-2. A myelogram confirmed dorsal spinal compression from T11 to L1. A cerebellomedullary cistern sample was taken 4 days postsurgery at the time of euthanasia. Pictured are two macrophages with large lipid-filled cytoplasmic vacuoles and basophilic ribbon material extracellularly. Necropsy confirmed a necrotic spinal cord in the areas shown compressed on the presurgery myelogram. (Wright-Giemsa; ×250.)

FIGURE 13–23. B, Myelin figures. CSF. Dog. Same case as in Figure 13–23A. Pictured are basophilic ribbon structures that likely represent phospholipids, derived from damaged cytomembranes. (Wright-Giemsa; ×250.)

spinal cord injury such as intervertebral disc herniation, neoplasia, inflammation, or degenerative conditions. Chronic hemorrhage will be indicated by the presence of hemosiderin-laden macrophages.

Homogeneous "ribbons" of basophilic material hypothesized to represent degenerated myelin, as myelin figures or myelin fragments (Fig. 13–23), have been reported in a postmortem collection of CSF from a dog (Fallin et al., 1996). Spinal cord infarction with diffuse myelomalacia in a dog resulted in the presence of foamy macrophages in the CSF (Mesher et al., 1996). Luxol fast blue staining of the amorphous eosinophilic material found within the macrophages was positive in this case, suggestive of myelin. Other demyelinating conditions such as degenerative myelopathy may present with free myelin (Fig. 13–24).

Another response to neural tissue injury in the brain and spinal cord is the proliferation and hypertrophy of the resident neuroglial cells, which include the astrocyte, a supporting cell with branched cellular projections (Fig. 13–25).

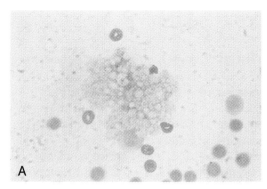

FIGURE 13–24. A, Myelin. CSF. Dog. Mixed-breed dog with a history of degenerative myelopathy with normal nucleated cell count and increased protein (62 mg/dl). Activated, phagocytic macrophages were present (not shown). Collections of eosinophilic foamy material are shown extracellularly. (Wright-Giemsa; ×250.)

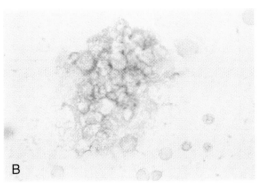

FIGURE 13–24. B, Same case as in Figure 13–24A. Extracellular material stained positive for myelin. Demyelination was suspected in this dog. (Luxol fast blue; ×250.)

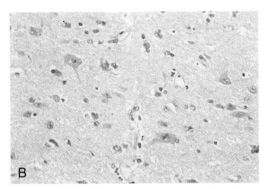

FIGURE 13–25. B, Same case as in Figure 13–25A. MRI revealed an intracranial mass. Tissue biopsy revealed normal gray matter with hypertrophied astrocytes, which is a nonspecific reaction. Although neoplastic cells were not found, adjacent neoplasia could not be ruled out. (H & E; ×125.)

With neoplasia, more often the protein concentration is elevated, with only occasional neoplastic cells present in the CSF. This will depend on the location of the mass with its proximity to the ventricle, its involvement with the meninges, or its com-

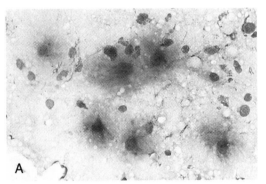

FIGURE 13–25. A, Astrocytosis. Brain aspirate. Cat. Six large cells with a wispy basophilic cytoplasm are evident in this aspirate from a cat with a 14-day progression of dementia and head pressing. Nuclei are round with a single small prominent nucleolus and the nuclear-to-cytoplasmic ratio is mildly increased. Cytologically, a neoplasm was suspected. (Wright-Giemsa; ×125.)

Cystic and Neoplastic Masses

Rare developmental defects have been demonstrated within the brain (Howard-Martin and Bowles, 1988) and in one case the CSF contained numerous mature squamous epithelium, consistent with an epidermoid cyst (Fig. 13–26).

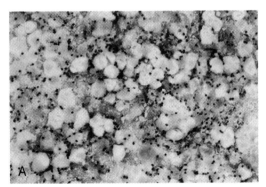

FIGURE 13–26. A, Epidermoid cyst. CSF. Dog. Direct smear of creamy opaque fluid with a nucleated cell count of 80,000/μl taken from the cerebellomedullary cistern of a dog with a 3-month duration of seizures. Numerous large blue-green cells are evident at low magnification. (Romanowsky-type stain; ×50.) (From a glass slide submitted by Joseph Spano to the 1988 ASVCP case review.)

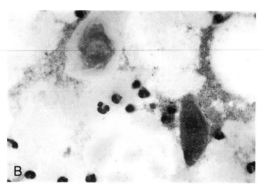

FIGURE 13–26. B, Same case as in Figure 13–26A. Squamous epithelium are present as keratinized (upper left) and intermediate (lower right) squamous epithelium along with numerous nondegenerate neutrophils. (Romanowsky-type stain; ×250.) (From a glass slide submitted by Joseph Spano to the 1988 ASVCP case review.)

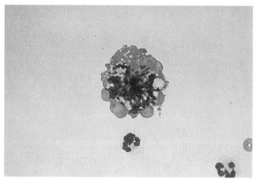

FIGURE 13–27. Abnormal mitotic figure. CSF. Dog. Fluid contained 142 nucleated cells/μl, protein 130 mg/dl, and mixed pleocytosis. Mitotic figures were present in low numbers in fluid taken from a dog with a focal intramedullary lesion at the thoracolumbar junction. Cytologically, neoplasia or reactive histiocytes was suspected. (Wright-Giemsa; ×250.) (Courtesy of Rick Alleman, Gainesville, FL.)

munication with the subarachnoid space in order to have access to the CSF. Some reparative or reactive processes may mimic malignancy. However, sufficient numbers of cells and their morphology, in combination with clinical history, presentation, diagnostic

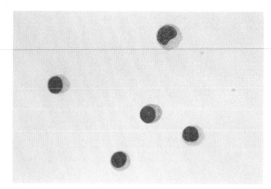

FIGURE 13–28. Lymphocytic pleocytosis. CSF. Cat. Cerebellomedullary collection contained 60 nucleated cells/μl, protein 140 mg/dl, and 80% lymphocytes in a cat with hindlimb paresis, urinary and fecal incontinence, and flaccid anal tone and tail. Intermediate-sized lymphocytes predominate in the field shown. Myelogram revealed a lumbar spinal cord mass that was cytologically diagnosed as large cell lymphoma. (Wright-Giemsa; ×250.) (Courtesy of Rick Alleman, Gainesville, FL.)

imaging (radiography, magnetic resonance imaging (MRI), and/or computed tomography (CT)), and results of other tests may be sufficient to provide a high degree of confidence that malignancy is present. These tests may be sufficiently specific as to suggest most likely cell type of origin (Roszel, 1972). Use of a membrane-filtration technique may increase the probability of demonstrating neoplastic cells in CSF preparations (Chrisman, 1994; Roszel, 1972).

The presence of mitotic cells in the CSF is unusual and often indicates a proliferative population such as a neoplasm (Fig. 13–27). The presence of immature lymphocytes is highly diagnostic for the presence of CNS lymphoma (Figs. 13–28 to 13–30). Well-differentiated lymphoid malignancies may not be readily distinguished from a lymphocytic pleocytosis (Fig. 13–31). Other round cell tumors are less common and include encephalic plasma cell tumors (Fig. 13–32)

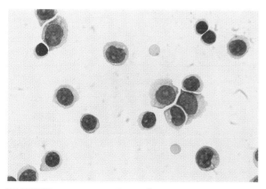

FIGURE 13–29. Lymphoma. CSF. Dog. Clinical signs involved a head tilt with ataxia of 3 months' duration. Increased protein (170 mg/dl) and pleocytosis (1417 cells/μl) were present in the clear fluid from the cerebellomedullary site. A mixed population of small well-differentiated lymphocytes and large lymphoid blast cells (greater than 50%) together accounted for 99% of the cell population. Blast cells often contain a single prominent nucleolus. (Wright-Giemsa; ×250.)

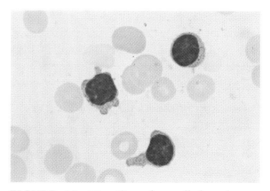

FIGURE 13–31. Granular cell lymphoma. CSF. Dog. Shown are three granular cell lymphocytes found in fluid collected from the cerebellomedullary cistern from a dog with granular cell lymphocyte leukemia that originated within the spleen. Two months later the dog presented with dementia and cerebellar signs. The fluid had moderate pleocytosis (32 cells/μl), increased protein (69 mg/dl), few erythrocytes (520/μl) with 91% lymphocytes. (Wright-Giemsa; ×500.)

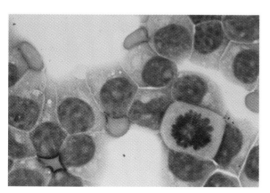

FIGURE 13–30. Lymphoma. CSF. Dog. Cream-colored CSF from the cerebellomedullary cistern of a dog with vestibular deficits. The fluid had marked pleocytosis of 109,400 nucleated cells/μl and increased protein of 220 mg/dl. A monomorphic population composing 92% of the cells involved large lymphoid blast cells with a prominent single nucleolus. Pictured are the blast cells along with a normal appearing mitotic figure. (Wright; ×500.)

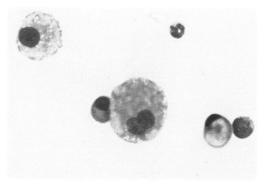

FIGURE 13–32. Plasma cell tumor. CSF. Dog. Two large mononuclear cells and two plasmacytoid cells are shown from the spinal fluid with marked mononuclear pleocytosis (27,600 nucleated cells/μl) and increased protein (greater than 2000 mg/dl). A primary encephalic plasma cell tumor involving the brainstem was diagnosed at necropsy with diagnostic support by electron microscopy and immunocytochemistry. (Wright-Giemsa; ×250.)

as described by Sheppard et al. (1997) and/ or histiocytic-appearing neoplasms (Fig. 13–33), which are difficult to distinguish from GME.

Neoplasms of the Meninges and Nerve Sheaths

Tumors that arise from the pia mater, arachnoid, or dura mater are termed *meningiomas.* These are the most common intracranial tumor in dogs and cats. The tumors are derived from leptomeningocytes that associate with neural crest tissue and have both epithelial and fibroblastic ultrastructural characteristics. As a result, these tumors have several variant forms that are found both in cervical and lumbar regions of the spinal cord as well as intracranially (Fingeroth et al., 1987; Zimmerman et al., 2000). Spinal cord meningiomas are mostly extramedullary but few reports note the ra-

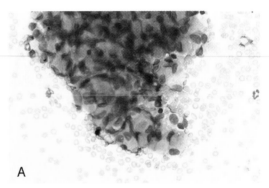

FIGURE 13–34. A, Meningioma. CSF. Dog. Large clump of cells in a sample taken from the cerebellomedullary cistern of a dog having a spinal cord lesion in the C1-2 region that presented with weakness. (Wright-Giemsa; ×125.)

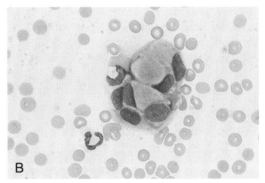

FIGURE 13–34. B, Same case as in Figure 13–34A. Higher magnification of the cell clusters showing plump cells with oval to round eccentric nuclei and occasional prominent nucleoli. The cytoplasm contains an eosinophilic secretory material. Necropsy confirmed the presence of a locally extensive meningioma. (Wright-Giemsa; ×250.)

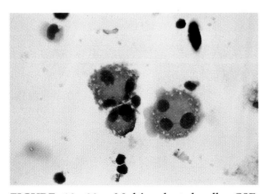

FIGURE 13–33. Multinucleated cells. CSF. Dog. A tumor of unknown origin in the area of the thalamus produced clinical signs of pain initially and later tetraparesis. The fluid had mild pleocytosis (21 nucleated cells/μl) and elevated protein (70 mg/dl). Large mononuclear cells (59%) predominated followed by lymphocytes (37%). The pleomorphism of the large mononuclear cells along with many giant multinucleated forms as shown supported a neoplastic process rather than an inflammatory disease. (Wright; ×100.)

diographic presentation of them as intramedullary (Hopkins et al., 1995; Hay et al., 1987). Of all primary brain tumors in dogs, meningiomas had the highest prevalence of pleocytosis, with a predominance of neutrophils often associated with necrosis (Bailey and Higgins, 1986). The meningioma was unique of all the tumors reviewed in this

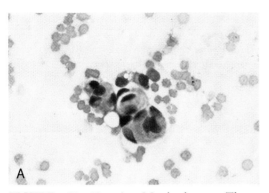

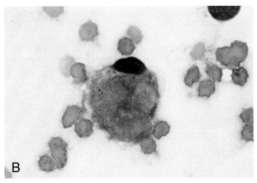

FIGURE 13–35. A, Meningioma. Tissue imprint. Dog. A spinal cord mass from a dog with a 2-year history of neck pain and front leg paresis was obtained at surgery. Cytologic features demonstrate cohesive ball formation with epithelial-like appearance. (Wright; ×100.)

FIGURE 13–35. B, Same case as in Figure 13–35A. Individual meningeal cell with histiocytic appearance. The cytoplasm is abundant with eosinophilic secretory material that was positive for acid mucopolysaccharides. (Wright; ×500.)

study being the only tumor with CSF nucleated cell counts greater than 50/μl. Myelography, MRI, and CT are imaging tools used currently to identify tumors of the brain and spinal cord. Fine-needle aspirations, crush preparations (Vernau et al., 1997), and incisional cutting needles (Dr. Simon Platt, personal communication, 2000) have been used to obtain cytologic and tissue samples for biopsy. The cytologic features of meningiomas have been discussed in several reports (Zimmerman et al., 2000; Hopkins et al., 1995; Altman et al., 1989; Raskin, 1984). Tumors with a sarcomatous appearance include one with a disseminated nature reported by Hay et al. (1987). Two examples of spinal cord meningiomas with a meningotheliomatous appearance are shown in Figures 13–34 and 13–35. One spinal cord meningioma with a spindle cell cytologic appearance having a psammomatous histologic appearance is shown in Figure 13–36.

Tumors of the nerve sheaths may be encountered in cytologic preparations. These are most often associated with peripheral nerve roots and include those of the neural crest-derived Schwann cell that assists in myelination and fibroblastic connective tissue cells that surround nerve bundles. A schwannoma is benign tumor that stains positive for S-100. A benign nerve sheath

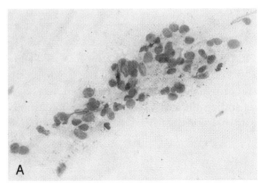

FIGURE 13–36. A, Meningioma. Tissue imprint. Dog. Progressive quadriparesis was present with a circular lesion on MRI suggesting an intramedullary disease. Large cellular aggregates of mesenchymal-appearing cells are shown against a pink finely granular background. (Wright-Giemsa; ×125.)

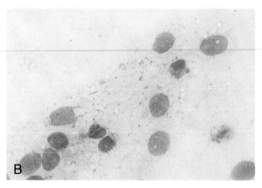

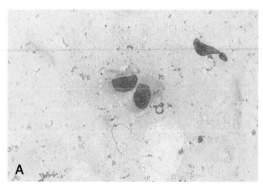

FIGURE 13–36. B, Same case as in Figure 13–36A. Higher magnification of a meningioma demonstrating the round to oval nucleus with finely granular chromatin, small nucleoli, and lightly basophilic cytoplasm that forms wispy tails. A finely granular eosinophilic material surrounds the cells and is seen within the cytoplasm as well. (Wright-Giemsa; ×250.)

FIGURE 13–37. A, Benign nerve sheath tumor. Tissue imprint. Dog. Two intact plump spindle cells demonstrate minimal anaplastic features. A compressive extradural lesion was found in the spinal canal at the nerve root region of C2-3. Clinical presentation included tetraparesis, ataxia, cervical pain, and Horner syndrome. (Wright-Giemsa; ×250.)

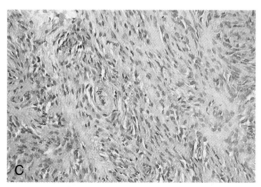

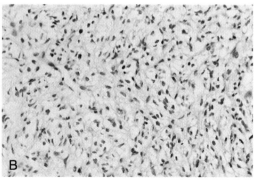

FIGURE 13–36. C, Same case as in Figure 13–36A. Interweaving bundles of spindle cells are prominent with dense collagenous bands separating the cells. A small psammoma body with presumed calcified center is present (left center). (H & E; ×100.)

FIGURE 13–37. B, Same case as in Figure 13–37A. Neoplastic mesenchymal cells with eosinophilic fibrillary cell borders are arranged loosely within a fibroblastic stroma. (H & E; ×125.)

tumor is shown in Figure 13–37. Malignant nerve sheath tumors may be locally extensive and recur more often. The histologic distinction between malignant fibroblasts and malignant Schwann cells is not readily discernible without immunohistochemistry and electron microscopy. A presumed neu-

rofibrosarcoma is shown in Figure 13–38. Cytologically, the benign nerve sheath cells are similar-appearing individualized, spindle or fusiform in shape with pale-blue cytoplasm that lacks well-defined cell borders. Nuclei are elongate to oval with small inconspicuous nucleoli. Malignant cells appear

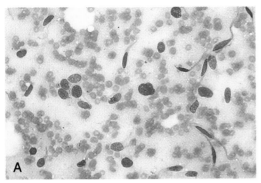

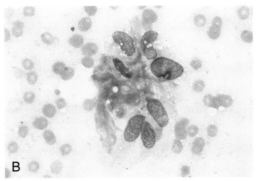

FIGURE 13–38. A, Malignant nerve sheath tumor. Tissue imprint. Dog. Clinical presentation included paraparesis that progressed to tetraparesis. A mass within the spinal canal at the C2-3 nerve root was resected but recurred 2 months later. Spindle cells predominate with two populations present. Some cells have elongated fusiform nuclei and others have plump round to oval nuclei. The cytoplasm forms tails more distinct on the more elongated cells. (Wright-Giemsa; ×125.)

FIGURE 13–38. B, Same case as in Figure 13–38A. Aggregate of neoplastic cells with associated amorphous eosinophilic collagenous stroma. Cells have oval nuclei with coarse chromatin, small distinct nucleoli, and vacuolated scant pale blue cytoplasm. Histologic diagnosis was neurofibrosarcoma. (Wright-Giemsa; ×250.)

oval to round with anisokaryosis, coarse chromatin, and prominent nucleoli, with frequent mitotic figures present.

Gliomas (Neoplasms of Neuroglial and Neuroepithelial Origin)

The neuroglial cells include the oligodendrocytes, astrocytes, and microglial cells. Tumors from these cells most often produce a normal CSF related to their deep parenchymal location (Bailey and Higgins, 1986). One report of oligodendrogliomas in cats described their cytologic features as they appeared in cytospin preparations of the CSF (Dickinson et al., 2000). Cells were large with nuclei four to six times the size of red cells. Nuclei were eccentric within a densely basophilic moderately abundant cytoplasm. An aspirate from a brain mass is shown in Figure 13–39. Normally these cells are responsible for myelination of neurons in the CNS and appear as small cells

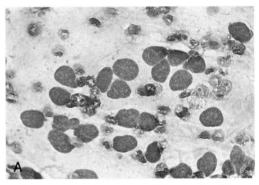

FIGURE   13–39.   A,   Oligodendroglioma. Tissue aspirate. Dog. This brain specimen was taken from a dog with demented behavior. MRI identified a 5-cm mass in the cerebrum that extended into the lateral ventricle. Nuclei measured two to three times a red cell and appeared free with clear area present around the cell when viewed against the proteinaceous background. Nuclei are round to oval with fine chromatin and indistinct nucleoli. (Wright-Giemsa; ×250.)

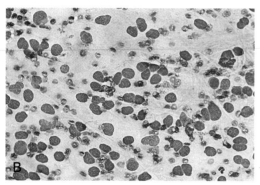

FIGURE 13–39. B, Same case as in Figure 13–39A. A monomorphic population of large mononuclear cells arranged in loose sheets or small clusters. (Wright-Giemsa; ×125.)

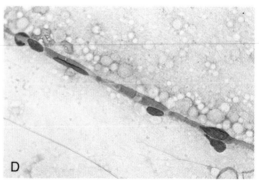

FIGURE 13–39. D, Capillary vessel. Tissue aspirate. Dog. Same case as in Figure 13–39A. Areas on the slide contained moderate numbers of blood vessels. Shown is a capillary filled with erythrocytes and lined by endothelium. (Wright-Giemsa; ×250.)

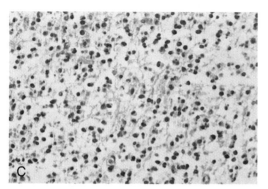

FIGURE 13–39. C, Same case as in Figure 13–39A. Tissue section showing linear arrays of round hyperchromatic cells surrounded by clear spaces producing a honeycomb appearance. (H & E; ×250.)

in Figure 13–25. Glial fibrillary acidic protein (GFAP) is a marker used to distinguish astrocytes from other neuroglial and meningeal cells but may sometimes yield a positive reaction in animals with neuroepithelial tumors, such as ependymoma and choroid plexus tumor (Fernandez et al., 1997).

Neuroepithelial cells include ependymal cells and choroid plexus cells. The ependymal cells line the ventricular system of the brain and central canal of the spinal cord. The ependymoma is a rare tumor that was reported in a cat with neoplastic cells found in the CSF with a moderately elevated protein content and mild pleocytosis with macrophages as the predominant cell type along with evidence of chronic hemorrhage (Ingwersen et al., 1989). The neoplastic cells were described as large cells having nuclear hyperchromasia, prominent nucleoli, and moderately abundant highly basophilic agranular cytoplasm appearing singly and in clusters. An anaplastic ependymoma in a dog was diagnosed from partial positive

with condensed chromatin. Tumors often demonstrate a unique honeycomb appearance and increased proliferation of blood vessels.

Astrocytes provide nutritional support to neurons, act as metabolic buffers or detoxifiers, and assist in repair and scar formation. They have been described as histiocytic in appearance (Fernandez et al., 1997). An example of reactive astrocytes is shown staining with GFAP and vimentin but a negative reaction with S100, CD3, and cytokeratin (Fernandez et al., 1997). The choroid plexus cells represent a highly vascular portion of the pia mater that projects into the ventricles of the brain and is thought to secrete the CSF. Positive cytokeratin staining is expected in choroid plexus tumors (Fernandez et al., 1997). A cytologic example of a choroid plexus tumor is shown in Figure 13–40 as an imprint of the tumor mass and within the CSF. The choroid plexus tumors were associated with an increased protein content and increased nucleated cell count in a study by Bailey and Higgins (1986). These cells appear similar to mesothelial cells in the CSF, having a large round nucleus with abundant well-defined deeply basophilic cytoplasm (Fig. 13–40C). A papillary appearance with epithelial features can be seen in cytologic preparations of choroid plexus papilloma (Fig. 13–40A).

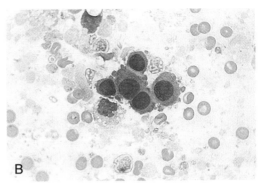

FIGURE 13–40. B, Same case as in Figure 13–40A. Higher magnification demonstrating the tight cohesion between cells. The nuclear-to-cytoplasmic ratio is high. The nucleus is round with finely granular chromatin and large prominent nucleoli. The cytoplasmic is basophilic and finely granular. (Wright-Giemsa; ×250.)

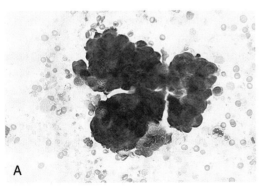

FIGURE 13–40. A, Choroid plexus papilloma. Tissue imprint. Dog. Seizure, dementia, ataxia, and tetraparesis were clinical signs present in this dog in which MRI diagnosed a ventricular mass. The sample was highly cellular with large dense cohesive clusters of cells having moderately abundant, deeply basophilic cytoplasm. (Wright-Giemsa; ×125.)

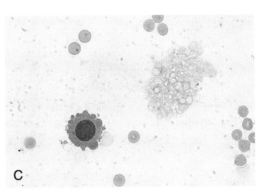

FIGURE 13–40. C, Choroid plexus papilloma with presumed myelin fragments. CSF. Dog. Same case as in Figure 13–40A. The fluid had increased protein (98 mg/dl) and a normal nucleated cell count. One neoplastic cell was present in two cytospin preparations. The nucleus is very large and round with dispersed chromatin and a single prominent nucleolus. The cytoplasmic is dark blue with smooth surface projections. To the right of the cell is granular gray-blue material consistent with myelin that suggests a degenerative process. (Wright-Giemsa; ×250.)

THE FUTURE OF NERVOUS SYSTEM CYTOLOGY

Cerebrospinal fluid cytology and fluid analysis are likely to continue to be an important part of the investigation of neurologic disease in dogs and cats. During the last decade, there has been an increased use of sophisticated imaging techniques with increased surgical investigation and surgical and medical treatment of neurologic disease. These trends indicate there may be opportunity to expand the use of nervous system cytology to include examination of fine-needle aspirates of lesions identified within the brain or spinal cord, ventricular fluids obtained by direct aspiration or by cannula, and squash preparations of small biopsy specimens or tissue fragments. All of these techniques are currently used in cytologic evaluations of human patients (Bigner, 1997) and to a limited extent in veterinary medicine (Vernau et al., 1997). There may be increased demand and/or need for development of special preparative techniques such as cell blocks and immunocytochemistry (Fernandez et al., 1997) for more precise identification of primary or metastatic tumors, inflammatory cell types, or immunophenotype of malignant or nonmalignant lymphoid proliferations. This has occurred in human medicine for the purpose of diagnosis, prognosis, and disease monitoring (Bigner, 1997). Recent studies have indicated diagnostic accuracy of 87.5% to 90% in diagnosis of intracranial masses sampled by fine-needle aspiration compared to histology of biopsy specimens (Mouriquand et al., 1987; Nguyen et al., 1989). Nguyen et al. (1989) reported impressive results with high correlation of cytologic and histologic diagnoses in 43 of 56 (77%) cases of neoplasia. New generations of diagnostic tests for detection of antibodies and antigens may provide new insights into the pathogenesis of neurologic disease. The future of veterinary nervous system evaluation may include types of collection, preparation, and analysis that differ significantly from those currently used.

SUMMARY

Cerebrospinal fluid evaluation is an important part of the investigation of neurologic disease. An alteration in CSF protein content, cell counts, or cytologic findings that provides a definitive diagnosis is infrequent. However, when considered in combination with clinical signs, presentation, history, and results of other tests, a high degree of confidence can be achieved in establishing a clinical diagnosis. Knowledge of methods of collection, sites of collection, methods for analysis, and possible contaminants is an important part of establishing expertise in laboratory and cytologic evaluation of the nervous system. In the future, emerging techniques, new testing methods, and new applications of current test methods may provide information different from or complementary to existing techniques.

References

Abate O, Bollo E, Lotti D, et al: Cytological, immunocytochemical and biochemical cerebrospinal fluid investigations in selected central nervous system disorder of dogs. Zentralbl Veterinarmed [B] 1998; 45:73–85.

Alleman AR, Christopher MM, Steiner DA, et al: Identification of intracytoplasmic inclusion bodies in mononuclear cells from the cerebrospinal fluid of a dog with canine distemper. Vet Pathol 1992; 29:84–85.

Altman D, Bolon B, Meyer DJ, et al: Cytologic features of a meningioma in a dog. Vet Clin Pathol 1989; 18:98–100.

Bailey CS, Higgins RJ: Characteristics of cerebrospinal fluid associated with canine granulomatous meningoencephalomyelitis: A retrospective study. J Am Vet Med Assoc 1986; 188:418–421.

Baker R, Lumsden JH: Color Atlas of Cytology of the Dog and Cat. CV Mosby, St. Louis, 2000, pp 95–115.

Baroni M, Heinold Y: A review of the clinical diagnosis of feline infectious peritonitis viral meningoencephalitis. Prog Vet Neurol 1995; 6: 88–94.

Berthelin CF, Legendre AM, Bailey CS, et al: Cryptococcosis of the nervous system in dogs, Part 2: Diagnosis, treatment, monitoring, and prognosis. Prog Vet Neurol 1994; 5:136–145.

Bichsel P, Vandevelde M, Vandevelde E, et al: Immunoelectrophoretic determination of albumin and IgG in serum and cerebrospinal fluid in dogs with neurologic diseases. Res Vet Sci 1984; 37:101–107.

Bigner SH: Central nervous system. In Bibbo M (ed): Comprehensive Cytopathology. WB Saunders, Philadelphia, 1997, pp 477–392.

Carmichael N: Nervous system. In Davidson M, Else R, Lumsden J (eds): Manual of Small Animal Clinical Pathology. British Small Animal Veterinary Association, Cheltenham, UK, 1998, pp 235–240.

Chrisman CL: Cerebrospinal fluid analysis. Vet Clin North Am Small Anim Pract 1992; 22: 781–810.

Christopher MM: Bone marrow contamination of canine cerebrospinal fluid. Vet Clin Pathol 1992; 21:95–98.

Christopher MM, Perman V, Hardy RM: Reassessment of cytologic values in canine cerebrospinal fluid by use of cytocentrifugation. J Am Vet Med Assoc 1988; 192:1726–1729.

Coles EH: Veterinary Clinical Pathology, 4th ed. WB Saunders, Philadelphia, 1986, pp 267–278.

Cook JR, DeNicola DB: Cerebrospinal fluid. Vet Clin North Am Small Anim Pract 1988; 18: 475–499.

Cordy DR, Holliday TA: A necrotizing meningoencephalitis of pug dogs. Vet Pathol 1989; 26:191–194.

Dickinson PJ, Keel MK, Higgins RJ, et al: Clinical and pathologic features of oligodendrogliomas in two cats. Vet Pathol 2000; 37:160–167.

Duncan JR, Prasse KW, Mahaffey EA: Veterinary Laboratory Medicine, 3rd ed. Iowa State University Press, Ames, 1994, pp 211–214.

Evans RJ: Ancillary diagnostic aids. In Wheeler SJ (ed): Manual of Small Animal Neurology. British Small Animal Veterinary Association, Cheltenham, UK, 1988, pp 47–62.

Fallin CW, Raskin RE, Harvey JW: Cytologic identification of neural tissue in the cerebrospinal fluid of two dogs. Vet Clin Pathol 1996; 25: 127–129.

Fenner WR: Diseases of the brain. In Ettinger SJ, Feldman EC (eds): Textbook of Veterinary Internal Medicine. WB Saunders, Philadelphia, 1995, pp 578–629.

Fernandez FR, Grindem CB, Brown TT, et al: Cytologic and histologic features of a poorly differentiated glioma in a dog. Vet Clin Pathol 1997; 26:182–186.

Fingeroth JM, Prata RG, Patnaik AK: Spinal meningiomas in dogs: 13 cases (1972–1987). J Am Vet Med Assoc 1987; 191:720–726.

Garma-Avina, Tyler JW: Large granular lymphocyte pleocytosis in the cerebrospinal fluid of a dog with necrotizing meningoencephalitis. J Comp Pathol 1999; 121:83–87.

Glass EN, Cornetta AM, deLahunta A, et al: Clinical and clinicopathologic features in 11 cats with Cuterebra larvae myiasis of the central nervous system. J Vet Intern Med 1998; 12:365–368.

Hay WH, Ogilvie GK, Parker AJ, et al: Disseminated meningeal tumor in a dog. J Am Vet Med Assoc 1987; 191:692–694.

Hoerlein BF: Canine Neurology, 2nd ed. WB Saunders, Philadelphia, 1971, p 19.

Hopkins AL, Garner M, Ackerman N, et al: Spinal meningeal sarcoma in a rottweiler puppy. J Small Anim Pract 1995; 36:183–186.

Howard-Martin M, Bowles MH: Intracranial dermoid cyst in a dog. J Am Vet Med Assoc 1988; 192:215–216.

Hurtt AE, Smith MO: Effects of iatrogenic blood contamination of results of cerebrospinal fluid analysis in clinically normal dogs and dogs with neurologic disease. J Am Vet Med Assoc 1997; 211:866–867.

Ingwersen W, Groom S, Parent J: Vestibular syndrome associated with an ependymoma in a cat. J Am Vet Med Assoc 1989; 195:98–100.

Jacobs RM, Cochrane SM, Lumsden JH, et al: Relationship of cerebrospinal fluid protein concentration determination by dye-binding and urinary dipstick methods. Can Vet J 1990; 31:587–588.

Jamison EM, Lumsden JH: Cerebrospinal fluid analysis in the dog: Methodology and interpretation. Semin Vet Med Surg (Small Anim) 1988; 3:122–132.

Keebler CM: Cytopreparatory techniques. In Bibbo M (ed): Comprehensive Cytopathology, 2nd ed. WB Saunders, Philadelphia, 1997, pp 889–917.

Kipar A, Baumgartner W, Vogl C, et al: Immunohistochemical characterization of inflammatory cells in brains of dogs with granulomatous meningoencephalitis. Vet Pathol 1998; 35:43–52.

Mandel NS, Senker EG, Bosler EM, et al: Intrathecal production of Borrelia burgdorferi-specific antibodies in a dog with central nervous system Lyme borreliosis. Compend Contin Educ Pract Vet 1993; 15:581–586.

Meadows RL, MacWilliams PS, Dzata G, et al: Diagnosis of histoplasmosis in a dog by cytologic examination of CSF. Vet Clin Pathol 1992; 21:122–125.

Meinkoth JH, Crystal MA: Cerebrospinal fluid analysis. In Cowell RL, Tyler RD, Meinkoth JH (eds): Diagnostic Cytology and Hematology of the Dog and Cat. CV Mosby, St. Louis, 1999, pp 125–141.

Meinkoth JH, Ewing SA, Cowell RL, et al: Morphologic and molecular evidence of a dual species ehrlichial infection in a dog presenting with inflammatory central nervous system disease. J Vet Intern Med 1998; 12:389–393.

Meric SM, Child G, Higgins RJ: Necrotizing vasculitis of the spinal pachyleptomeningeal arteries in three Bernese mountain dog littermates. J Am Anim Hosp Assoc 1986; 22:459–465.

Mesher CI, Blue JT, Guffroy MRG, et al: Intracellular myelin in cerebrospinal fluid from a dog with myelomalacia. Vet Clin Pathol 1996; 25:124–126.

Mouriquand C, Benabid AL, Breyton M: Stereotaxic cytology of brain tumors. Review of an eight-year experience. Acta Cytol 1987; 31:756–764.

Munana KR, Luttgen PJ: Prognostic factors for dogs with granulomatous meningoencephalo-myelitis: 42 cases (1982–1996). J Am Vet Med Assoc 1998; 212;1902–1906.

Nguyen GK, Johnston ES, Mielke BW: Cytology of neuroectodermal tumors of the brain in crush preparations. Acta Cytol 1989; 33:67–73.

Oliver JE, Lorenz MD, Kornegay JN: Handbook of Veterinary Neurology. WB Saunders, Philadelphia, 1997, pp 89–108.

Parent JM, Rand JS: Cerebrospinal fluid collection and analysis. In August JR (ed): Consultations in Feline Internal Medicine 2, WB Saunders, Philadelphia, 1994, pp 385–392.

Rand JS: The analysis of cerebrospinal fluid in cats. In Bonagua JD, Kirk RW (eds): Kirk's Current Veterinary Therapy XII. Small Animal Practice. WB Saunders, Philadelphia, 1995, pp 1121–1126.

Rand JS, Parent J, Jacobs R, et al: Reference intervals for feline cerebrospinal fluid: Cell counts and cytological features. Am J Vet Res 1990; 51:1044–1048.

Rand JS, Parent J, Percy D, et al: Clinical, cerebrospinal fluid and histological data from thirty-four cats with primary noninflammatory disease of the central nervous system. Can Vet J 1994; 35:174–181.

Raskin RE: An atypical spinal meningioma in a dog. Vet Pathol 1984; 21:538–540.

Roszel JF: Membrane filtration of canine and feline cerebrospinal fluid for cytologic evaluation. J Am Vet Med Assoc 1972; 160:720–725.

Roszel JF, Steinberg SA, McGrath JT: Periodic acid–Schiff-positive cells in the cerebrospinal fluid of dogs with globoid cell leukodystrophy. Neurology 1972; 22:738–740.

Schultze AE, Cribb AE, Tvedten HW: Eosinophilic meningoencephalitis in a cat. J Am Anim Hosp Assoc 1986; 22:623–627.

Sheppard BJ, Chrisman CL, Newell SM, et al: Primary encephalic plasma cell tumor in a dog. Vet Pathol 1997; 34:621–627.

Smith-Maxie LL, Parent JP, Rand J, Wilcock BP, et al: Cerebrospinal fluid analysis and clinical outcome of eight dogs with eosinophilic meningoencephalomyelitis. J Vet Intern Med 1989; 3:167–174.

Sorjonen DC: Total protein, albumin quota and electrophoretic patterns in cerebrospinal fluid of dogs with central nervous system disorders. Am J Vet Res 1987; 48:301–305.

Sorjonen DC: Clinical and histopathological features of granulomatous meningoencephalomyelitis in dogs. J Am Anim Hosp Assoc 1990; 26: 141–147.

Sorjonen DC, Cox NR, Swango LJ: Electrophoretic determination of albumin and gamma globulin concentrations in the cerebrospinal fluid of dogs with encephalomyelitis attributable to canine distemper virus infection: 13 cases (1980–1987). J Am Vet Med Assoc 1989; 195: 977–980.

Stalis IH, Chadwick B, Dayrell-Hart B, et al: Necrotizing meningoencephalitis of maltese dogs. Vet Pathol 1995; 32:230–235.

Thomson CE, Kornegay JN, Stevens JB: Analysis of cerebrospinal fluid from the cerebellomedullary and lumbar cisterns of dogs with focal neurologic disease: 145 cases (1985–1987). J Am Vet Med Assoc 1990; 196:1841–1844.

Tipold A, Fatzer R, Jaggy A, et al: Necrotizing encephalitis in Yorkshire terriers. J Small Anim Pract 1993; 34:623–628.

Tipold A, Vandevelde M, Zurbriggen A: Neuroimmunological studies in steroid-responsive meningitis-arteritis in dogs. Res Vet Sci 1995; 58: 103–108.

Tyler JW, Cullor JS: Titers, tests, and truisms: Rational interpretation of diagnostic serologic testing. J Am Vet Med Assoc. 1989; 194:1550–1558, 1989.

Uchida K, Hasegawa T, Ikeda M, et al: Detection of an autoantibody from pug dogs with necrotizing encephalitis (pug dog encephalitis). Vet Pathol 1999; 36:301–307.

Vernau KM, Higgins RJ, LeCouteur RA, et al: Cytological characteristics of brain tumors in dogs and cats using crush preparations. (Abstract) 15th Proceedings of the Am Coll Vet Intern Med Forum, Lake Buena Vista, FL, 1977, p 665.

Wilson JW, Stevens JB: Effects of blood contamination on cerebrospinal fluid analysis. J Am Vet Med Assoc. 1977; 171:256–258.

Zimmerman KL, Bender HS, Boon GD, et al: A comparison of the cytologic and histologic features of meningiomas in four dogs. Vet Clin Pathol 2000; 29:29–34.

Chapter 14

Eyes and Adnexa

Rose E. Raskin

Cytologic examination of the eye and surrounding structures is frequently helpful in determining general categories of pathology prior to performing more invasive or expensive procedures. The following cytodiagnostic categories apply to the various anatomic sites of the eye. It should be noted that more than one presentation might occur in a specimen at a time.

General Cytodiagnostic Groups for Ocular Cytology

- Normal tissue
- Cystic or hyperplastic tissue
- Inflammation
- Neoplasia
- Response to tissue injury

Cytologic Biopsy Considerations

Aspiration of focal and diffuse lesions is recommended for the lesions of the eyelid, eye, and other associated structures. The thinner conjunctival tissue requires scraping with a blunt instrument such as an ophthalmic spatula or the use of a soft brush. The use of a brush was shown to reduce cellular clumping of samples and provide less cellular distortion (Willis et al, 1997). Exudate material, duct washings, and aspirate material can be used as specimens of the nasolacrimal apparatus.

EYELIDS

Normal Histology and Cytology

The dorsal and ventral eyelids are thin skin extensions of facial skin that meet at the lateral and medial margins, called canthi. Two to four rows of lashes are found on the upper eyelid at the free margin of the dog, while the cat has a row of cilia (Samuelson, 1999). The outermost layer resembles typical skin, with keratinized squamous epithelium and numerous hair follicles that lie in close association with sebaceous and modified sweat glands. Striated muscle fibers course through the deeper layers. The innermost layer, the palpebral conjunctiva, is lined by pseudostratified columnar epithelium containing numerous goblet cells. Near the margins of both eyelids at the posterior end are the meibomian or tarsal glands. These large sebaceous glands lie adjacent to the palpebral conjunctiva and contribute to the lipid component of the tear film.

Inflammation

Blepharitis refers to inflammatory conditions of the eyelid. Cytologically it is characterized by the predominant cell type. Neutrophilic or purulent blepharitis most often involves bacteria such as *Staphylococcus* and *Streptococcus* sp, however, immune-mediated disease or foreign body reactions may result in purulent inflammation. Eosinophilic inflammation should be considered for allergic reactions, some autoimmune conditions, parasitic migration (*Cuterebra* sp), or conditions associated with collagen degeneration. Dermatophytosis or other fungal infections may be associated with granulomatous inflammation containing macrophages alone or mixed with other cell types.

Neoplasia

Diffuse neoplasms of the eyelids involve squamous cell carcinoma (especially in cats), sarcoma, mast cell tumor, and lymphoma. Focal presentations involve sebaceous gland adenoma/adenocarcinoma, pilloma, mast cell tumor, melanoma, squamous cell carcinoma, and histiocytoma. Benign tumors predominate but occasionally malignant tumors such as apocrine sweat gland tumors can invade the globe and extensively damage the eye (Hirai et al, 1997).

Cyst

Chalazion refers to the granuloma formed as a result of retained meibomian secretions. The leakage of meibomian cyst material incites an inflammatory response similar to a foreign body reaction. In this situation, numerous foamy macrophages, few giant cells, neutrophils, lymphocytes, amorphous debris, and sebaceous epithelium are present.

CONJUNCTIVAE

Normal Histology and Cytology

The palpebral conjunctiva is lined by a pseudostratified columnar epithelium with numerous goblet cells. Goblet cells appear as distended cells with an eccentric nucleus. The cytoplasm may contain clear vacuoles or red-blue granules. Mucus is common on cytologic specimens, appearing as lightly basophilic amorphous strands. The bulbar conjunctiva is the reflected conjunctiva onto the globe that is continuous with corneal epithelium. It consists of sheets of stratified nonkeratinized squamous epithelium that lacks goblet cells. The junction of the two conjunctivae creates a sac termed the *fornix;* this blind sac is lined by stratified cuboidal epithelium containing many goblet cells. Cytologically, sheets of uniform polygonal basophilic cells with large round nuclei are present without significant numbers of inflammatory cells.

Hyperplasia

Conditions such as keratoconjunctivitis sicca, vitamin A deficiency, chronic disease, and trauma from mechanical irritants result in increased cell numbers sometimes with evidence of metaplasia. These specimens

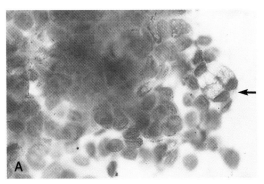

FIGURE 14–1. A. Goblet cell hyperplasia. Conjunctival scraping. Cat. Chronic conjunctival disease in this animal resulted in increased numbers of goblet cells. Two are shown (*arrow*) characterized by columnar shape, eccentric nucleus, and pale foamy cytoplasm. (Wright-Giemsa; ×250.)

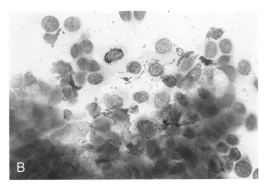

FIGURE 14–1. B. Pigmentation and hyperplastic epithelium. Conjunctival scraping. Same case as in Figure 14–1A. Two cells are present with abundant fine black-green cytoplasmic granules. Also note the hyperplastic epithelium with increased nuclear-to-cytoplasmic ratio. (Wright-Giemsa; ×250.)

contain many keratinized epithelial cells and goblet cells (Fig. 14–1A) (Murphy, 1988). Increased pigmentation of the epithelium may also occur such that the cytoplasm contains numerous fine black-green melanin granules (Fig. 14–1B).

Inflammation

The predominant cell type present characterizes the conjunctivitis. Neutrophilic conjunctivitis may be associated with infectious agents such as bacteria and viruses as well as noninfectious causes. One should suspect a bacterial origin if degenerative changes are present. With viruses such as feline herpesvirus and chronic canine distemper virus, nondegenerate neutrophils predominate (Fig. 14–2). Multinucleated epithelial cells (Fig. 14–3) were found in approximately half of the cases with feline herpesvirus (FHV-1) infection diagnosed by culture or immunofluorescent assay (Naisse et al, 1993). Intranuclear inclusions in FHV-1 infection are not found in conjunctival

smears but may be seen in histologic sections. A polymerase chain reaction (PCR) test has greater sensitivity for detection of the virus than other tests (Stiles et al, 1997). Canine distemper inclusions appear pink with alcohol-based Romanowsky stains but purple with aqueous-based Wright stains.

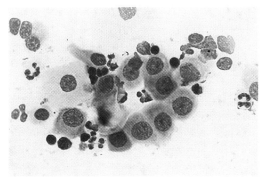

FIGURE 14–2. Suppurative conjunctivitis. Conjunctival scraping. Cat. The bulbar conjunctiva is hyperplastic with many nondegenerate neutrophils and few lymphocytes present in this young cat with chronic conjunctivitis. Infection with feline herpesvirus (FHV-1) was suspected. (Aqueous-based Wright; ×250.)

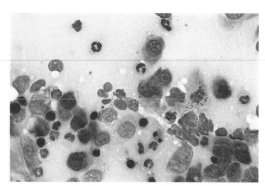

FIGURE 14–3. Herpesvirus infection with suppurative conjunctivitis. Conjunctival scraping. Cat. Many nondegenerate neutrophils are present along with reactive epithelium, including multinucleation (center). This case was confirmed previously for herpesvirus infection by polymerase chain reaction. One pigmented epithelial cell is also noted. (Wright-Giemsa; ×250.)

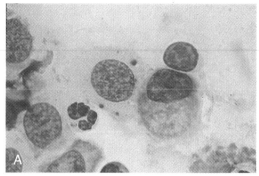

FIGURE 14–4. A. Chlamydiosis. Conjunctival scraping. Cat. Three small basophilic initial bodies are present in the cytoplasm of one epithelial cell of this 10-month-old kitten. (Wright-Giemsa; ×500.)

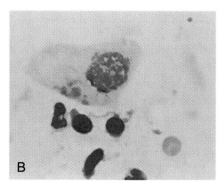

FIGURE 14–4. B. Chlamydiosis. Conjunctival scraping. Same case as in Figure 14–4A. Degenerating epithelial cells contain several small basophilic granular initial bodies. Another cat in the house and the owner have conjunctivitis. Nondegenerate neutrophils and small lymphocytes are also present in this sample. (Wright-Giemsa; ×500.)

Other infectious causes include feline chlamydiosis, which presents as variably sized discrete basophilic bodies in the cytoplasm of epithelium within first 2 weeks of infection. Small elementary bodies (0.3 μm) are shed which infect new cells and grow into larger (0.5 to 1.5 μm) initial bodies (Greene, 1998). The initial bodies (Fig. 14–4A & B) proliferate to become a large, membrane-bound reticulate body containing many elementary bodies (Fig. 14–5). In the Naisse et al study (1993), visible epithelial inclusions were present in only a third of the cases identified as *Chlamydia psittaci* positive by immunofluorescent assay. Besides fluorescent antibody detection, cell inoculation or PCR procedures may be used. In one case reported, infection of *C. psittaci* in a cat was possibly transmitted from a macaw (Lipman et al, 1994). Infection with feline *Mycoplasma* sp presents as small basophilic granules similar to the elementary bodies of chlamydial infections with the exception that they are adherent to the surface membrane (Fig. 14–6A & B). One study from Belgium indicated mycoplasmal infection had an incidence of 25% in cats with conjunctivitis (Haesebrouck et al, 1991).

Noninfectious causes include keratoconjunctivitis sicca and allergic conditions. Eosinophilic conjunctivitis has been associated

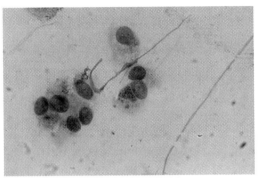

FIGURE 14–5. Chlamydiosis. Conjunctival scraping. Cat. One week earlier this cat developed pyrexia, conjunctivitis, rhinitis, and oral ulcers. The cell in the center contains a perinuclear reticulate body filled with numerous elementary bodies. Diagnosis was confirmed by fluorescent antibody testing. (Wright.) (Photo courtesy of John Kramer, Washington State University; presented at the 1989 ASVCP case review session.)

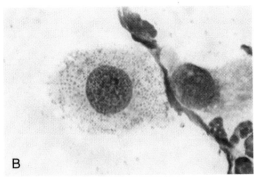

FIGURE 14–6. B. Mycoplasmosis. Conjunctival scraping. Same case as in Figure 14–6B. Note the numerous organisms over the cytoplasm and nucleus. These granules are adherent to the surface membrane and extend into the background. (Wright-Giemsa; ×500.)

with a hypersensitivity reaction in the cat (Pentlarge, 1991). In this situation eosinophils are seen commonly (Fig. 14–7A). Mast cell infiltrates may also be so numerous that there is concern for a conjunctival mast cell tumor (Fig. 14–7B). Lymphocytes and plasma cells have been associated with allergic conditions as well as with early canine distemper infection or with chronic inflammation of the conjunctiva.

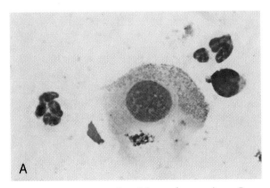

FIGURE 14–6. A. Mycoplasmosis. Conjunctival scraping. Goat. This animal had keratoconjunctivitis clinically. Numerous small gray granules are associated with the cell and few organisms are found extracellularly in the background. Nondegenerate neutrophils are frequent. Stain precipitate or cellular debris is present below the cell. (Wright-Giemsa; ×500.)

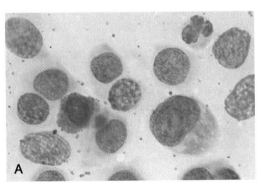

FIGURE 14–7. A. Eosinophilic conjunctivitis. Conjunctival scraping. Cat. Bilateral conjunctivitis is present in this animal. An eosinophil is shown at the upper right and a mast cell is at left center. Note the mast cell granules in the background. This response is associated with a hypersensitivity reaction. (Wright-Giemsa; ×500.)

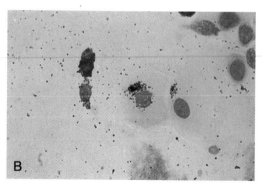

FIGURE 14–7. B. Eosinophilic conjunctivitis. Conjunctival scraping. Same case as in Figure 14–7A. Many mast cell granules are free in the background. Two mast cells are noted left of center and two pigmented epithelial cells are present in the center. The numerous mast cells present cause concern for a mast cell tumor, but they appear benign. (Wright-Giemsa; ×500.)

Neoplasia

Epithelium is frequently atypical and hyperplastic as a result of severe inflammation, therefore neoplasia may be difficult to diagnose confidently. Neoplasms found associated with the conjunctival area include squamous cell carcinoma, papilloma, melanoma, lymphoma, hemangiosarcoma, and mast cell tumor. An uncommon location of transmissible venereal tumor has been the conjunctivae of the upper and lower eyelids (Boscos et al, 1998).

Miscellaneous Finding

Large amorphous basophilic inclusions within the cytoplasm of squamous epithelium have been attributed to ophthalmic ointment use, particularly those medications containing neomycin (Prasse and Winston, 1999).

NICTITATING MEMBRANE
Normal Histology and Cytology

The third eyelid, or nictitating membrane, is a large fold of conjunctiva protruding from the medial canthus. It contains a T-shaped cartilaginous plate surrounded by glandular epithelium that is serous in the cat and seromucoid in the dog (Samuelson, 1999). The palpebral and bulbar surfaces are covered by nonkeratinized stratified squamous epithelium. The free margin of the membrane is pigmented and cytologically, fine green-black melanin granules can be found within the epithelium. Variably sized lymphoid aggregates are located within the stroma associated with the bulbar surface of the nictitating membrane. The stroma also contains fibrous connective tissue.

Inflammation

With follicular conjunctivitis there is a mixed population of lymphoid cells that re-

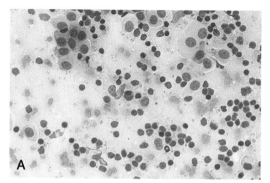

FIGURE 14–8. A. Follicular hyperplasia. Nictitating membrane. Cat. Numerous small lymphocytes predominant. (Aqueous-based Wright; ×125.)

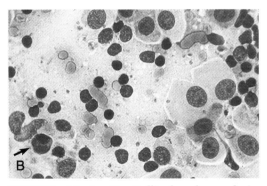

FIGURE 14–8. B. Follicular hyperplasia. Nictitating membrane. Same case as in Figure 14–8A. Higher magnification to demonstrate the presence of a plasma cell (*arrow*) and several intermediate lymphocytes in addition to the small lymphocytes. (Aqueous-based Wright; ×250.)

Neoplasia

These are similar to those seen in the conjunctivae. Adenocarcinomas, papillomas, and malignant melanomas are most common in dogs. A report of an adenocarcinoma affecting the gland of the nictitating membrane in a cat demonstrated the presence of malignant epithelial cells from impression smears of excisional biopsy material (Komaromy et al, 1997). Squamous cell carcinoma when present on the nictitating membrane is considered an extension from the eyelid. It appears similar to those found in the skin often with nonseptic purulent inflammation (Fig. 14–9A–E).

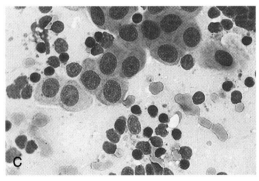

FIGURE 14–8. C. Follicular hyperplasia. Nictitating membrane. Same case as in Figure 14–8A. Reactive epithelium accompanies the reactive lymphoid population. (Aqueous-based Wright; ×250.)

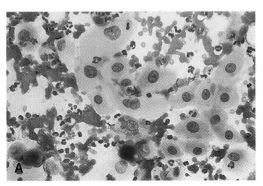

FIGURE 14–9. A. Squamous cell carcinoma. Nictitating membrane. Cat. Several weeks duration of erythema and edema along with proliferative lesions on the conjunctiva and third eyelid were present in this 14-year-old cat. Sheets of epithelium appear with some features of malignancy, including anisokaryosis, multinucleation, variable nucleocytoplasmic ratio, and coarse chromatin. Many nondegenerate neutrophils are noted without evidence of sepsis. (Aqueous-based Wright; ×125.)

sembles a hyperplastic lymph node (Figs. 14–8A–C). Plasma cell infiltrates (plasmacytic conjunctivitis or plasmoma) have been seen in German shepherd dogs. These thickened depigmentating lesions are composed of numerous well-differentiated plasma cells.

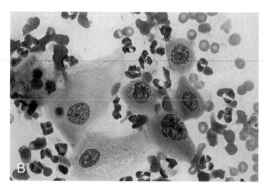

FIGURE 14–9. B. Squamous cell carcinoma. Nictitating membrane. Same case as in Figure 14–9A. In addition to the previously mentioned malignant features there is perinuclear vacuolation, a feature often associated with malignant squamous epithelium. The presence of severe suppurative inflammation likely accounts for some of the dysplastic changes in the epithelium. (Aqueous-based Wright; ×250.)

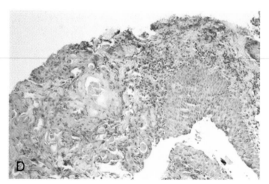

FIGURE 14–9. D. Squamous cell carcinoma. Nictitating membrane. Same case as in Figure 14–9A. This section is taken from the junction between the palpebral conjunctiva on the left and the nictitating membrane on the right. Note the marked disorganization of the mucous membrane and dermis. This tumor is thought to originate from the eyelid with extension to the nictitating membrane. (H & E; ×50.)

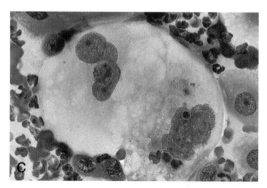

FIGURE 14–9. C. Squamous cell carcinoma. Nictitating membrane. Same case as in Figure 14–9A. Two giant epithelial cells with multiple nuclei. The presence of very bizarre morphologic changes and the absence of sepsis further supports the malignant, not dysplastic nature of the epithelium. (Aqueous-based Wright; ×250.)

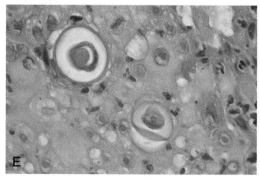

FIGURE 14–9. E. Squamous cell carcinoma. Nictitating membrane. Same case as in Figure 14–9A. Two keratin pearls that are often associated with malignant squamous epithelium appear in the center and help to identify the neoplasm. (H & E; ×250.)

SCLERA

Normal Histology and Cytology

The sclera is a fibrous covering of the globe that merges with the peripheral cornea and bulbar conjunctiva at the limbus, where it is pigmented. Pigment is found in all layers of the limbus except the superficial squamous cells. The underlying stroma contains dense collagen fibers, elastic fibers, fibrocytes, melanocytes, and blood vessels. Aspirates may be poorly cellular, with mostly collagen present and occasional melanocytes.

Inflammation

Nodular fasciitis is a dome-shaped lesion composed of lymphoid cells, macrophages, plasma cells, fibroblasts, and few neutrophils. Melanocytes may be seen.

Neoplasia

Neoplasms present in the sclera include melanoma, mast cell tumor, lymphoma, and sarcoma.

CORNEA

Normal Histology and Cytology

The surface of the cornea is composed of nonkeratinized stratified squamous epithelium (Fig. 14–10A). Below this surface is a thick layer of parallel bundles of collagenous stroma (Fig. 14–10B) with infrequent intermixed fibrocytes called *keratocytes.* Deeper to the stroma is a basement membrane, termed *Descemet's membrane,* composed of fine collagen fibrils. The deepest

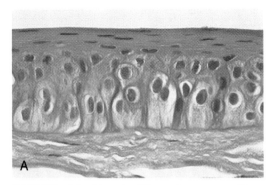

FIGURE 14–10. A. Normal cornea. Dog. The outer surface is composed of nonkeratinized stratified squamous epithelium. (H & E; ×250.)

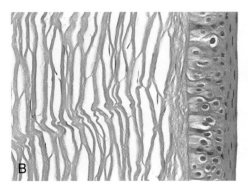

FIGURE 14–10. B. Normal canine cornea. Same case as in Figure 14–10A. Below the surface epithelium is a thick layer of parallel bundles of collagenous stroma. (H & E; ×125.)

---

layer consists of a single layer of flattened endothelium. Cytologically, basal and intermediate squamous epithelial cells that normally lack pigmentation predominate.

Inflammation

Infectious keratitis involves bacterial and fungal agents. Bacterial agents such as *Pseudomonas* sp, *Streptococcus* sp, and *Staphylococcus* sp produce suppurative responses with degenerative neutrophils. Fungal agents commonly isolated in mycotic keratitis are *Aspergillus* sp, *Fusarium* sp, and *Candida* sp (Fig. 14–11). These infections produce mostly neutrophilic infiltration, but macrophages are common with occasional eosinophils. Hyphal elements are best seen with stains such as Gomori's methenamine silver. Samples should be obtained from deep within the lesion or at its edge. When used together with microbial culture, cytologic evaluation of scrapings from corneal ulcers has resulted in a maximal identification of infectious ulcerative keratitis (Massa et al, 1999).

Eosinophilic keratitis is a raised vascular lesion with white granular surface seen in cats. It is composed of squamous epithe-

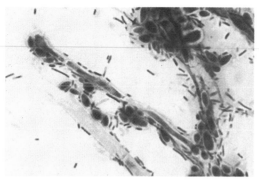

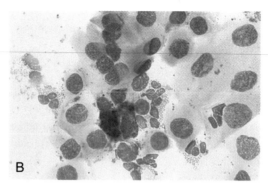

FIGURE 14–11. Mycotic keratitis. Corneal scraping. Dog. There is a 1-week history of raised white punctate masses on the cornea. Against the background of extracellular rod-shaped bacteria are hyphal elements and many spore forms. Infection with *Candida* sp was suspected. Neutrophils were present in other fields of the specimen. (Aqueous-based Wright; ×500.)

FIGURE 14–12. B. Eosinophilic keratitis. Corneal scraping. Same case as in Figure 14–12A. This sample was likely taken from deeper into the cornea since it contains many more eosinophils than mast cells. (Wright-Giemsa; ×250.)

lium, cellular debris, including eosinophil granules, and numerous mast cells with lower numbers of intact eosinophils (Fig. 14–12A). Deeper scrapings contain predominantly eosinophils and lymphoid cells (Fig. 14–12B) (Prasse and Winston, 1999).

The histopathology and cytology have been well described in an article by Prasse and Winston (1996) in which they demonstrate that mast cells are most frequent in scrapings that avoid the white surface exudate.

Pannus, or chronic superficial keratitis, is a common condition seen in German shepherds that reflects a chronic progressive disease. It initially appears at the limbus as a red, vascularized lesion that progresses centrally, becoming flesh-like and later pigmented and scarred. Initially it appears cytologically as mixed inflammation with plasma cells, lymphocytes, macrophages, and neutrophils.

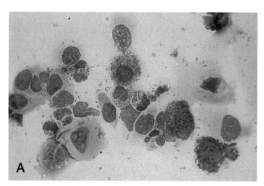

FIGURE 14–12. A. Eosinophilic keratitis. Corneal scraping. Cat. There was a gritty white proliferative mass at the lateral limbus of this animal with recurrent keratitis. Note the mixture of eosinophils and many mast cells along with corneal epithelium. Surface granular material often contains high numbers of mast cells in addition to eosinophils. (Wright-Giemsa; ×250.)

Response to Tissue Injury

Noninflammatory opaque corneal lesions may result from disease. Lipid corneal degeneration may be seen in old dogs with renal disease. Cytologically, only normal epithelium is seen. Another condition is mineralization, which appears as a granular plaque. On cytology, nonstaining crystalline material is found which often stains positive for calcium using the von Kossa stain.

Neoplasia

Squamous cell carcinoma, papilloma, melanoma, and sarcoma are the predominant tumor types, although tumors of the cornea are rare.

IRIS AND CILIARY BODY

Normal Histology and Cytology

The iris and ciliary body are termed the *anterior uvea*. The uvea is highly vascular and often pigmented. The anterior border layer contains a single layer of fibroblasts with several underlying layers of melanocytes (Samuelson, 1999). These melanocytes in the dog and cat contain lanceolate to oval brown melanin granules. The iris stroma consists of fine collagenous fibers along with blood vessels and nerves. Unstriated muscle fibers within the stroma help to dilate the iris. The posterior iridal surface is covered by pigmented epithelium that is continuous with the ciliary body (Fig. 14–13). As an extension of the choroid layer,

the ciliary body provides nutrients and removes wastes for the cornea and lens through formation of the aqueous humor. The main portion of the ciliary body consists of smooth muscle along with vascular sinuses and heavily pigmented epithelium at the surface.

Inflammation

Pyogranulomatous or granulomatous inflammation may occur with fungal infections such as coccidioidomycosis, blastomycosis, cryptococcosis, and histoplasmosis. Feline infectious peritonitis may also produce an anterior uveitis with pyogranulomatous iridocyclitis (Fig. 14–14). Lens-induced uveitis may produce a lymphocytic–plasmacytic infiltration consistent with immune reactivity to lens proteins.

Neoplasia

Melanomas are the most common primary intraocular tumor in the dog, with the anterior uvea more often affected. When mela-

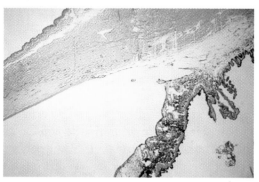

FIGURE 14–13. Normal anterior uvea. Dog. Present in this view is the cornea near the limbus where the iris and ciliary body attach at the iridocorneal angle. Portions of both the anterior and posterior chambers of the anterior humor compartment are shown. (H & E; ×10.)

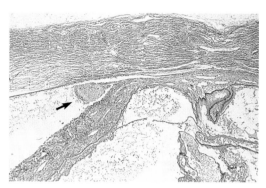

FIGURE 14–14. Pyogranulomatous iridocyclitis. Cat. Note the presence of an anterior uveitis with accumulation of inflammatory cells in the iridocorneal angle (*arrow*) and in the junction between the iris and ciliary body in this animal with confirmed feline infectious peritonitis. (H & E; ×10.)

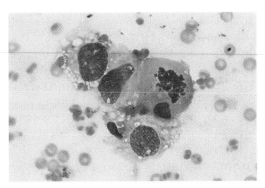

FIGURE 14–15. Ciliary body adenocarcinoma. Tissue aspirate of an ocular mass extending from the iris. Dog. Shown is a tight cluster of epithelial cells with high nuclear-to-cytoplasmic ratio, coarse chromatin, anisokaryosis, and a mitotic figure. The cytoplasm is foamy with numerous discrete vacuoles. (Wright-Giemsa; ×250.)

noma occurs in the cat, it involves more often the iris and ciliary body. Ocular melanoma is more common than oral and dermal melanomas in the cat (Patnaik and Mooney, 1988). Ocular melanoma is also more malignant than dermal melanoma,

with higher rates of mortality and metastasis. Aspiration of the neoplasm may be accomplished through the anterior chamber using a 25-gauge or smaller needle. Cytologic features of mitotic index, nuclear size and pleomorphism, and degree of pigmentation are helpful for prognostic purposes in the dog but not in the cat. The presence of anisokaryosis, variable nuclear-to-cytoplasmic ratio, and prominent nucleoli should help to distinguish malignant melanocytes from melanophages.

Ciliary neoplasms such as iridociliary adenoma and adenocarcinoma are the second most common primary intraocular tumors in the dog (Fig. 14–15). These tumors are rare in the cat.

Lymphoma has been recognized as the most frequent intraocular tumor in cats (Glaze and Gelatt, 1999). It occurs as a diffuse or nodular iris lesion. Evidence of ocular lymphoma often suggests this is metastatic from a primary site that should be found. Cytologic changes are similar to lymphoid neoplasms in other sites (Fig. 14–16).

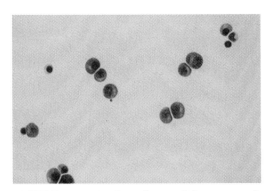

FIGURE 14–16. Lymphoma. Iris mass aspirate. Large discrete round cells with plasmacytoid features are prominent in this neoplasm. Lymphoma is the most frequent intraocular tumor in cats. (Romanowsky; ×250.)

AQUEOUS HUMOR

Normal Cytology and Collection

When aqueous humor is cloudy, cytologic evaluation of the fluid may help to diagnose the presence of infectious agents or neoplasms. Fine-needle aspiration is conducted under anesthesia using a 25-gauge or smaller needle by entering at the limbus through the bulbar conjunctiva. A small amount of fluid is removed which is then evaluated immediately. A direct cell count using a hemocytometer is performed followed by sedimentation of the fluid for smear or cytospin preparation. Additional fluid is used to measure total protein by a microprotein technique. Normal aqueous humor in the dog has a direct cell count mean of 8.2/μl (range 0 to 37) and protein mean of 36.4 mg/dl (range 21 to 65). Normal aqueous humor in the cat has a direct cell count mean of 2.2/μl (range 0 to 15) and protein mean of 43.7 mg/dl (range 22 to 75) (Hazel et al, 1985). Cytologically, the low-protein fluid is acellular with only occasional free melanin granules or melanin-containing cells.

This clear fluid originates from the vascular sinuses within the folds and processes of the posterior portion of the ciliary body. The humor flows from the posterior chamber of the anterior compartment through the pupil, then into the anterior chamber to the filtration angle. Excess fluid is removed at the iridocorneal angle through a vascular meshwork.

Inflammation

Anterior uveitis most often produces a neutrophilic infiltrate. Infectious causes to consider include bacteria, *Blastomyces* sp, *Prototheca* sp, and *Leishmania* sp.

Hemorrhage

Hyphema may present as acute or chronic hemorrhage. Acute hemorrhage may be indicated by the presence of platelets and erythrophagocytosis, by macrophages. Chronic hemorrhage is indicated by the presence of hemosiderin-laden macrophages.

Neoplasia

Metastatic tumors rarely exfoliate, with the exception of lymphoma.

RETINA

Normal Histology and Cytology

The retina is composed of 10 classical layers, which include the retinal pigment epithelium, rod and cone layer, outer limiting membrane, outer nuclear layer, outer plexiform layer, inner nuclear layer, inner plexiform layer, ganglion cell layer, nerve fiber layer, and inner limiting membrane (Fig. 14–17A). External to the retina and closely adherent to the retinal pigment epithelium is the choroid, also termed the *posterior uvea*. The retinal pigment epithelium is continuous with the outer layer of the ciliary body and is highly pigmented except in the region of the tapetum lucidum. Melanin granules within the pigmented retinal epithelial cells are lanceolate or elongated. The outer nuclear layer in dogs and cats contains predominately rod nuclei, which are small, round, dense, and very distinctive in appearance (Fig. 14–17B).

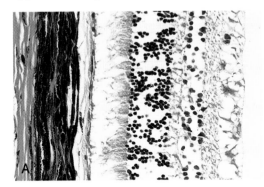

FIGURE 14–17. A. Normal retina. Dog. Shown are the layers of the retina beginning externally at the left side adjacent to the pigmented choroid. They are the retinal pigment epithelium, rod and cone layer, outer limiting membrane (not visible), outer nuclear layer, outer plexiform layer, inner nuclear layer, inner plexiform layer, ganglion layer, nerve fiber layer, and inner limiting membrane. (H & E; ×125.)

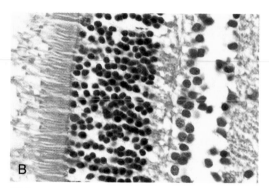

FIGURE 14–17. B. Normal canine retina. Same case as in Figure 14–17A. Higher magnification to better demonstrate from left to right, the rod and cone layer, outer nuclear layer, outer plexiform layer, and inner nuclear layer. The outer nuclear layer in dogs and cats contains predominately rod nuclei, which are small, round, dense and very distinctive in appearance when found in vitreal aspirates. (H & E; ×250.)

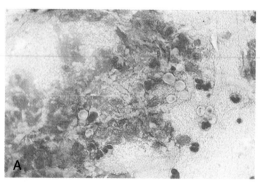

FIGURE 14–18. A. Aspergillosis. Vitreocentesis. Dog. This German shepherd dog had a history of paraplegia related to discospondylitis. Bilateral uveitis was present along with other systemic signs of infection. The background is eosinophilic and granular with degenerate neutrophils. Against this proteinaceous material are the clear-staining hyphae and round spores of this fungal agent, which were cultured and identified as *Aspergillus terreus*. (Wright-Giemsa; ×250.)

Response to Tissue Injury

Retinal detachment may produce a subretinal cavity that contains only normal retinal cells, as was demonstrated in one feline case (Knoll, 1990).

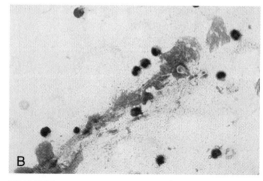

FIGURE 14–18. B. Aspergillosis. Vitreocentesis. Same case as in Figure 14–18A. Hyphae are more visible in this field. Aspergillosis is a common cause of infectious endophthmalitis. (Wright-Giemsa; ×250.)

VITREOUS BODY

Normal Cytology and Collection

Vitreocentesis may be attempted under general anesthesia using a 23-gauge or smaller needle to extract 0.2 to 0.5 ml of fluid from a region 6 to 8 mm caudal to the limbus. It is important to direct the needle caudad within the center of the globe but avoid the lens. The fluid is a transparent jellylike material that is primarily water with the remainder composed of collagen and hyaluronic acid (Samuelson, 1999). The humor is likely formed by the nonpigmented epithelium of the ciliary body. In dogs and cats the vitreous humor is dense in the center of the cavity and fluid at the periphery, unlike in primates. It is acellular except for hyalocytes, a type of histiocyte. In addition to hyalocytes, fibrocytes and glial cells make

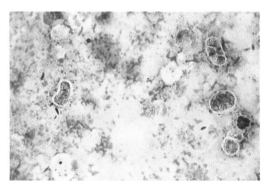

FIGURE 14–19. Protothecosis. Vitreocentesis. Dog. Shown present against the eosinophilic granular vitreal material are four sporulating forms of *Prototheca zopfii*. Also present in the background are several lanceolate melanin granules typical of the retina melanocytes. One condensed neutrophil is also seen. (Wright-Giemsa; ×330.) (Photo courtesy of A. Eric Schultze, University of Tennessee.)

up a small portion of the vitreal cells found in the fluid. Occasional lanceolate or caraway seed-shaped melanin granules may be present that are likely retinal in origin.

Inflammation

Infectious causes of endophthmalitis include bacteria, aspergillosis (Gelatt et al, 1991) (Fig 14–18A & B), blastomycosis, cryptococcosis, histoplasmosis, and protothecosis (Fig. 14–19).

Response to Tissue Injury

Hemorrhage appears similar to that found in the aqueous humor. Lens fibers may be seen with primary lens disease or secondary to accidental puncture during sample collection. They appear as uniform amorphous basophilic strands or ribbon structures (Fig. 14–20A & B). Their degeneration may induce a neutrophilic inflammatory response. Retinal cells, when present, are usually the

result of inadvertent aspiration. Photoreceptor and ganglion cells have been rarely identified on cytology; photoreceptor cells have tightly clumped nuclei with central cleavage (Knoll, 1990).

Neoplasia

This is rarely seen on cytology, but will be diagnostic when found.

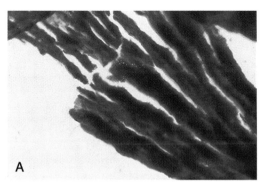

FIGURE 14–20. A. Lens fibers. Vitreocentesis. Dog. Dark basophilic staining fibers appear in parallel fashion. A mononuclear infiltrate of small lymphocytes (not shown) is present in low numbers in the vitreous humor, suggesting the presence of the lens fibers was the result of inadvertent puncture of the lens. (Wright-Giemsa; ×125.)

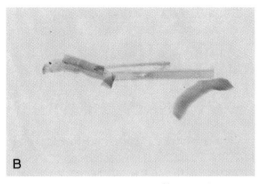

FIGURE 14–20. B. Lens fibers. Vitreocentesis. Same case as in Figure 14–20A. Isolated lightly basophilic lens fibers are recognized by the rectangular sharp outlines and ribbon-like appearance. (Wright-Giemsa; ×250.)

ORBITAL CAVITY

The orbit has bony borders but may be approached through several sites. The most direct routes are the lateral and medial canthi by fine-needle aspiration biopsy (FNAB). Another route is the insertion of a needle behind the last upper molar into the retrobulbar space. One study compared the usefulness of FNAB in conjunction with ultrasonography in the diagnosis of clinical exophthalmos (Boydell, 1991). The procedure was diagnostic in 34 of 35 cases.

Inflammation

Bacterial infection is likely to induce a purulent response resulting in cellulitis or abscess formation. Periorbital masses may arise from fungal infections such as cryptococcosis (Fig. 14–21). Inflammation may also result from a mucocele from the zygomatic gland. The material obtained is often clear and viscid, consistent with saliva.

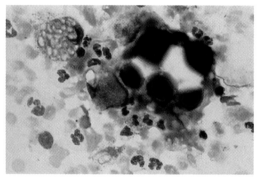

FIGURE 14–21. Cryptococcosis. Tissue aspirate of periorbital mass. Dog. This animal presented with protuberance of the frontal bone and blindness. Pyogranulomatous reaction occurred in response to the dark spherical yeast forms of *Cryptococcus neoformans*. (Wright-Giemsa; ×250.)

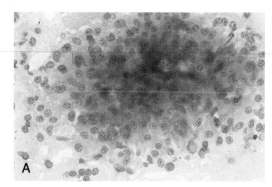

FIGURE 14–22. A. Salivary/lacrimal gland adenocarcinoma. Tissue aspirate of retrobulbar mass. Dog. Dense cluster of a monomorphic population of epithelial cells having high nuclear-to-cytoplasmic ratios and anisokaryosis. The exact origin was not clear on histopathology. It produced minor degenerative changes to the retina but did not invade the globe. (Wright-Giemsa; ×125.)

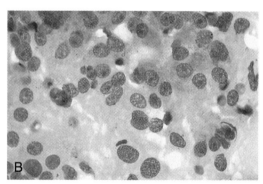

FIGURE 14–22. B. Salivary/lacrimal gland adenocarcinoma. Tissue aspirate. Same case as in Figure 14–22A. Higher magnification demonstrates an acinus (upper right corner) and the foamy secretory appearance of the cytoplasm. Several nuclear features of malignancy are present, including high nuclear-to-cytoplasmic ratio, anisokaryosis, coarse chromatin, prominent nucleoli, and multinucleation. (Wright-Giemsa; ×250.)

Neoplasia

Neoplasms involving the orbit include lymphoma, melanoma, mast cell tumor, squamous cell carcinoma, adenocarcinoma of the lacrimal or salivary glands (Fig. 14–22A–B), chondrosarcoma, and other sarcomas. In one case, FNAB of a suspected neoplasm posterior to the eye resulted in inadvertent aspiration of normal retinal epithelium with resultant intraocular hemorrhage (Roth and Sisson, 1999).

NASOLACRIMAL APPARATUS

Normal Histology and Cytology

Tears are formed in part by the lipid secretions of sebaceous glands such as the meibomian glands, by mucin from conjunctival goblet cells, and by seromucoid secretions from the gland of the nictitating membrane, but are predominantly formed by the aqueous fluid from the lacrimal gland located dorsolateral to the globe. The lacrimal gland is composed of serous gland epithelium in the cat but is seromucoid in the dog. Ducts are lined by flattened, cuboidal epithelium.

Inflammation

Inflammation of the lacrimal sac, or *dacryocystitis,* is frequently bacterial in origin and neutrophil exudates result obstructing the ducts.

Cyst

A cyst arising within the duct of the lacrimal gland is termed *dacryops* and contains serous or seromucoid material of low cellularity. It may be mixed with few neutrophils and macrophages (Prasse and Winston, 1999).

References

Boscos CM, Ververidis HN, Tondis DK, et al: Ocular involvement of transmissible venereal tumor in a dog. Vet Ophthalmol 1998; 1:167–170.

Boydell P: Fine needle aspiration biopsy in the diagnosis of exophthalmos. J Sm Anim Pract 1991;32:542–546.

Gelatt KN, Chrisman CL, Samuelson DA, et al: Ocular and systemic aspergillosis in a dog. J Am Anim Hosp Assoc 1991;27:427–431.

Glaze MB, Gelatt KN: Feline ophthalmology. In Gelatt KN (ed): Veterinary Ophthalmology. 3rd ed. Lippincott Williams & Wilkins, Philadelphia, 1999, pp 997–1052.

Greene CE: Chlamydial infections. In Greene CE (ed): Infectious Diseases of the Dog and Cat. 2nd ed. WB Saunders, Philadelphia, 1998, pp 172–174.

Haesebrouck F, Devriese LA, van Rijssen B, et al: Incidence and significance of isolation of *Mycoplasma felis* from conjunctival swabs of cats. Vet Microbiol 1991;26:95–101.

Hazel SJ, Thrall MAH, Severin GA, et al: Laboratory evaluation of aqueous humor in the healthy dog, cat, horse, and cow. Am J Vet Res 1985;46:657–659.

Hirai T, Mubarak M, Kimura T, et al: Apocrine gland tumor of the eyelid in a dog. Vet Pathol 1997;34:232–234.

Knoll JS: What is your diagnosis? Vet Clin Pathol 1990;19:32–34.

Komaromy AM, Ramsey DT, Render JA, et al: Primary adenocarcinoma of the gland of the nictitating membrane in a cat. J Am Anim Hosp Assoc 1997; 33:333–336.

Lipman NS, Yan L-L, Murphy JC: Probable transmission of *Chlamydia psittaci* from a macaw to a cat. J Am Vet Med Assoc 1994;204:1479–1480.

Massa KL, Murphy CJ, Hartmann FA, et al: Usefulness of aerobic microbial culture and cytologic evaluation of corneal specimens in the diasnosis of infectious ulcerative keratitis in animals. J Am Vet Med Assoc 1999;215:1671–1674.

Murphy JM: Exfoliative cytologic examination as an aid in diagnosing ocular diseases in the dog and cat. Semin Vet Med Surg (Sm Anim) 1988; 3:10–14.

Naisse MP, Guy JS, Stevens JB, et al: Clinical and laboratory findings in chronic conjunctivitis in cats: 91 cases (1983–1991). J Am Vet Med Assoc 1993;203:834–837.

Patnaik AK, Mooney S: Feline melanoma: a comparative study of ocular, oral, and dermal neoplasms. Vet Pathol 1988;25:105–112.

Pentlarge VW: Eosinophilic conjunctivitis in five cats. J Am Anim Hosp Assoc 1991;27:21–28.

Prasse KW, Winston SM: Cytology and histopathology of feline eosinophilic keratitis. Vet Comp Opthalmol 1996;6:74–81.

Prasse KW, Winston SM: The eyes and associated structures. In Cowell RL, Tyler RD, Meinkoth JH (eds): Diagnostic Cytology and Hematology of the Dog and Cat, 2nd ed. CV Mosby, St Louis, 1999, pp 68–82.

Roth L, Sisson A: Aspirate of a mass posterior to the eye. Vet Clin Pathol 1999;28:89–90.

Samuelson DA: Ophthalmic anatomy. In Gelatt KN (ed): Veterinary Ophthalmology, 3rd ed. Lippincott Williams & Wilkins, Philadelphia, 1999, pp 31–150.

Stiles J, McDermott M, Bigsby D, et al: Use of nested polymerase chain reaction to identify feline herpesvirus in ocular tissue from clinically normal cats and cats with corneal sequestra or conjunctivitis. Am J Vet Res 1997;58:338–342.

Willis M, Bounous DI, Hirsh S, et al: Conjunctival brush cytology: evaluation of a new cytological collection technique in dogs and cats with a comparison to conjunctival scraping. Vet Comp Ophthalmol 1997;7:74–81.

CHAPTER 15

Endocrine System

A. Rick Alleman

The endocrine system consists of the thyroid, parathyroid, adrenal cortex, and pancreatic islet cells. These highly integrated, highly vascularized glands have sinusoids that are closely associated with secretory parenchymal cells from which hormones are produced. Also included within the endocrine system are paraganglionic cells, which are neuroendocrine cells that synthesize and secrete both catecholamines and other regulatory peptides. The neuroendocrine cells involve those of the adrenal medulla and extra-adrenal sites that are derived from neuroectoderm. The extra-adrenal paraganglionic cells include the aortic and carotid bodies, which have chemoreceptor activity in the blood gas regulation, as well as others found in the gastrointestinal tract and lung.

Disease involving the endocrine system may involve hyperplasia, hypoplasia, inflammation, and neoplasia, with the latter condition of most interest to the cytopathologist. Endocrine system tumors are often very cellular, with the exception of aspirates from some thyroid tumors, which are often

blood contaminated. Tumors of endocrine glands and neuroendocrine cells share a characteristic cytologic feature. Slide preparations appear as naked nuclei or free nuclei embedded in a background of pale cytoplasm with few distinct cytoplasmic borders. This is an artifact of aspiration and slide preparation that results from the fragile nature of the cells from these organs. This cytologic feature should not be confused with poorly prepared samples from other tissues, where cell lysis occurs when excessive pressure is applied to the slides during sample preparation. In the later case, cell damage such as nuclear lysis and nuclear streaming will also be evident.

Although neuroendocrine tumors share common characteristics, they can often be distinguished from each other by the location of the lesion and distinctive cytologic features that may be present. Identification of the tissue of origin of the tumor is important in predicting the biologic behavior since the cytologic criteria for malignancy are not easily interpreted with these neoplasms. If criteria of malignancy are present, the tumors are likely to metastasize or locally invade surrounding structures. However, nuclei from neuroendocrine tumors often do not display anaplastic features, even when there is a likelihood of metastasis or local invasion. Thus, tumor identification and knowledge of the malignant potential of the specific neoplasms in different species is critical for prognosticating tumors of endocrine and neuroendocrine origin. This is true of all the endocrine system tumors, but is particularly important when evaluating thyroid tumors, the most commonly encountered endocrine system lesion.

THYROID TUMORS

The thyroid is composed of variably sized follicles lined by simple epithelium. Squamous to low cuboidal epithelium is present in the resting stage and cuboidal to columnar epithelium is found in the active stage (Fig. 15–1). The follicular colloid contains the thyroglobulin, from which thyroid hormone is produced. Follicles are separated by

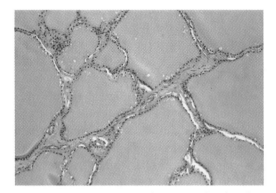

FIGURE 15–1. Normal active gland. Thyroid. Cat. Variably sized follicles that contain colloid are lined by cuboidal epithelium. Vacuoles are present adjacent to epithelium related to active endocytosis of thyroglobulin. (H & E; ×50.) (Courtesy of Rose Raskin, Gainesville, FL.)

delicate fibrous septa with an abundant vascular supply. The active follicle has vacuoles adjacent to the epithelium as evidence of the endocytosis of thyroglobulin.

Thyroid tumors occur most frequently in the dog, cat, and horse (Capen, 1990). They often present clinically as a subcutaneous mass located on the neck, usually lateral to the trachea, or near the thoracic inlet. Ectopic thyroid tumors may occasionally be found in the cranial thoracic cavity, at the base of the heart, or even in the oral cavity at the base of the tongue (Lantz and Salisbury, 1989). There is marked species variation regarding the biologic behavior of thyroid tumors. Therefore, the features of these lesions will be described as they relate to the dog and the cat.

Canine Thyroid Tumors

Thyroid tumors represent from 1.2% to 3.7% of all canine tumors (Harari et al., 1986). No sex predilection has been established, however, a breed predilection has been suggested for boxers, beagles, and golden retrievers (Harari et al., 1986). Approximately 90% to 95% of the thyroid tumors identified clinically in the dog are carcinomas (Ogilvie, 1996). Aspirates from thyroid tumors, particularly carcinomas, may contain a large amount of blood contamination (Harari et al., 1986). Clusters or sheets of epithelial cells are typically seen scattered throughout the preparations. These clumps will appear as free nuclei embedded in a background of pale-blue cytoplasm, with infrequent appearance of cytoplasmic membranes or borders (Fig. 15–2A). Dark-blue to black pigment is sometimes seen in the cytoplasm of epithelial cells (Fig. 15–2B). Although not definitively identified as such, this pigment is thought to represent tyrosine-containing granules (Maddux and Shull, 1989). Amorphous

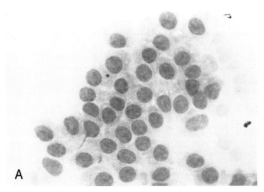

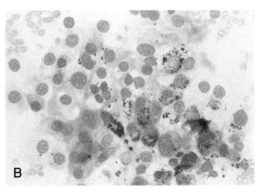

FIGURE 15–2. A, Adenocarcinoma. Thyroid. Dog. Tissue aspirate taken from a subcutaneous mass located on the neck. A fairly uniform cluster of cells have pale, lightly granular cytoplasm with poorly defined cytoplasmic borders, typical of an endocrine tumor. (Wright-Giemsa; ×250.)

FIGURE 15–2. B, Same case as Figure 15–2A. The cytoplasm of the cells has poorly defined borders and pink colloid is observed within the cluster. The dark, cytoplasmic pigment (bottom) is believed to contain tyrosine granules. The nuclei have moderate anisokaryosis. (Wright-Giemsa; ×125.)

pink material representing colloid may be associated with some clusters (Fig. 15–3). Colloid and/or pigmented granules, along with the naked nuclei appearance of the cells, are used to definitively identify the tissue as thyroid in origin.

The nuclei of most tumors are round to oval with minimal anaplastic features. Most thyroid tumors, even adenocarcinomas, will be composed of a fairly uniform population of cells, displaying few if any criteria of malignancy (Figs. 15–2 and 15–3). There may be mild to moderate anisokaryosis (Fig. 15–4) and small indistinct nucleoli may occasionally be seen in some tumors. However, as previously mentioned, approximately 90% to 95% of the canine thyroid tumors are adenocarcinomas. Therefore, anytime a canine tumor is identified as thyroid in origin, it should be regarded as a probable carcinoma until histopathologic confirmation is obtained.

The biologic behavior of canine thyroid tumors is well characterized. Thyroid adenocarcinomas are invasive and will metastasize if given sufficient time. The prognosis

and the potential for metastasis may depend on tumor size. In one study, 14% of dogs with tumor volumes less than 20 cm^3 had evidence of metastasis, whereas a metastatic rate of 75% to 100% was seen in dogs with

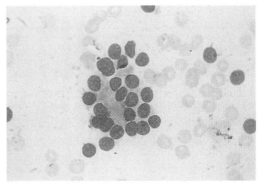

FIGURE 15–3. Adenocarcinoma. Thyroid. Dog. Tissue aspirate taken from a subcutaneous mass located on the neck. A cluster of cells has pale cytoplasm and poorly defined cytoplasmic borders. Nuclei are fairly uniform with only mild anisokaryosis. A small amount of amorphous eosinophilic material or colloid can be seen within the cluster of cells. (Wright-Giemsa; ×250.)

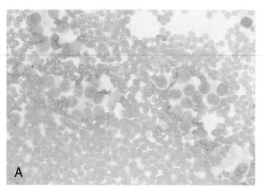

FIGURE 15–4. A, Adenocarcinoma. Thyroid. Dog. This animal had an intermittent honking cough. On physical examination, a 2- to 3-cm firm, round, moveable mass was found lateral to the trachea at mid-neck. Present are groups of loosely adherent cells appearing as naked nuclei against a blood-contaminated background. (Wright-Giemsa; ×125.) (Courtesy of Rose Raskin, Gainesville, FL.)

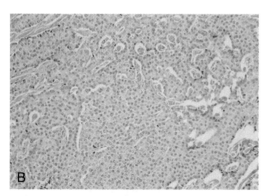

FIGURE 15–4. B, Same case as Figure 15–4A. Variably sized compact nests and diffuse sheets of neoplastic cells efface the gland leaving normal thyroid gland with small follicles at the periphery. (H & E; ×50.) (Courtesy of Rose Raskin, Gainesville, FL.)

tumor volumes between 21 and 100 cm³ (Leav et al., 1983). The earliest and most frequent site of metastasis is the lungs, resulting from invasion of tumor cells into the thyroid or jugular vein (Capen, 1990). When possible, surgical resection is the treatment of choice, however, carcinomas

are rapidly invasive and may involve vital structures such as the jugular vein, carotid artery, and esophagus. In dogs, hypersecretion of thyroid hormones in association with thyroid tumors is rare (Ogilvie, 1996).

Feline Thyroid Tumors

Thyroid tumors in the cat are cytologically identical to those seen in the dog (Figs. 15–5 and 15–6). However, unlike in the dog, the vast majority of tumors in the cat are benign adenomas, also known as adenomatous hyperplasia. Both thyroid glands are involved in about 70% of the cases (Peterson et al., 1983; Peterson and Turrel, 1986). Functional adenocarcinomas occur in only 1% to 2% of cats presenting with clinical signs of hyperthyroidism (Peterson et al., 1983; Peterson and Turrel, 1988). In the cat, if cytologic preparations contain a very uniform population of nuclei with no criteria for malignancy, the thyroid tumor is considered most likely benign. It is not possible to cytologically differentiate between

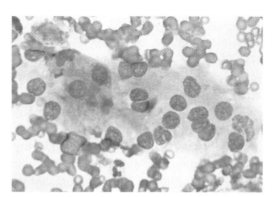

FIGURE 15–5. Adenoma. Thyroid. Cat. Tissue aspirate taken from a subcutaneous mass located on the neck of a cat. The cytoplasm of the cells has poorly defined borders and pink colloid is observed within the cluster. The nuclei are uniform. (Wright-Giemsa; ×250.)

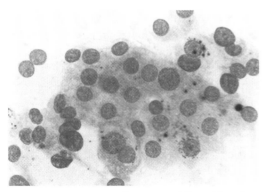

FIGURE 15–6. Adenoma. Thyroid. Cat. Tissue aspirate from an animal with clinical hyperthyroidism of 3 years' duration. Cat was treated 3 months earlier with radioactive iodine and now presents with reoccurrence of hyperthyroidism. Cytologically, several binucleated forms are present along with black granular cytoplasmic inclusions. Moderate degree of anisocytosis and anisokaryosis are noted. (Wright-Giemsa; ×250.) (Courtesy of Rose Raskin, Gainesville, FL.)

adenomas and adenocarcinomas. However, histologic evaluation of capsular or lymphatic invasion is often required to distinguish adenomas from adenocarcinomas (Capen, 1990; Turrel, et al., 1988).

Unlike the canine, most thyroid adenomas in the cat actively secrete thyroid hormones. Adenomas are usually well encapsulated and the prognosis is excellent with surgical removal. If bilateral thyroidectomy is performed, the patient must be monitored for signs of hypothyroidism or hypocalcemia resulting from removal of the parathyroid glands (Capen, 1990). Adenocarcinomas are locally invasive and often metastasize to regional lymph nodes. Metastatic disease has been reported in up to 71% of cats with adenocarcinomas (Turrel et al., 1988).

Treatment may consist of antithyroid drugs, which are not cytotoxic but are used to reduce the metabolic effects of thyrotoxicosis prior to surgery. Radiotherapy with

Iodine 131 (^{131}I) can alternatively be performed to reduce the neoplasm, especially for cats with hyperfunctional ectopic thyroid tissue.

PARATHYROID TUMORS

Parathyroid tumors are uncommon neoplasms in domestic animals. Most reported cases involve dogs (Berger and Feldman, 1987; DeVries et al., 1993) or cats (den-Hertog et al., 1997; Kallet et al., 1991). There may be a breed predisposition in the Keeshond (Berger and Feldman, 1987). The tumors are usually recognized in older animals, for example, dogs 7 years of age or older and cats 8 years of age or older (Berger and Feldman, 1987; den-Hertog et al., 1997; DeVries et al., 1993; Kallet et al., 1991).

The most frequently reported parathyroid tumor is the adenoma of the parathyroid chief cells. Parathyroid carcinomas are rare, but have been diagnosed in older dogs and cats (Capen, 1990, Kallet et al., 1991, Marquez et al., 1995). Cytologic evaluation of parathyroid tumors in the dog is usually performed on surgically removed specimens since tumors are usually too small to be detected by cervical palpation (Ogilvie, 1996). However, in one report, four of seven cats with primary hyperparathyroidism had palpable cervical masses (Kallet et al., 1991). In these cases, cytologic evaluation has been useful in making a diagnosis (den-Hertog et al., 1997). Chief cells aspirated from parathyroid adenomas have a typical naked nuclei appearance on cytologic preparations. Cells appear as free nuclei in a lightly eosinophilic background of cytoplasm. Nuclei are round to oval and fairly uniform in size and shape. Parathyroid adenocarcinomas typically are larger than adenomas, however, they may appear similar cytologically. The diagnosis of adenocarcinoma is made when there is histologic or gross evidence of capsular invasion, invasion into surrounding structures, or metastasis to regional lymph or lungs (Capen, 1990).

Since parathyroid tumors, especially adenomas, are often not palpable, the presurgical diagnosis frequently relies on recognition of clinical signs and characteristic laboratory findings. The vast majority of parathyroid tumors actively secrete inappropriate amounts of parathormone, and most cases are presented for clinical signs associated with increased hormonal activity. Although some species variation may exist with regard to the frequency of observance of specific clinical signs, similarities in clinical and laboratory findings exist in all species. Commonly reported abnormalities include hypercalcemia (the most common finding), polydipsia and polyuria, muscle weakness, skeletal abnormalities, and cystic calculi (DeVries, et al., 1993; Ogilvie 1996; Klausner et al., 1986; Klausner et al., 1987; Marquez et al., 1995).

Surgical exploration of the cervical area is warranted if laboratory and clinical findings establish a diagnosis of primary hyperparathyroidism. Parathyroid adenomas are well encapsulated and can be surgically removed by blunt dissection (Ogilvie, 1996). Patients must be monitored closely for the rapid development of postsurgical hypocalcemia (Berger and Feldman, 1987; Capen, 1990; Ogilvie, 1996). The long-term prognosis for patients with parathyroid adenomas is good.

TUMORS OF THE ENDOCRINE PANCREAS

The most frequently diagnosed tumor of endocrine pancreas is the insulinoma, a tumor of the beta islet cells (β-cells). These lesions have been referred to as insulinomas, insulin-producing pancreatic tumors, insulin-producing islet cell tumors, islet cell tumors, and β-cell tumors (Ogilvie, 1996). They most commonly occur in dogs, generally large breeds over 5 years of age (Capen, 1990; Ogilvie, 1996). Commonly affected breeds include boxers, German shepherd dogs, Irish setters, standard poodles, fox terriers, collies, and Labrador retrievers (Ogilvie, 1996). These tumors have also been identified with some frequency in the ferret and rarely in the cat (Hawks, 1992; Ogilvie, 1996).

The cytologic appearance of insulinomas is typical of other endocrine tumors, with most preparations being fairly cellular, containing mostly naked nuclei embedded in a background of lightly basophilic cytoplasm. In many instances, the cytoplasm of the cells contains numerous, small, punctate, clear vacuoles (Fig. 15–7). There may be a mild to moderate anisokaryosis and nuclei may contain a single prominent nucleolus, typical of some endocrine tumors. Although most β-cell tumors in the dog are carcinomas, nuclear features of malignancy are inconsistently seen, and as with other endocrine tumors, it is often difficult to predict the biological behavior of these lesions based on the histologic or cytologic characteristics of the cells (Capen, 1990; Ogilvie, 1996). Therefore, some pathologists prefer to identify these lesions as islet cell tumors unless there is evidence of invasion into surrounding structures, lymphatics, or metastatic disease. If the criteria for malignancy are met, a diagnosis of adenocarcinoma can reliably be made; however, the lack of anaplastic features cannot be used to predict the biologic behavior. Even small tumors composed of well-differentiated β-cells have been known to metastasize (Capen, 1990).

The biologic behavior of these lesions is well characterized. Unlike in humans, in

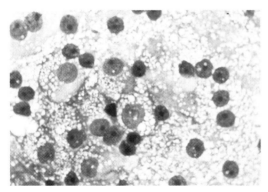

FIGURE 15–7. Insulinoma (β-cell tumor). Pancreatic mass. Dog. Tissue imprint taken from an intra-abdominal mass located in the pancreas of a hypoglycemic dog. The cytoplasmic borders of the cells are indistinct and contain numerous punctate, clear vacuoles. There is moderate anisokaryosis and a prominent, usually singular nucleolus, typical of some neuroendocrine/endocrine tumors. (Wright-Giemsa; ×250.)

whom 90% of the pancreatic islet cell tumors are adenomas, most islet cell tumors in the dog are adenocarcinomas (Capen, 1990). Metastasis is via lymphatics with involvement of regional lymph nodes and liver in about 50% of the cases (Ogilvie, 1996). Metastatic disease has been documented in other sites as well. Most tumors actively secrete inappropriate amounts of insulin, resulting in profound hypoglycemia. Because of the low blood glucose, patients often present with neuromuscular signs such as seizures, hind-limb weakness, ataxia, muscle tremors, and generalized weakness (Ogilvie, 1996). Although not exclusively associated with insulinomas, most all dogs with the disease have Whipple's triad, which consists of (1) clinical signs associated with hypoglycemia, (2) fasting blood glucose less than 40 mg/dl, and (3) alleviation of clinical signs by the administration of dextrose.

A tentative diagnosis of β-cell tumor can be made by demonstrating profound hypoglycemia and an abnormal insulin-to-glucose ratio. Confirmation can be made by exploratory celiotomy or ultrasound-guided, fine-needle aspiration if the lesion is large enough. One report suggests that once a tentative diagnosis is made, exploratory celiotomy and partial pancreatectomy are indicated in dogs since surgery significantly increases the mean survival time from 74 days (medical or dietary management) to 381 days (surgery plus medical or dietary management) (Tobin et al., 1999).

CHEMORECEPTOR TUMORS

Chemoreceptor tumors are generally referred to as *chemodectomas* or *nonchromaffin paragangliomas*. Although chemoreceptor tissue is found in several areas of the body, tumors of chemoreceptor cells are primarily found in the aortic bodies or the carotid bodies (Capen, 1990). They are uncommon tumors of the dog and have rarely been reported in cats (Ogilvie, 1996; Tillson et al., 1994). Most dogs affected are between 10 and 15 years of age, and there is a higher incidence of these tumors in brachycephalic breeds, particularly boxers and Boston terriers (Capen, 1990; Ogilvie, 1996). The majority (80% to 90%) of chemoreceptor tumors reported in animals have originated from the aortic bodies, however, there are rare reports of carotid body tumors in the dog (Obradovich et al., 1992; Ogilvie, 1996).

The aortic body tumor or heartbase tumor generally occurs as a single mass within the pericardial sac at or near the base of the heart (Capen, 1990). Presenting clinical signs are usually those associated with cardiac decompensation, particularly right heart failure resulting from significant pericardial effusion. Cytologic evaluation of the pericardial effusion rarely allows identification of tumor cells. Reactive mesothelium often associated with the fluid may be mistaken for neoplastic cells (see Chapter 6). Unlike the pericardial fluid, ultrasound-guided, fine-needle aspirates taken directly from the lesions are usually very cellular and are often diagnostically rewarding. Care must be taken when performing this procedure because of the close association of aortic body tumors with the atria and major vessels.

Cytologically, aspirates and imprints taken from these lesions are usually quite cellular. The typical naked nuclei appearance with free nuclei in a background of cytoplasm is a prominent feature (Fig. 15–8A). Nuclei are round with clumped chromatin and usually contain a single, prominent nucleolus (Fig. 15–8B) typical of neuroendocrine cell tumors. Both benign and malignant forms occur and anaplastic features of ani-

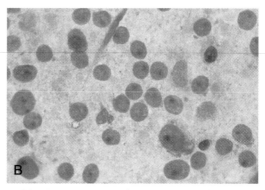

FIGURE 15–8. B, Same case as in Figure 15–8A. Cells display a moderate degree of anisokaryosis along with prominent, usually singular nucleoli. (Wright-Giemsa; ×250.)

sokaryosis and multiple, variable nucleoli are not reliable indicators of the malignant potential. Both adenomas and adenocarcinomas have scattered areas of the tumor that contain larger more pleomorphic cells (Fig. 15–8A) and bizarrely shaped giant cells (Capen, 1990). Carcinomas are identified by invasion into the surrounding capsule, blood vessels, lymphatics, or adjacent structures (Capen, 1990). Aortic body tumors may be difficult to distinguish from ectopic thyroid tumors, which may appear cytologically similar and may on occasion occur in the same area. The identification of colloid or pigment granules would help to identify the tissue as thyroid in origin.

Most aortic body tumors in the dog are benign adenomas (Capen, 1990). They are usually well encapsulated and are slow growing with low metastatic potential, however, they are expansive lesions and will eventually compress the atria or vena cavae. With adenomas, surgical resection is the treatment of choice; however, long-term success is limited because complete resection is difficult to achieve owing to the close association of these neoplasms with major vessels. The role of chemotherapy in

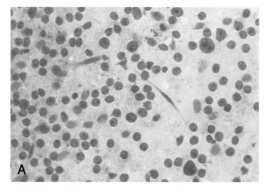

FIGURE 15–8. A, Aortic body tumor (chemodectoma). Thoracic mass. Dog. Tissue aspirate taken from a mass located in the thoracic cavity, just dorsal to the base of the heart. The cells appear as naked nuclei or free nuclei within a background of lightly basophilic cytoplasm without distinct cell borders, typical of neuroendocrine tumors. There is moderate anisokaryosis and a prominent, usually singular nucleolus. (Wright-Giemsa; ×125.)

the treatment of these lesions is unknown (Ogilvie, 1996). Malignant forms or carcinomas are invasive and may spread locally to veins, lymphatics, or myocardium (Capen, 1990, Zimmerman et al., 2000). When distant metastasis occurs it is usually to the lung or the liver, but a number of organs may be involved. The prognosis for cats with chemodectomas may be worse because of the frequent invasive nature of the tumor in this species (Tillson, 1994).

Carotid body tumors are rare neoplasms that are located in the neck, near the angle of the jaw, at the bifurcation of the common carotid artery (Capen, 1990, Obradovich, et al., 1992). Cytologically they appear similar to aortic body tumors (Fig. 15–9). The location of carotid body tumors also necessitates differentiation from thyroid tumors. Identification of colloid or pigment granules would help to identify tissue as thyroid in origin. Although case reports are

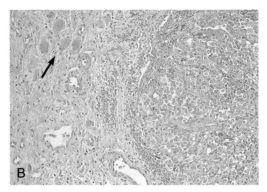

FIGURE 15–9. B, Same case as in Figure 15–9A. Section contains dense sheets of neoplastic cells (right side) adjacent to fibrovascular stroma (left side) and nerve cell bodies *(arrow)*. Tumor emboli occur with blood vessels (not shown) demonstrating the invasive nature of the tumor. (H & E; ×50.) (Courtesy of Rose Raskin, Gainesville, FL.)

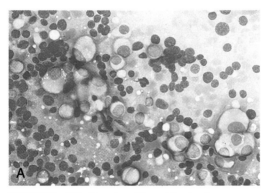

FIGURE 15–9. A, Carotid body tumor (chemodectoma). Cervical mass. Dog. Surgical excision imprint from an animal that presented with a head tilt. Magnetic resonance imaging indicated the presence of the mass in the neck region near the tympanic bulla. Cytologically, there are numerous free nuclei with a small number of variably sized intact cells. Anisocytosis and anisokaryosis are marked. (Aqueous-based Wright; ×250.) (Courtesy of Rose Raskin, Gainesville, FL.)

limited, these tumors are more likely to be malignant than are aortic body tumors, and they are characterized by local tissue invasion and a tendency to metastasize to multiple sites in the body (Capen, 1990; Obradovich, et al., 1992). Metastasis usually occurs late in the course of the disease, primarily to the liver, mediastinum, brain, heart, and lungs. Early surgical excision is the treatment of choice (Obradovich, et al., 1992; Ogilvie, 1996). The role of chemotherapy in the treatment of these tumors has not been evaluated.

ADRENAL GLAND TUMORS

Enlargement of the adrenal gland may arise from either the conical or the medullary areas of this gland. Those enlargements originating within the cortex often result in the excessive production of corticosteroids and the clinical condition of hyperadrenocorticism. Tumors of the adrenal medulla

cause the paroxysmal release of catecholamines, primarily norepinephrine.

Tumors of the Adrenal Medulla

The most common tumor of the adrenal
medulla is the pheochromocytoma, also
called *chromaffin paraganglioma,* or *chromaffin cell tumor.* Rarely, other tumors,
such as neuroblastomas and ganglioneuromas, may arise from the primitive neuroectodermal cells in this area (Capen, 1990).
Neuroblastomas are often seen in very
young animals, resulting in large intra-abdominal masses, which often metastasize to
peritoneal surfaces. Ganglioneuromas are
small benign tumors in the adrenal medulla.

Pheochromocytomas are tumors of the
chromaffin cells of the adrenal medulla.
They occur most frequently in middle-aged
to older dogs with no apparent gender or
breed predilection and are rarely reported
in cats (Barthez et al., 1997; Ogilvie, 1996;
Patnaik et al., 1990; Henry et al., 1993).
Clinical evidence of this tumor is usually
seen upon release of large amounts of catecholamines from the neoplasm. However,
clinical signs are varied and vague, and in
one study, 57% of the cases were diagnosed
as incidental findings (Barthez et al., 1997).
Two cases of pheochromocytoma in dogs
presented with paraparesis related to their
invasion into the spinal canal (Platt et al.,
1998). In addition, a large number of patients with pheochromocytomas have concurrent diseases, including other neoplasms
originating from other tissues (Barthez et
al., 1997; Bouayad et al., 1987). This further
complicates the clinical presentation of patients and makes it difficult to conclude
which clinical signs are attributable to the
release of catecholamines from the adrenal
tumor and which signs are the result of
concurrent diseases.

Abdominal ultrasonography is able to

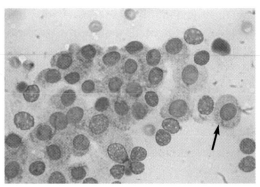

**FIGURE 15–10. Pheochromocytoma. Ab-
dominal mass. Dog.** Tissue aspirate taken
from an intra-abdominal mass located in the
adrenal gland. The cluster of cells contains pale
cytoplasm with occasional distinct cytoplasmic
borders. Fine, pale, basophilic, intracytoplasmic
granules can be seen in the cells *(arrow).*
There is mild anisokaryosis but no significant
criteria for malignancy, however, local invasion
into the caudal vena cava was detected ultrasonographically and histologically. Surgical excision resulted in complete removal of the tumor. (Wright-Giemsa; ×250.)

detect adrenal pheochromocytomas in approximately 50% of the cases (Barthez et al.,
1997). In these situations, ultrasound-
guided, fine-needle aspiration may be used
to make a more definitive diagnosis. Care
must be taken during the sampling procedure since manipulation of the affected
adrenal gland could cause the paroxysmal
release of catecholamines, resulting in hypertension, tachycardia, and/or arrhythmias.
In addition, many of these lesions are
closely associated with the caudal vena cava
and, in fact, may invade this vessel.

The cytologic appearance of pheochromocytomas is typical of other neuroendocrine
tumors. Much of the preparation may appear as naked nuclei against a background
of cytoplasm, however, intact cells are usually identified in most carefully prepared
specimens (Fig. 15–10). The cytoplasm of
the cells is lightly basophilic to amphophilic

with faint granules sometimes visible using Romanowsky-type stains (Fig. 15–10). Nuclei are round to oval and a single, small nucleolus may occasionally be observed. Both benign and malignant forms of the tumor exist. Nuclear features of malignancy are unreliable in predicting the biologic behavior of the lesion since even small tumors with well-differentiated cells are known to metastasize or invade surrounding structures (Capen, 1990; Bouayad et al., 1987). The presence of nuclear criteria of malignancy would strongly suggest a high potential for local invasion or metastasis (Fig. 15–11).

Pheochromocytomas may be recognized clinically upon the release of large quantities of catecholamines, primarily norepinephrine, which often results in a variety of clinical signs related to the cardiovascular

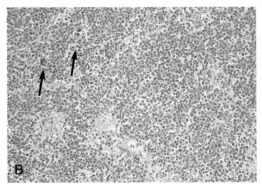

FIGURE 15–11. B, Same case as in Figure 15–11A. The mass is composed of pleomorphic neoplastic cells arranged in a dense lobular formation separated by fibrovascular septa. Occasional multinucleate cells *(arrows)* are seen. (H & E; ×50.) (Courtesy of Rose Raskin, Gainesville, FL.)

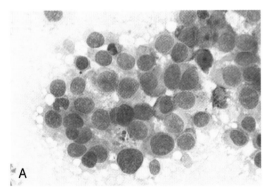

FIGURE 15–11. A, Pheochromocytoma. Abdominal mass. Dog. This animal presented with cervical and thoracic pain that progressed rapidly to paraparesis. A myelogram revealed an epidural mass at L1-2 and ultrasound examination indicated an abdominal mass. A tissue aspirate of the abdominal mass contained large round to oval loosely adherent cells with several criteria of malignancy including anisokaryosis, variable nuclear-to-cytoplasmic ratios, multiple prominent nucleoli, multinucleation (lower left) and coarse chromatin pattern. (Wright-Giemsa; ×250.) (Courtesy of Rose Raskin, Gainesville, FL.)

system and nervous system. Immunocytochemical stains (see Chapter 16) such as chromogranin A and synaptophysin on cytologic specimens may be used to support the diagnosis of a medullary tumor. Ultrastructural studies of pheochromocytomas are helpful to demonstrate the cytoplasmic neurosecretory granules.

The prognosis for patients is guarded to poor since 50% or more of these tumors are nonresectable owing to early invasion of the venous system and distant metastasis via the caudal vena cava (Barthez et al., 1997; Bouayad et al., 1987; Capen, 1990). However, with complete surgical excision long-term survival can be obtained. Several reports indicate a greater than 50% frequency of concurrent neoplasia of patients with pheochromocytomas, many of which are endocrine in origin (Barthez et al., 1997; Bouayad et al., 1987; Capen, 1990; von Dehn et al., 1995). The concurrent finding of pituitary adenoma or adrenocortical neoplasia resulted in a significant number of the dogs with pheochromocytomas having concurrent hyperadrenocorticism (Barthez et al., 1997; von Dehn et al., 1995).

Adrenocortical Disease

Hyperadrenocorticism is a common endocrinopathy in the dog and is rarely seen in the cat. In the dog, the condition is most often the result of a pituitary tumor, however, between 10% and 20% of the cases are associated with adrenocortical neoplasia (Ogilvie; 1996). In 89 reported cases of dogs with adrenocortical tumors, adenocarcinomas were diagnosed in 53 dogs and adenomas were found in 36 dogs (Penninck et al., 1988; Reusch and Feldman, 1991; Scavelli et al., 1986). The mean age was approximately 11 years (range 5 to 16 years). There appeared to be no significant breed or sex predilection. Both adrenocortical adenomas and edenocarcinomas have rarely been reported in the cat (Jones et al., 1992; Nelson et al., 1988).

Patients with adrenocortical tumors usually present with clinical and laboratory signs of hyperadrenocorticism. Once a diagnosis of hyperadrenocorticism is made, discriminatory tests such as the high-dose dexamethasone suppression test, measurement of endogenous adrenocorticotropic hormone (ACTH) concentrations, and abdominal ultrasonography should be used to distinguish pituitary-dependent hyperadrenocorticism (PDH) from adrenal tumors (AT). In contrast to PDH, which causes bilateral adrenal enlargement, AT typically cause asymmetrical enlargement of the one adrenal gland and atrophy of the contralateral adrenal (Nelson, 1992). In one study, abdominal ultrasonography detected 18 of 25 dogs (72%) with AT (Reusch et al., 1991). In this situation, an ultrasound-guided, fine-needle aspiration of the affected adrenal gland can be performed for cytologic evaluation of the lesion.

Cytologically, aspirates taken from adrenocortical adenomas contain cells resembling normal secretory cells from the zona fasiculata or zona reticularis (Capen, 1990). Preparations are typical of other endocrine tumors with most cells appearing as naked nuclei in a background of abundant cytoplasm. The cytoplasm is moderately basophilic and often contains abundant, clear, lipid vacuoles (Fig. 15–12A). Nuclei of adenomas are round and uniform in size. They may contain a prominent, often singular nucleolus (Fig. 15–12C). Focal areas of hematopoiesis, adipocytes, and mineral deposits may be found in some cortical adenomas (Fig. 15–12B) (Capen, 1990). It should be noted that cells aspirated from adrenal glands that are hyperplastic, as seen in dogs with PDH, and cells from adrenal adenomas are cytologically indistinguishable. Therefore, cytology cannot be used as a tool

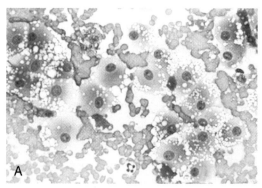

FIGURE 15–12. A, Adrenocortical adenoma. Adrenal mass. Dog. Tissue aspirate taken from an single nodule off the cranial pole of the adrenal gland noted on ultrasound examination of a dog with probable hyperadrenocorticism. The cluster of uniform cells contains abundant, amphophilic cytoplasm with mostly indistinct cytoplasmic borders. The cytoplasm contains numerous, clear, punctate vacuoles. (Wright-Giemsa; ×125.) (Courtesy of Peter Fernandes, Gainesville, FL.)

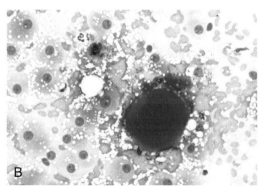

FIGURE 15–12. B, Same case as in Figure 15–12A. A large megakaryocyte (center) indicates the presence of extramedullary hematopoiesis, which is sometimes seen in tumors of the adrenal cortex. Evidence of chronic hemorrhage is indicated by the hemosiderin-laden macrophage (dark cell in upper center). (Wright-Giemsa; ×125.) (Courtesy of Peter Fernandes, Gainesville, FL.)

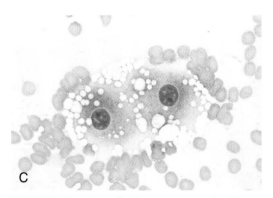

FIGURE 15–12. C, Same case as in Figure 15–12A. Two adrenocortical cells with small nuclei and prominent, usually singular nucleoli. The cytoplasm contains variably sized punctate vacuoles located predominately at the periphery of the cell. (Wright-Giemsa; ×250.) (Courtesy of Rose Raskin, Gainesville, FL.)

to distinguish between PDH and hyperadrenocorticism associated with AT.

Tumor cells from adrenocortical adenocarcinomas may be more pleomorphic compared with those from adenomas (Ca-

pen, 1990). Adenocarcinomas may display features of anaplasia, including anisokaryosis and multiple nucleoli. However, since some adenocarcinomas may contain well-differentiated cells, histologic evaluation of invasion into the capsule, adjacent structures, or vessels is the preferred method of distinction between adenomas and adenocarcinomas. Therefore, if the cytologic criteria of malignancy are fulfilled, a diagnosis of adenocarcinoma can reliably be made, however, in the absence of such criteria, caution should be used in making a firm diagnosis.

Adenomas of the zona fasiculata or zona reticularis are usually small and do not metastasize. Surgical resection is treatment of choice for adenomas; however, operative and postoperative complications involving the removal of the gland are frequently seen. Approximately half of the dogs with adrenocortical adenocarcinomas have gross evidence of local invasion into the caudal vena cava or renal artery, or distant metastasis, primarily to the liver, lung, or kidney (Ogilvie, 1996; Scavelli et al., 1986). Surgical resection of adenocarcinomas is difficult and as with adrenal adenomas, the incidence of postoperative complications is high (Scavelli et al., 1986). Treatment of adenocarcinomas with o,p-DDD (Lysodren, Bristol Laboratories, Syracuse, NY) or ketoconazole (Nizoral, Janssen Pharmaceutica Inc., Piscataway, NJ) has had very limited success (Ogilvie, 1996).

SUMMARY

Lesions involving endocrine glands and neuroendocrine tissues are a varied group of conditions that may arise from a number of specialized organs. Even so, these lesions share cytologic features, including the appearance of naked nuclei within a background of lightly basophilic cytoplasm with indistinct borders. In addition, as a group, it is difficult to predict the biologic behavior of these lesions based solely on abnormal nuclear features. Location of the lesion and distinguishing cytologic features must be used to identify the tissue of origin. The potential biologic behavior should be evaluated based on the specific tumor type and the species involved, along with histologic and/or clinical evidence of invasion.

References

Barthez PY, Marks, SL, Woo J, et al: Pheochromocytoma in dogs: 61 cases (1984–1995). J Vet Intern Med 1997; 11:272–278.

Berger B, Feldman EC: Primary hyperparathyroidism in dogs: 21 cases (1976–1986). J Am Vet Med Assoc 1987; 191:350–356.

Bouayad H, Feeney DA, Caywood DD, et al: Pheochromocytoma in dogs: 13 cases (1980–1985). J Am Vet Med Assoc 1987; 191:1610–1615.

Capen CC: Tumors of the endocrine glands. In Moulton JE (ed): *Tumors in Domestic Animals*, 3rd ed. University of California Press, Berkeley, 1990, pp 583–628.

den-Hertog E, Goossens MM, van-der-Linde-Sipman JS, et al: Primary hyperparathyroidism in two cats. Vet Q 1997; 19:81–84.

DeVries SE, Feldman EC, Nelson RW, et al: Primary parathyroid gland hyperplasia in dogs: Six cases (1982–1991). J Am Vet Med Assoc 1993; 202: 1132–1136.

Harari J, Patterson JS, Rosenthal RC: Clinical and pathologic features of thyroid tumors in 26 dogs. J Am Vet Med Assoc 1986; 188:1160–1164.

Hawks D, Peterson ME, Hawkins KL, et al: Insulin-secreting pancreatic (islet cell) carcinoma in a cat. J Vet Intern Med 1992; 6:193–196.

Henry CJ, Brewer WG, Montgomery RD, et al: Adrenal pheochromocytoma. J Vet Intern Med 1993; 7:199–201.

Jones CA, Refsal KR, Stevens BJ, et al: Adrenocortical adenocarcinoma in a cat. J Am Anim Hosp Assoc 1992; 28:59–62.

Kallet AJ, Richter KP, Feldman EC, et al: Primary hyperparathyroidism in cats: Seven cases (1984–1989). J Am Vet Med Assoc 1991; 199:1767–1771.

Klausner JS, O'Leary TP, Osborne CA: Calcium urolithiasis in two dogs with parathyroid adenomas. J Am Vet Med Assoc 1987; 191:1423–1426.

Klausner JS, Fernandez FR, O'Leary TP, et al: Canine primary hyperparathyroidism and its association with urolithiasis. Vet Clin North Am Small Anim Pract 1986; 16:227–239.

Lantz GC, Salisbury SK: Surgical excision of ectopic thyroid carcinoma involving the base of the tongue in dogs: Three cases (1980–1987). J Am Vet Med Assoc 1989; 195:1606–1608.

Leav I, Schillert AL, Rijnberk A, et al: Adenomas and adenocarcinomas of the canine and feline thyroid. Am J Pathol 1983; 83:61–93.

Maddux JM, Shull RM: Subcutaneous glandular tissue: Mammary, salivary, thyroid, and parathyroid. *In:* Cowell RL, Tyler RD (eds): *Diagnostic Cytology of the Dog and Cat.* American Veterinary Publications, Inc., Goleta, CA, 1989, pp 83–92.

Marquez GA, Klausner JS, Osborne CA: Calcium oxalate urolithiasis in a cat with a functional parathyroid adenocarcinoma. J Am Vet Med Assoc 1995; 206:817–819.

Nelson RW, Feldman EC, Smith MC: Hyperadrenocorticism in cats: Seven cases (1978–1987). J Am Vet Med Assoc 1988; 193:245–250.

Nelson RW: Disorders of the adrenal gland. *In:* Nelson RW, Couto CG (eds): *Essentials of Small Animal Internal Medicine.* Mosby-Year Book, St. Louis, 1992.

Obradovich JE, Withrow SJ, Powers BE, et al: Carotid body tumors in the dog: Eleven cases (1978–1988). J Vet Intern Med 1992; 6:96–101.

Ogilvie GK: Tumors of the endocrine system. *In:* Withrow SJ, MacEwen EG (eds): *Small Animal Clinical Oncology*, 2nd ed, WB Saunders, Philadelphia, 1996, pp 316–346.

Patnaik AK, Erlandson RA, Leiberman PH, et al: Extra-adrenal pheochromocytoma (paraganglioma) in a cat. J Am Vet Med Assoc 1990; 197: 104–106.

Penninck DG, Feldman EC, Nyland TG: Radiographic features of canine hyperadrenocorticism caused by autonomously functioning adrenocortical tumors: 23 cases (1978–1986). J Am Vet Med Assoc 1988; 192:1604–1608.

Peterson ME, Kintzer PP, Cavanagh PG, et al: Feline hyperthyroidism: Pretreatment clinical and laboratory evaluations of 131 cases. J Am Vet Med Assoc 1983; 183:103–110.

Peterson ME, Turrel JM: Feline hyperthyroidism. *In:* Kirk RW (ed): *Current Veterinary Therapy IX.* WB Saunders, Philadelphia, 1986, pp 1026–1033.

Platt SR, Sheppard BJ, Graham J, et al: Pheochromocytoma in the vertebral canal of two dogs. J Am Anim Hosp Assoc 1998; 34:365–371.

Reusch CE, Feldman EC: Canine hyperadrenocorticism due to adrenocortical neoplasia. J Vet Intern Med 1991; 5:3–10.

Scavelli TD, Peterson ME, Matthiesen DT: Results of surgical treatment of hyperadrenocorticism caused by adrenocortical neoplasia in the dog: 25 cases (1980–1984). J Am Vet Med Assoc. 1986; 189:1360–1364.

Tillson DM, Fingland RB, Andrews GA: Chemodectoma in a cat. J Am Anim Hosp Assoc 1994; 30:586–590.

Tobin RL, Nelson RW, Lucroy MD, et al: Outcome of surgical versus medical treatment of dogs with beta cell neoplasia: 39 cases (1990–1997). J Am Vet Med Assoc 1999; 215:226–230.

Turrel JM, Feldman EC, Nelson RW, et al: Thyroid carcinoma causing hyperthyroidism in cats: 14 cases (1981–1986). J Am Vet Med Assoc 1988; 193:359–364.

von Dehn BJ, Nelson RW, Feldman EC, et al: Pheochromocytoma and hyperadrenocorticism in dogs: Six cases (1982–1992). J Am Vet Med Assoc 1987; 207:322–324.

Zimmerman KL, Rossmeisl JH, Thorn CE, et al: Mediastinal mass in a dog with syncope and abdominal distension. Vet Clin Pathol 2000; 29: 19–21.

CHAPTER 16

Advanced Diagnostic Techniques

JANICE M. ANDREWS

DAVID E. MALARKEY

Cytopathology is a highly useful noninvasive method for diagnosis of malignant vs. benign conditions and identification of infectious agents. However, a number of problems confront the cytopathologist on a daily basis because of limitations of conventional cytologic features. Adjunct techniques can be utilized to give additional information, which allows one to reach a definitive diagnosis. These techniques must be used in parallel with conventional cytologic features and include immunodiagnostics, special stains, flow cytometry, image analysis, electron microscopy, and molecular diagnostics. They aid in determining the primary cell of origin or presence and type of infectious agent. In this chapter, we discuss adjunct diagnostic techniques and focus on both their applications in cytopathology and histopathology.

IMMUNODIAGNOSIS

Since the development of monoclonal antibodies, the immunolocalization of cellular specific antigens has become increasingly popular in diagnostic cytology and histopathology. In particular, it is used to determine the histogenesis of neoplasms or cellular phenotyping of lymphomas/leukemias. The approach is based on the assumption that neoplastic cells can express the same antigens as from the tissues they originate. Immunohistochemistry (IHC) and immunocytochemistry (ICC) are applications of immunodiagnostics in histopathology and cytopathology, respectively. The use of ICC techniques with cytologic specimens has been limited in comparison to histologic specimens.

Application of ICC in cytopathology is

TABLE 16–1	Intermediate Filament Proteins Used to Distinguish Tissue of Origin
Intermediate Filament	**Source**
Cytokeratin	Epithelial, mesothelial
Desmin	Muscle; smooth, skeletal, cardiac
Glial fibrillary acidic protein	Glia (astrocytes, ependymal cells, oligodendrocytes)
Neurofilament	Neurons
Vimentin	Connective tissue cells, melanocytes, lymphocytes

TABLE 16–2	Tumor Markers Used in Immunocytochemistry and Immunohistochemistry
Cellular Marker	**Source**
Actin	
sarcomeric	Skelelal muscle
smooth muscle	Smooth muscle, myofibroblast, myoepithelial cells
Alpha-1-antichymotrypsin	Monocyte/macrophage lineage
Alpha-1-antitrypsin	Monocyte/macrophage lineage
Alpha fetoprotein	Fetal liver cells, yolk sac
Calcitonin	Thyroid C cells
Carcinoembryonic antigen	Fetal epithelial cells
Chromogranin	Neuroendocrine
Epithelial membrane antigen	Epithelial, mesothelial cells, plasma cells
Factor VIII-related antigen	Endothelial cells, platelets, megakaryocytes, mast cells
HMB 45	Melanocytes
Immunoglobulin	Plasma cells
Leukocyte common antigen (CD45)	Lymphocyte, monocytes, granulocytes
Lymphocyte subset markers	Lymphocytes
Lysozyme	Monocyte/macrophage lineage
Myelin basic protein	Oligodendrocytes, Schwann cells
Myoglobin	Muscle: skeletal, cardiac
Myosin	Muscle: skeletal, cardiac
Neuron-specific enolase	Neuroendocrine cells, neurons
Parathyroid hormone	Parathyroid
Prostatic acid phosphatase	Prostate
Prostate-specific antigen	Prostate
Protein gene peptide 9.5	Neuroendocrine cells, melanocytes
S-100	Melanocytes, neuroendocrine, glial cells, Schwann cells
Serotonin	Neuroendocrine
Synapsin	Neuroendocrine
Synaptophysin	Neuroendocrine
Thyroglobulin	Thyroid follicle cells

only helpful if an adequate specimen is obtained. Three types of specimens are most commonly used: direct smears, cytocentrifuge preps, and embedded cell blocks. Cytocentrifuge preparations are advantageous in that more preparations can generally be made, fewer reagents are required, and background staining is minimal. Most methods employ immunoperoxidase staining techniques to visualize the antigen. Immunoperoxidase techniques are favorable in that the preparations can be examined under a light microscope and cellular morphology is easily recognized. When evaluating results one must distinguish positively stained cells from nonspecific staining or background. In cytologic samples, nonspecific staining may occur at cell edges or folds. In addition, necrotic tissue, degenerated cells, and crushed cells can nonspecifically absorb antibodies, resulting in false-positive staining. Attention to technical detail, blocking techniques, and appropriate dilution of antibodies can reduce false positives, thus increasing specificity. Detailed methodology is beyond the scope of this chapter and the reader should refer to other resources (Krausz et al., 1993).

ICC and IHC are most commonly used in the subtyping of neoplasms. Poorly differentiated tumors may look similar with routine staining techniques and do not mimic the appearance of the tissue of origin. One of the most common problems is distinguishing among anaplastic carcinomas, lymphomas, and sarcomas. Antibodies that identify the five classes of intermediate filament proteins are frequently used in these situations (Table 16–1). Intermediate filaments are a group of cytoskeletal proteins expressed in virtually all eukaryotic cells and in most cases are cell type specific. Because of this cell-type specificity intermediate filaments are useful in the characterization of tumors, particularly to identify the cell origin of poorly differentiated neoplasms. In addition to intermediate filaments, many other tumor markers are available for subtyping of neoplasms, including antibodies restricted to particular structures found only in differentiated cells. Table 16–2 lists tumor markers available for ICC and IHC in differentiating malignancies. Table 16–3 lists examples of major tumor categories, which may present cytologic and/or histologic diagnostic dilemmas that can be clarified by ICC or IHC. This should be used only as a guideline with the

TABLE 16–3	**ICC and IHC for the Differential Diagnosis of Major Tumor Categories**					
	Keratin	**Vimentin**	**Common Leukocyte Antigen***	**S-100**	**Lysozyme**	**Neuron-Specific Enolase**
Carcinoma	+	−	−	−	−	−
Sarcoma	−	+	−	−†	−	−†
Lymphoma	−	+	+	−	−	−
Neuroendocrine	−	−	−	+	−	+
Melanoma	−	+	−	+	−	+

ICC, immunocytochemistry; IHC, immunohistochemistry; + positive staining; − negative staining.
* CD45.
† Unless neurogenic in origin.

clear understanding there are exceptions to these general rules. Poorly differentiated tumors may gain or lose antigens that are normally present, co-express markers, or differentiate toward multiple tissue types. For example, mesotheliomas and synovial cell sarcomas can dually express keratin and vimentin and thyroid carcinomas can demonstrate osseous differentiation. In these situations other tumor markers along with overall cytologic/histologic impression should be utilized to reach a definitive diagnosis.

The specificity of tumor markers should be regarded with caution, with the understanding that a perfect tumor marker does not exist. Reliability of results is determined by the ability of the pathologist to interpret the staining patterns. The proper interpretation of ICC and IHC depends on being aware of factors that cause false-positive and false-negative results. Positive and negative controls should be included with each antibody. A definitive diagnosis should never be made on the result of a single antibody. A preliminary differential diagnosis should first be developed based on cytologic/histologic impression and available clinical data, and then a panel of tumor markers selected to evaluate based on suspected tumor types. Only proper technique and interpretation can allow one to use ICC and IHC reliably as an important diagnostic adjunct.

SPECIAL STAINS

The morphologic identification of specific substances or organisms can increase the accuracy of cytologic and histologic diagnoses. Identification of organisms (Table 16–4) or specific substances (Table 16–5) is based on the use of special stains, which depends on chemical, enzymatic, or dye-binding characteristics of the substance of interest. The common special stains for histopathology can be used for cytologic specimen with minor modifications (Luna, 1968).

ELECTRON MICROSCOPY

Electron microscopy (EM) is used to morphologically characterize cells by magnification many times greater than with routine light microscopy. Histogenesis of neoplastic cells can be determined by ultrastructural

TABLE 16–4	Special Stains for Diagnosing Infectious Agents
Stain	**Infectious Agent**
Giemsa	*Rickettsia*, bacteria, *Leishmania*
Gram stain	Bacteria
Grocott's methenamine silver (GMS)	Fungi
Macchiavello	Chlamydiae
Mucicarmine	*Cryptococcus* (capsule only)
Periodic acid–Schiff (PAS)	Fungi
Steiner and Steiner, Warthin-Starry	*Campylobacter*, spirochetes, *Helicobacter*, *Bartonella*
Ziehl-Neelsen acid-fast	*Mycobacterium*

TABLE 16-5	Special Stains for the Diagnosis of Intracellular and Extracellular Substances
Stain	**Substance or Structure**
Acid phosphatase	Prostate
Alcian Blue	Mucin, hyaluronic acid, chondroitin sulfate
Alizarin Red S	Calcium
Azure A	Mast cells
Best's Carmine	Glycogen
Bielschowsky	Axons
Congo red	Amyloid
Cresyl Violet	Nissl bodies
Feulgen	DNA
Fontana-Masson	Melanin
Gremlins	Argyrophilic granules
Hall's Bilirubin	Bile
Luxol Fast Blue	Myelin
Methyl green pyronin	Nucleic acids
Mucicarmine	Mucin
Oil Red 0	Fat
PAS	Glycogen, mucin
Phosphotungstic Acid Hematoxylin (PTAH)	Muscle, fibrin, glial cell processes
Prussian Blue	Iron
Rubeanic	Copper
Schmorl's Reaction	Melanin, lipofuscin
Sudan Black B	Fat
Toluidine blue	Mast cells
Trichrome stains	Collagen
Von Kossa	Calcium

examination for unique cellular organelles or features. Although immunodiagnostics is becoming increasing popular as the ancillary method of tumor subtyping, EM is still useful in particular situations and can be complementary. These situations occur when available tumor markers are not specific enough for a definitive diagnosis, tumor markers have not been diagnostic, or a sufficient amount of material is not available for a panel of markers. Intracellular and nuclear structures present in normal cells are usually present in their malignant counterparts, allowing for tumor classification. In addition to tumor subtyping, EM can be used to identify infectious agents, in particular viruses (Cheville, 1994). Table 16-6 outlines some useful ultrastructural features unique to specific cell types in which EM is a value.

TABLE 16–6   Distinguishing Ultrastructural Features of Different Cell Types

Cell Type	Ultrastructural Features
Epithelial (glandular)	Lumina, microvilli (short and blunt), ± secretory granules
Epithelial (nonglandular)	Desmosomes, tonofilaments
Mesothelial cells	Desmosomes, microvilli (long and slender)
Myocytes	Myofibrils, Z-lines, mitochondria
Neuroendocrine	Neurosecretory granules
Melanoma	Melanosomes
Leukocytes	Pseudopods, primary and secondary granules
Plasma Cells	Abundant endoplasmic reticulum, Golgi complex, filopodia

FLOW CYTOMETRY

Flow cytometry is a rapid, sensitive, quantitative method of automated cell analysis. Cellular parameters that can be measured include surface marker analysis, DNA and RNA content, and DNA synthesis (S-phase fraction). In the veterinary clinical setting, flow cytometry is used primarily to determine cellular phenotypes in hemolymphatic disorders, and to a limited extent in quantitative measurement of DNA content. Cellular morphology and cytochemistry are the traditional methods to characterize and classify hemolymphatic neoplasms (Jain et al., 1991; Raskin et al., 2000). Cellular phenotypes by flow cytometry are determined by using monoclonal antibodies tagged to fluorochromes directed against surface molecules expressed on leukocytes. Examples include lymphomas, which may be subclassified as B- or T-cell type, and monocytic vs. granulocytic proliferations, which may also be distinguished from lymphoid cells. Additionally, clonality can be determined, which is used as an indicator of malignancy. There are numerous antibodies available to phenotypically characterize lymphomas/leukemias (see also Chapter 4). The clinical flow cytometry antibody panel currently used at the North Carolina State University College of Veterinary Medicine

TABLE 16–7   Clinical Immunology Flow Cytometry Panel Used at the North Carolina State University College of Veterinary Medicine

Cellular Phenotype	Dog Marker	Cat Marker
Pan T Lymphocyte	CD3	1.572*
T helper subset	CD4	CD4
T cytotoxic or suppressor subset	CD8	CD8
B cell	Surface IgG, CD21, B5*	CD21
Monocyte progenitors	CD14	CD14 (occasionally)

* Antibody developed at NCSU, antigen unknown.

for subtyping clinical samples is listed in Table 16–7. Cellular phenotyping in hematopoietic neoplasms has been found to not only guide therapeutic decisions but also to provide prognostic information in both human and veterinary medicine (Ruslander et al., 1997).

The DNA content of neoplastic cells as determined by flow cytometric analysis is used as a marker of malignancy in oncology (Hellmen and Lindgren, 1989). The DNA content or cellular ploidy determines if tumor cells contain a normal (diploid) or abnormal (aneuploid) number of chromosomes. The assumption is that benign tissues are diploid and high-grade malignancies are aneuploid. Human and animal studies have shown that aneuploidy may be useful in providing prognostic information and directing the course of therapy.

IMAGE ANALYSIS

Complementary to flow cytometry is image analysis. Image analysis is the measuring and counting of microscopic images in order to obtain information of diagnostic importance. Although image analysis has existed for some time, the advent of computer-assisted analysis has led to a more rapid, sensitive, and quantitative method of evaluation (Meijer et al., 1997). Typically, a television camera receives images from a light microscope. These signals are converted into digits by an interfaced computer, creating digitized cell images that can be displayed on a monitor.

Image analysis can be divided into three different areas, for example, cellular morphometry, counting cellular components, and cytometry. Morphometry is the quantitative description of geometric features of cellular structures of any dimension. The counting of cellular components or object counting is usually applied to the assess-

ment of cell kinetics by evaluating proliferative markers in tumors. This allows for the quantitation of the proliferative fraction or number of mitoses in a cell population, which has been shown to be useful for evaluation of the biologic behavior of tumors. Proliferation markers include bromodeoxyuridine (BrdU), proliferating cell nuclear antigen (PCNA), Ki67, and AgNOR method.

DNA cytometry is the measurement of DNA content in tumor cells and is used as a marker of malignancy in oncology. Image cytometry is used to measure the amount of ICC- or IHC-stained proteins in cells.

Laser scanning cytometry is a newer technology in which cells on a slide are scanned and then evaluated by flow cytometry-type analysis (Darzynkiewicz et al., 1999). Laser cytometry permits the observer to view cells and correlate flow cytometry data directly with cells measured and classify those cells by standard morphologic criteria.

MOLECULAR DIAGNOSTICS

In recent years there has been an explosion of molecular techniques available to aid in the diagnosis and treatment of infectious, hereditary, and neoplastic diseases in humans and animals. Most of the molecular methods are based on the principles of nucleic acid hybridization, such as Southern blotting and *in situ* hybridization (ISH), or nucleic acid amplification by the polymerase chain reaction (PCR). In conjunction with the traditional assays, the aims of the molecular techniques are to increase the sensitivity and specificity of disease diagnosis, identify prognostic factors, and potentially gauge therapeutic response. Although these new methods offer promise and are useful, there are also limitations to the interpretation and application of the results in a clin-

TABLE 16-8	Infectious Agents Studied Using Molecular Techniques	
Bacteria	**Viruses**	**Protozoal**
Bartonella	Adenovirus	Neospora
Borrelia	Canine distemper	Sarcocystis
Campylobacter		Toxoplasma
Chlamydia	FeLV	
Clostridium	FIP	
Ehrlichia	FIV	
Helicobacter	Herpes	
Mycobacterium	Parvovirus	
Mycoplasma	Rabies	
Rickettsia		

FeLV, feline leukemia virus; FIP, feline infectious peritonitis; FIV, feline immunodeficiency virus.

ical setting. This section presents an overview of the basis for many of the molecular techniques, their applications in disease diagnosis, and advantages or disadvantages of these tools.

There are many nucleic acid probes and PCR protocols available for the direct detection of many important pathogens in veterinary medicine (Table 16–8). Because the sensitivity often exceeds that of culture or serologic tests, the assays are useful for identifying organisms that are difficult or impossible to culture and detecting latent infections or infection in seronegative animals. ISH allows for localization of infection to affected tissues and cells.

Interpretation of the results for infectious diseases must be regarded with caution because of the occurrence of false-positive results (usually due to contamination) or identification of organisms that are not causing clinical disease. Results should always be evaluated in conjunction with other

clinical findings and results from other tests. PCR-positive results have been obtained in samples from clinically unaffected animals, from nonviable organisms, or after vaccination with strains of live or inactivated viruses. As for preventing contamination, strict precautions are recommended during collection, submission, and processing of samples. Furthermore, routine measures should be taken to chemically and enzymatically inactivate PCR products that can be found on lab equipment and in reagents, or be in airborne droplets in the laboratory. Even very low false-positive rates impact on the reliability of a test and this must be overcome before PCR becomes widely used and replaces current testing methods.

The specificity of many PCR-based assays for the identification of infectious agents should also be regarded with caution. For bacteria, the specificity of the tests are dependent on the degree of variability in the primary nucleotide sequences of the 16S ribosomal RNA (rRNA) or other genes. These sequences are nearly identical in phylogenetically closely related bacteria.

Molecular techniques are also being employed to identify animals at risk of developing or afflicted with specific hereditary or neoplastic diseases. Mutations have been identified and used in the diagnosis of diseases such as muscular dystrophy, hemophilia, pyruvate kinase deficiency, malignant hyperthermia, phosphofructokinase deficiency, progressive retinal atrophy, and myelination disorders.

Applications in oncology are examining the utility of molecular methods for the early detection of tumor recurrence, the diagnosis of lymphoma, involvement of oncogenes and tumor suppressor genes in carcinogenesis, identifying prognostic factors, and evaluating therapeutic response to chemotherapy. Clonality analysis of lymphocytes by molecular techniques is now a commonly used method to aid in the diagnosis human B- and T-cell lymphomas (Greiner, 1999; Signoretti et al., 1999; Chen et al., 1994) and is being developed by some investigators in the dog (Burnett et al., 1998). The diagnosis and lineage assignment of lymphoma in dogs is usually uncomplicated, however, for a minority of cases lymphoma is difficult to distinguish from benign hyperplasia. Current diagnosis of canine lymphoma relies primarily on histopathology, cytopathology, and/or ancillary tests such as flow cytometry or ICC/IHC to aid in the determination of cell lineage. Hybridization and PCR-based assays are designed to assess for the presence of a clonally expanded population of lymphocytes based on analysis for gene rearrangement of the immunoglobulin gene for B lymphocytes and T-cell receptor gene for T lymphocytes. The assays are based on the principle that there is imprecise joining of the V–D–J region of the immunoglobulin gene or T-cell receptor gene. It has been shown that during the V–D–J joining process, short segments of DNA are inserted or deleted in the V–D and D–J junctions. The insertions and deletions act to expand the normal immunoglobulin repertoire and contribute to the variations in the overall size of the V–D–J segment in B-cells. Primers are designed to amplify this segment and the PCR products are analyzed by gel electrophoresis. Monoclonal B-cell populations would be characterized by a discrete band, while polyclonal populations would show a smear pattern. This strategy has been applied with success to analyses of peripheral blood, lymph nodes, lymph node aspirates, cytology specimens, and formalin-fixed paraffin-embedded tissues. Most human studies report a high specificity for the assay, however, occasional false-positive results occur in reactive or hyperplastic lymph nodes. False-positive results are reported to be low for routine surgical biopsy specimens. False negative results have been reported. These results may be related to suboptimal annealing of the primers, detrimental effects of fixation, translocations of the Ig locus, mixture of neoplastic cells with polyclonal populations of lymphocytes, and limits of sensitivity using ethidium bromide/gel electrophoresis detection system, and occasionally there can be a polyclonal pattern in B-cell lymphomas.

It is true that many of these molecular biology advances will greatly impact diagnostic pathology and pathogenesis studies, but we should be cautious in our interpretation of the results, mainly because of the occurrence of false-positive results. The information obtained from these techniques should be in conjunction with the results of other diagnostic assays. With continued development, molecular diagnostic techniques will become more automated, reliable, and cost effective and eventually supplement and replace many current diagnostic tests.

References

Burnett R, Vernau B, Moore PF, Avery A: Abstract: Diagnosis of canine lymphocytic neoplasia using clonal rearrangements of antigen receptor genes. Proceedings of the International Meeting on Canine Immunogenetics, Davis, CA, 1998.

Chen Y, Whitney KD, Chen Y: Clonality analysis of B-cell lymphoma in fresh-frozen and paraffin-embedded tissues: The effects of variable PCR parameters. Mod Pathol 1994; 7(4):429–434.

Cheville NF: *Ultrastructural Pathology. An Introduction to Interpretation.* Iowa State University Press, Ames, 1994, pp 490–615.

Darzynkiewicz Z, Bedner E, Li X, et al: Laser-scanning cytometry: A new instrumentation with many applications. Exp Cell Res 1999; 249: 1–12.

Greiner TC: Advances in molecular hematopathology: T-cell receptor γ and bcl-2 genes. Am J Path 1999; 154(1):7–9.

Hellmen E., Lindgren A: The accuracy of cytology in diagnosis and DNA analysis of canine mammary tumours. J Comp Path 1989; 101:443–450.

Jain NC, Blue JT, Grindem CB, et al: A report of the animal leukemia study group: Proposed criteria for classification of acute myeloid leukemia in dogs and cats. Vet Clin Pathol 1991; 20: 63–81.

Krausz T, Schofield JB, Van Noorder S, et al: In Young JA (ed): *Fine Needle Aspiration Cytopathology.* Oxford Univ. Press, Boston, 1993, pp 310–347.

Luna LG (ed): *Manual of Histologic Staining Methods of the Armed Forces Institute of Pathology,* 3rd ed., McGraw-Hill, New York, 1968, pp 72–240.

Meijer GA, Belien JAM, van Diest PJ, Bank JPA: Image analysis in clinical pathology. J Clin Pathol 1997; 50:365–370.

Raskin RE, Valenciano A: Cytochemical tests for diagnosis of leukemia. In: Feldman BF, Zinkl JG, Jain NC (eds): *Schalm's Veterinary Hematology,* 5th ed. Williams & Wilkins, Baltimore, 2000, pp 755–763.

Ruslander DA, Gebhard DH, Tompkins MB, et al: Immunophenotypic characterization of canine lymphoproliferative disorders. In Vivo 1997; 11: 169–172.

Signoretti S, Murphy M, Cangi MG, et al: Detection of clonal T-cell receptor γ gene rearrangements in paraffin-embedded tissue by PCR and nonradioactive SSCP analysis. Am J Pathol 1999; 154(1):67–75.

Index

Note: Page numbers in *italics* refer to illustrations; page numbers followed by t refer to tables.